Springer Series on Life Styles and Issues in Aging

Editor
Bernard D. Starr, PhD
Director, Gerontology Program
Marymount Manhattan College
New York, NY

Advisory Board

Robert C. Atchley, PhD
Director, Scripps Foundation
Gerontology Center
Miami University
Oxford, OH

Marjorie Cantor, PhD (Hon)
Research Director, University
Center for Gerontology
Fordham University and School of
Social Science at Lincoln Center
New York, NY

M. Powell Lawton, PhD
Director, Behavioral Center
Philadelphia Geriatric Center
Philadelphia, PA

Harvey L. Sterns. PhD
University of Akron Institute of Life
Span Development and
Gerontology
Akron, OH

Volumes

1993
Retirement Counseling: A Handbook for Gerontology Practitioners
Virginia E. Richardson, PhD

1994
Aging and Quality of Life
Ronald P. Abeles, PhD, Helen C. Gift, PhD, and Marcia G. Ory, PhD, MPH

Ronald P. Abeles, PhD, is the Associate Director for Behavioral and Social Research at the National Institute on Aging (BSR/NIA), where he served as the Deputy Associate Director from 1980 to 1991. He received his doctoral degree in Social Psychology (with a minor in sociology) from the Department of Social Relations, Harvard University in 1971. His experience as a Staff Associate at the Social Science Research Council (1974–1978) for the Committee on Work and Personality in the Middle Years and the Committee on Life Course Development stimulated his interest in life course issues. Dr. Abeles has held elected offices in the aging sections of the American Sociological Association (ASA) and the American Psychological Association (APA). Recently he received the National Institutes of Health Award of Merit for "leadership and contributions to the advancement of behavioral and social research on aging."

In addition to his duties at the National Institute on Aging, Dr. Abeles has been instrumental in fostering behavioral and social research throughout the National Institutes of Health. Since 1980 he has served as the Executive Secretary and Acting Chair of the ad hoc NIH Working Group on Health and Behavior and is now Vice Chair of the newly established NIH Health and Behavior Coordinating Committee.

Helen C. Gift, PhD, is the Chief of the Disease Prevention and Health Promotion Branch, Epidemiology and Oral Disease Prevention Program, of the National Institute of Dental Research, National Institutes of Health. She received her masters and doctoral degrees in sociology from Emory University in 1969 and 1971, respectively. Since then, she has been an active researcher and has published research papers on social and behavioral factors in oral health and disease and in health promotion and disease prevention in special populations, especially older adults. Dr. Gift was the recipient of the NIH Director's Award in 1990.

Marcia G. Ory, PhD, MPH, is Chief, Social Science Research on Aging, Behavioral and Social Research Program, National Institute on Aging, National Institutes of Health, Bethesda, MD. She holds a doctorate from Purdue University and a Masters of Public Health from The Johns Hopkins University. Dr. Ory is very active in professional organizations and serves on several national task forces and advisory boards dealing with aging and health issues. She has published widely in her main areas of interest, which include aging and health care, health and behavior research, and gender differences in health and longevity.

Aging and Quality of Life

RONALD P. ABELES, PhD
HELEN C. GIFT, PhD
MARCIA G. ORY, PhD
EDITORS

DONNA M. COX, PhD
EDITORIAL ASSISTANT

**SPRINGER PUBLISHING COMPANY
NEW YORK**

Copyright © 1994 by Springer Publishing Company, Inc.

All rights reserved

No part of this publication may be reproduced, stored in a retrieval system, or transmitted in any form or by any means, electronic, mechanical, photocopying recording, or otherwise, without the prior permission of Springer Publishing Company, Inc.

Series design by Holly A. Block

Springer Publishing Company, Inc.
536 Broadway
New York, NY 10012

94 95 96 97 98 / 5 4 3 2 1

Library of Congress Cataloging-in-Publication Data

Aging and Quality of life / Ronald P. Abeles, Helen C.
Gift, Marcia G. Ory, editors
    p. cm. — (Springer series on life styles and issues in aging)
    Includes bibliographical references and index.
    ISBN 0-8261-8430-8
    1. Gerontology   2. Aging.   3. Aged—Health and hygiene.
4. Quality of life.   I. Abeles, Ronald P., 1944–   II. Gift, Helen C.   III. Ory, Marcia G.   IV. Series.
HQ1061.A4567   1994
305.26—dc20   94-6081
                                                                       CIP

Printed in the United States of America

Contents

Foreword   ix
   James O. Mason, MD, DrPH

Acknowledgments   xiii

Contributors   xv

Introduction: Aging and Quality of Life—Celebrating New Discoveries   1
   Marcia G. Ory, PhD, MPH, Donna M. Cox, PhD,
   Helen C. Gift, PhD, and Ronald P. Abeles, PhD

Part I: Background Perspectives

Chapter 1   Historical Perspective on Aging and Quality of Life   19
   Robert N. Butler, MD

Chapter 2   Conceptualizing and Measuring Quality of Life
in Older Populations   27
   Anita L. Stewart, PhD, and Abby C. King, PhD

Part II: Life Style and Quality of Life

Chapter 3   Behavioral and Social Factors in Healthy Aging   57
   George A. Kaplan, PhD, and
   William J. Strawbridge, PhD

Chapter 4   Disability in Late Life   79
   Lois M. Verbrugge, PhD, MPH

Chapter 5	Self-Care and Quality of Life in Old Age Gordon H. DeFriese, PhD, Thomas R. Konrad, PhD, Alison Woomert, PhD, Jean E. Kincade Norburn, PhD, and Shulamit Bernard, RN, MS	99

Part III: Physical Health, Quality of Life, and Aging

Chapter 6	Rehabilitation in Old Age T. Franklin Williams, MD	121
Chapter 7	Psychosocial Status in Cancer Patients Barrie R. Cassileth, PhD	133
Chapter 8	Biopsychosocial Risks for Cardiovascular Disease in Spouse Caregivers of Persons with Alzheimer's Disease Peter P. Vitaliano, PhD, Cynthia M. Dougherty, PhD, RN, and Ilene C. Siegler, PhD, MPH	145

Part IV: Older People and Their Environments

Chapter 9	Social Support: Content, Causes, and Consequences Robert L. Kahn, PhD	163
Chapter 10	Aging Well and Institutional Living: A Paradox? Margret M. Baltes, PhD	185
Chapter 11	Human Factors and Aging: The Operator–Task Dynamic Robin A. Barr, DPhil	202
Chapter 12	Maintaining a Sense of Control in Later Life Margie E. Lachman, PhD, Mauri A. Ziff, MA, and Avron Spiro III, PhD	216

Part V: Social Structures, Quality of Life, and Aging

Chapter 13	The Changing Structure of Work Opportunities: Toward an Age-Integrated Society Matilda White Riley, DSc and Karyn A. Loscocco, PhD	235

Chapter 14	Socioeconomic Status and Health over the Life Course *Stephanie A. Robert, MSW, and James S. House, PhD*	253
Chapter 15	New Directions in Socioeconomic Research on Aging *James P. Smith, PhD*	275
Chapter 16	Minority and Socioeconomic Status: Impact on Quality of Life in Aging *H. Asuman Kiyak, PhD and Nancy R. Hooyman, MSW, PhD*	295

Part VI: Policy Implications

Chapter 17	Public Policy and Long-Term Care *Carroll L. Estes, PhD, and Liz Close, MS*	319
Chapter 18	Changing the Social Environment to Promote Health *Lennart Levi, MD, and Donna M. Cox, PhD*	336
Chapter 19	Exploring the Future of Health Care for Older People *Robert H. Binstock, PhD, Dennis W. Jahnigen, MD, and Stephen G. Post, PhD*	350

Index   *367*

Foreword

The oldest quests of the human race have been to lengthen life, to improve its quality, and to reduce burdens of social conditions and diseases. Over the centuries, science explorers have searched new frontiers to reach these goals. Spectacular progress has been made, but challenges and frontiers in aging continue. They are: to further increase the span of healthy and productive life; to investigate issues and find resolutions which will lift the spirit, alleviate illness and diseases; and to elevate the quality of life.

This volume addresses critical components of the scientific frontier of aging research—the social, psychological, and economic issues in health and the quality of life. Most of these chapters were an integral part of a larger research agenda that was addressed in a conference, "Aging: The Quality of Life," held as part of the Christopher Columbus Quincentenary Jubilee in February, 1992.

Columbus's explorations in the 15th and 16th centuries resulted in social, cultural, and scientific revolutions. In the coming millennium, a demographic revolution of comparable consequence will result in the graying of a very diverse world population. The social and cultural issues of this change will require a great deal of attention. The promise of biology, biotechnology, and our unlimited imagination will challenge our determination to explore anew biomedical ethics, quality of life, as well as to use appropriately human and technological resources.

Today, in industrial societies the populations are graying. The world's geriatric population is currently growing at a rate of 3% a year. There are 352 million persons age 65 and older now, and it is expected that there will be 417 million by the year 2000. Explorers landing on the North American continent today would certainly find a very different demographic mix in the residents, perhaps believing that the age profile represented the presence of a "fountain of longevity" rather than a "fountain of youth."

Persons age 80 and over constitute more than 16% of the world's elderly. According to Census Bureau projections, by the year 2000, 26% of the U.S. population will be 80 years of age or older. This longevity is both a promise and a challenge. The challenge for research is to broaden the promise of quality life to those in this age group.

Most older people living in developed countries today are reasonably healthy and are living independently within their community. However, 80% of those over 65 experience at least one chronic illness, and multiple comorbidities are commonplace. Five to seven percent over the age of 65 and 40% over the age of 85 need some type of help in their daily functioning. As the number of older people continues to grow, and disease and disabilities accumulate in old age, the demand for acute and long-term care will increase unless dramatic successes can be achieved in preventing or treating the disabilities associated with old age. Some hope such success can be found in current research.

In light of these demographic and epidemiological facts, a number of important and promising directions in research and services confront us. At the basic level a better understanding of the effects of biological aging, as distinguished from the effects of diseases, is needed. On the social, psychological, and economic fronts, far more needs to be understood about interventions that can improve functioning and quality of life across the entire spectrum of life, but especially in old age.

A first step is to answer "What is aging?" It is essential to have much better understanding of what aging is and what older people are capable of doing to develop social policy, assure adequate living standards, provide adequate health care services, and project and control costs.

Scientists, public leaders, and lay people must dispel old stereotypes of aging and use only accurate knowledge--knowledge that is changing rapidly. The best evidence today suggests that there is surprisingly little so called "inevitable decline" in function with age. Contrary to popular belief and even many standard tests, many people maintain excellent function, as measured by almost any standard, into their eighties and nineties. Even though more people are entering old age in better health and with greater resources, we need to extend "successful aging" to greater numbers of older people. The prevailing thought that all people age more or less alike is also contrary to scientific knowledge. Older people are in fact more varied than any age group in society. They bring a whole lifetime of health behaviors and experience to aging, making the answers to questions such as "What is aging?" or "Who is old?" elusive. The thoughtful contributions in this volume provide a significant basis for moving toward improved quality of life for the older generations now and in the future.

JAMES O. MASON, M.D., Dr. Ph.H.
Former Assistant Secretary of Health,
Vice President for Development and Planning
Uniformed Services University of the Health Sciences

---

*Based on "Opening Remarks and Overview" for Aging: The Quality of Life Conference, Washington, D.C., February 10–12, 1992.

Acknowledgments

We are pleased to acknowledge the National Institutes of Health Planning Committee for the Conference on Aging: The Quality of Life Conference for developing the concept for and organizing the program that served as the original basis for this book. We are especially appreciative of the efforts of George Galasso and Sue Ohata in this regard.

We owe a debt of gratitude to Matilda White Riley and H. Asuman Kiyak for their encouragement and to Jayne Lura-Brown and Jeanette Wilson for their secretarial assistance.

Contributors

Margret M. Baltes, PhD
Freie Universität Berlin
Psychiatrische Klinik [WE 12]
Abteilung für Gerontopsychiatrie
Berlin, Germany

Robin A. Barr, DPhil
Behavioral and Social Research
National Institute on Aging
Bethesda, MD 20892

Shulamit Bernard, RN, MS
Health Services Research Center
University of North Carolina
  at Chapel Hill
Chapel Hill, NC 27599

Robert H. Binstock, PhD
Department for Epidemiology and
  Biostatistics
School of Medicine
Case Western Reserve University
Cleveland, OH 44106

Robert N. Butler, MD
Department of Geriatrics and Adult
  Development
Mount Sinai Medical Center
New York, NY 10029

Barrie R. Cassileth, PhD
Behavioral Resources Corporation
Chapel Hill, NC 27516

Liz Close, MS
Department of Social and Behavioral
  Sciences
School of Nursing
University of California
San Francisco, CA 94143

Donna M. Cox, PhD
School of Medicine
University of Maryland Long Term
  Care Project
Baltimore, MD 21201

Gordon H. DeFriese, PhD
Health Services Research Center
University of North Carolina at
  Chapel Hill
Chapel Hill, NC 27599

Cynthia M. Dougherty, PhD, RN
Department of Psychiatry and
  Behavioral Sciences
University of Washington
Seattle, WA 98195

Carroll L. Estes, PhD
Department of Social and
  Behavioral Sciences
School of Nursing
University of California
San Francisco, CA 94143

CONTRIBUTORS

Nancy R. Hooyman, MSW, PhD
School of Social Work
University of Washington
Seattle, WA 98195

James S. House, PhD
Survey Research Center
Institute for Social Research
University of Michigan
Ann Arbor, MI 48106

Dennis W. Jahnigen, MD
Health Sciences Center
University of Colorado
Denver, CO 80262

Robert L. Kahn, PhD
Survey Research Center
Institute for Social Research
University of Michigan
Ann Arbor, MI 48106

George A. Kaplan, PhD
Human Population Laboratory
California Department of Health
  Services
Berkeley, CA 94704

Abby C. King, PhD
Stanford Center for Research and
  Disease Prevention
Stanford University School of Medicine
Palo Alto, CA 94304

H. Asuman Kiyak, PhD
Department of Oral and Maxillofacial
  Surgery
University of Washington
Seattle, WA 98195

Thomas R. Konrad, PhD
Health Services Research Center
University of North Carolina at
  Chapel Hill
Chapel Hill, NC 27599

Margie E. Lachman, PhD
Department of Psychology
Brandeis University
Waltham, MA 02254

Lennart Levi, MD
Department of Stress Research
WHO Psychosocial Center
Stockholm, Sweden

Karyn A. Loscocco, PhD
Department of Sociology
State University of New York–Albany
Albany, NY 12222

James O. Mason, MD, DrPH
Farmington, UT 84025

Jean E. Kincade Norburn, PhD
Health Services Research Center
University of North Carolina at
  Chapel Hill
Chapel Hill, NC 27599

Stephen G. Post, PhD
Department for Epidemiology and
  Biostatistics
School of Medicine
Case Western Reserve University
Cleveland, OH 44106

Matilda White Riley, DSc
Senior Social Scientist
National Institute on Aging
Bethesda, MD 20892

Stephanie A. Robert, MSW
Institute for Social Research
University of Michigan
Ann Arbor, MI 48106

Ilene C. Siegler, PhD, MPH
Duke University Medical Center
Duke University
Durham, NC 27705

James P. Smith, PhD
The Rand Corporation
Santa Monica, CA 90407

CONTRIBUTORS

Avron Spiro III, PhD
Normative Aging Study
Veterans Administration Medical Center
Bedford, MA 01730

Anita L. Stewart, PhD
Institute for Health and Aging
University of California, San Francisco
San Francisco, CA 94143

William J. Strawbridge, PhD
Human Population Laboratory
California Department of Health
 Services
Berkeley, CA 94704

Lois M. Verbrugge, PhD, MPH
Institute of Gerontology
University of Michigan
Ann Arbor, MI 48109

Peter P. Vitaliano, PhD
Department of Psychiatry and
 Behavioral Sciences
University of Washington
Seattle, WA 98195

T. Franklin Williams, MD
University of Rochester
School of Medicine and Dentistry
Rochester, NY 14620

Alison Woomert, PhD
Health Services Research Center
University of North Carolina at
 Chapel Hill
Chapel Hill, NC 27599

Mauri A. Ziff, MA
Department of Psychology
Brandeis University
Waltham, MA 02254

Introduction

Aging and Quality of Life: Celebrating New Research Discoveries

Just as Christopher Columbus sailed forth in search of new lands, members of the research community chart new territories in their search for information that can be applied to assure individuals an opportunity to live longer, fuller lives. During this century, modern societies have witnessed an unprecedented increase in the number of people who live to the age of 65 and beyond. Whereas only one of 25 Americans reached age 65 at the turn of this century, one of every eight Americans was at least 65 years old in 1990. By the year 2030, the number of older Americans will nearly double and make up 20% of the entire population. The fastest growing portion of the aged population is the oldest-old (85+), a group expected to almost triple in size between now and 2030 (Aging America, 1991; U.S. Bureau of the Census, 1993).

These dramatic increases in U.S. life expectancy in the latter part of the twentieth century are largely caused by declines in mortality among the middle-aged and elderly populations. In 1900 a person aged 65 could expect to live nearly 12 more years; today, a 65-year-old person can expect to live more than 17 additional years (U.S. Bureau of the Census, 1993). Yet, decreases in mortality are not without consequences. Although most older people are not frail and dependent as depicted by aging stereotypes (NCHS, 1991; 1993), with increased longevity, chronic illnesses are increasingly more prevalent. They are now a major cause of death and disability in old age (Institute of Medicine, 1991). In the past decade, the number of multiple chronic conditions reported by older people has increased notably. Most older people now report two or more chronic conditions. Moreover, older women, in contrast to older men, are especially likely to experience multiple chronic conditions (Guralnik, La Croix, Everett, & Kovar, 1989). The increases in chronic conditions often translate into functional disability and need for some type of assistance (Verbrugge, 1990). Approximately 7 million Americans over the age of 65 depend on others for help with some basic task of daily living (Hing & Bloom, 1990; Ory & Duncker, 1992).

Projections of life expectancy now differentiate years of active life expectancy or healthy years of life from the number of *expected* years of life. For example, a healthy man who reaches age 65 can expect to live at least 15 more years, with good health and independence expected for 13 of those extra years (Suzman, Willis & Manton, 1992). A healthy woman, on the other hand, can expect to live as many as 20 more years after reaching age 65, but she may enjoy good health for just 16 years.

The ill health of older persons is not necessarily a fixed intrinsic process related to biological senescence. Rather it is the result of cumulative exposures to risk (Suzman et al., 1992). Research on aging includes the identification of ways to enhance life rather than to simply extend it (Riley & Riley, 1989). Behavioral geriatrics research is documenting the link between health and behavior and identifying points of intervention for both health promotion and disability prevention across the life course (Ory, Abeles, & Lipman, 1992).

A fundamental question remains: Does increased longevity translate into a greater burden of disability, or will changes in life styles, medical care and technology result in a compression of morbidity and disability (Fries, Green, & Levine, 1989; Schneider & Brody, 1983)? Recent findings show that population aging does not inevitably lead to increases in disability rates.

Strong support for a compression of morbidity hypothesis is found by Manton and colleagues (1993a) in their longitudinal analysis of older people's health and functional status. Despite a 14.7% increase in the number of older people between 1982 and 1989, fewer people were disabled or institutionalized in 1989. After adjusting the data to account for the more rapid growth in the number of very old people age 85 and over, the decline in disability rate reached about 7%, or about 540,000 fewer disabled people in 1989 than would have been expected. Various types of disability were examined, by identifying the number of people who had difficulty performing specific daily activities, such as eating, bathing, and dressing, as well as instrumental activities such as cooking, shopping, and managing finances. Some decline in disability was demonstrated for nearly every activity (Manton, Corder, & Stallard, 1993b).

Manton and colleagues (1993b) also noted changes in services used by people once they became disabled. For example, substantial increases were found in the use of certain equipment, such as raised toilets (+148%), shower seats, and tub stools (+65.9%). At the same time the use of personal assistance fell by more than 9% for both older men and women. This research indicates the importance of the social and physical environment in determining whether particular functional impairments and disabilities are translated into handicaps.

Decreases in disability noted by Manton and colleagues reflect changes in the older population overall. Specific groups distinguished by demographic and social factors, such as race, gender, and socioeconomic factors, may not experience the same level of change, if any. In addition to the dramatic growth in the older population, American society is becoming more racially and ethnically diverse, with life long patterns of health and health care being quite dissimilar in different segments of the American population (U.S. Bureau of the Census, 1993). This heterogeneous nature of the older population points to variable needs. Research is needed that focuses on reducing frailty and disability in groups that are not experiencing the same improvements in health and functioning as the older population overall.

Industrialized nations today are wrestling with a complex array of issues in their efforts to provide for variable needs of an increasingly diverse and aging population. Five hundred years after Columbus' voyage, information from research and new scientific tools makes it possible to address these needs. Questions of critical importance center on how society can foster an individual's quality of life, particularly as that person ages and faces the possibility of increased frailty and dependence. Even before societies can take steps to enhance the quality of life in all segments of the older population, however, answers are needed to questions that until recently have been left primarily to philosophers. Research on aging has only recently begun to grapple with the problems associated with defining and measuring the nebulous concept of "quality of life."

Defining and Measuring Quality of Life

Quality of life is a multidimensional concept that refers to an individual's overall life satisfaction and total well-being. Lawton (1983, 1991) identifies four dimensions in his conceptualization of quality of life: (1) behavioral competence is the socio-normative evaluation of the person's functioning in the health, cognitive, time-use, and social dimensions; (2) perceived quality of life refers to the person's subjective evaluation of function in any of the behavior competence dimensions; (3) environment affords or hinders particular behaviors and influences perceived quality of life; and (4) psychological well-being is the weighted evaluated level of the person's competencies and perceived quality in all domains of contemporary life and encompasses what is usually thought of as mental health. Careful definition and measurement of quality of life is of special significance in light of medical and technological advances that affect not only disease processes but also the kind of lives people subsequently lead (Stewart & King, 1991).

A notable factor affecting an individual's quality of life is his or her health and ability to function. As this nation ponders how to reform the U.S. health care system, an important challenge for researchers and policymakers alike is to find ways to maintain optimal functioning and decrease disablement in the face of acute and chronic disease and disabilities (Institute of Medicine, 1991). Therefore, health-related quality of life has become an increasingly important measure in assessing the impact of disease and its treatment on individuals and their families.

The domains commonly thought to comprise health-related quality of life are: physical health functioning, emotional health, cognitive function, sexual functioning, social role performance and work productivity, and life satisfaction (Stewart & Ware, 1992). Thus, health-related quality of life assessments offer a broad view of health that is consistent with the World Health Organization's (WHO) conceptualization of health as a state of complete physical, mental, and social well-being and not merely the absence of disease or infirmity (WHO, 1946).

At all ages, quality of life is clearly influenced by psychological, social, and economic factors. However, the weight of any one factor in assessing quality of life changes with life situations. Conditions or events of limited importance to younger people may be more critical to an older person's quality of life when trying to maintain integrity, independence, and autonomy (Patrick & Bergner, 1990; Shumaker,

Anderson, & Czajkowski, 1990; Schumacher, Olschewski, & Schulgen, 1991). For example, although mobility may be taken for granted by young adults, mobility is often an overriding concern for older adults, particularly for those who live alone.

With older people expecting to live well into their 80s, there are multiple opportunities for intervention across the full spectrum of health and illness (Omenn, 1992). Therefore, the crux of the issue is how research can be directed toward understanding health behaviors for the purpose of developing interventions that keep older people healthy and independent for as long as possible. It is this issue that forces attention to the difficult but important concept of quality of life.

Genesis and Purpose of the Book

The basis of this volume was a conference, "Aging: The Quality of Life," held by the Christopher Columbus Medical Sciences Committee of the National Institutes of Health in February 1992. The conference was one part of the Christopher Columbus Quincentenary Jubilee Presidential Commission established by Congress to coordinate the celebration of 500 years since Columbus landed in America.

The conference had a multidisciplinary focus, highlighting the contributions of science to the study of aging. Ranging from basic science to applications, the program was organized into seven tracks: cardiovascular, brain, cancer, osteoporosis, nutrition and obesity, diabetes, and healthy aging. The editors of this volume were active on the conference planning committee and instrumental in planning and implementing the track on healthy aging, which set out to address quality of life issues as they relate to normal functioning of the aging individual.

The strength of the program lay in the multidisciplinary framework within which quality of life and healthy aging were addressed. Functioning was related to demographic, economic, psychosocial and political factors. Positive aging (the process of adapting to the interactions of aging, changing health status, self, family, and society) was the primary focus of discussion.

All but one of the presenters in the healthy aging track of the conference, in addition to the two keynote speakers and other psychosocial researchers from other components of the conference, made contributions to this volume. Also included were several chapters specially commissioned to provide additional information on health-related quality of life and age-related chronic illnesses and disabilities. Thus, this volume represents a continuation of the science transfer process by bringing the benefits of research and conference discussion to a broader audience.

The underlying purpose of this volume is to review what is known about aging and quality of life. Greater understandings of how aging affects and is affected by quality of life are quests as integral to the gerontological research community as Columbus' desire for riches and fame were to his quest for the new world. This volume attempts to push new research frontiers in the behavioral sciences by defining quality of life and identifying the complexities associated with its measurement, such as understanding how quality of life changes over time and within specific social and cultural groups. The ultimate implications of this volume are to link what has been learned about aging and quality of life with the development of interventions that enhance an individual's opportunity to age successfully.

Part I: Background Perspectives

The foreword by James O. Mason directs attention to the significance of the "graying" of the world's population and stresses the need for more research that distinguishes aging from disease processes. Mason reviews the importance of aging research within the context of the Christopher Columbus Quincentenary Conference. His remarks underscore the volume theme of charting new territories in behavioral sciences research. Two introductory chapters in Part I, Background perspectives, review advances made in the field of gerontology and quality of life research. Robert Butler's reflections on the rise of modern science sets the stage for this volume. In his thoughtful essay, Butler highlights critical scientific advances since the days of Columbus, with special attention to aging and longevity. Additionally, several research priorities for improving current understanding and enhancing older people's quality of life are identified. The importance of collaboration at the disciplinary as well as at the research funding level is stressed.

Although there is general popular agreement about what constitutes quality of life, there is still debate in the scientific community over its precise conceptualization and measurement. Even less is known about the influence of interacting aging processes. Therefore, the chapters in this volume address some fundamental quality-of-life research issues: Is there a universal definition of quality of life? Are older people's evaluations of their quality of life modified by their expectations and life experiences?

Anita Stewart and Abby King provide a conceptual framework for defining and using "quality of life" as a meaningful construct for research and practice. Their chapter reviews various domains of quality of life, highlights different approaches for measuring quality of life, and draws attention to common measurement issues. Several fundamental research issues are discussed in relation to defining and measuring quality of life. These include: health-related concepts (e.g., physical and cognitive functioning) as a component of quality of life versus a predictor of quality of life; definitions of quality of life and differences in conceptions between the young and the old; and the selection of domains and content areas for particular subgroups of the aged population.

The remainder of this volume is organized into four substantive parts and one policy-oriented part. Each of these substantive parts addresses a major area of research on aging and quality of life, with an emphasis on factors that distinguish quality of life in the aged and its subpopulations from that of younger populations. The final and sixth part of this volume emphasizes public policy implications in light of research advances and a changing health care environment. It frames research and policy agendas for the future. Common themes in aging and quality of life research will be highlighted throughout the following brief chapter reviews.

Part II: Life Style and Quality of Life

Part II presents an epidemiological perspective on the health and functioning of older Americans, identifying factors that can modify linkages between health, disease, and disability. It focuses on lifestyles and social, behavioral, and physical factors that can detract from or enhance an older person's quality of life. The variability in aging processes, the continued impact of behavioral or social risk factors in late life, and the potential for modifiability of risk factors in old age are highlighted in this section.

George Kaplan discusses the need for an expanded definition of "healthy aging" set within a socioenvironmental context. His chapter focuses on the importance of behavioral and social factors (e.g., smoking, physical activity, social participation, socioeconomic status) as determinants of longevity and functioning in later life. The substantial body of epidemiological evidence demonstrating the salience of interacting behavioral and social processes is summarized. Kaplan suggests several pathways through which social and behavioral factors modify the impact of disease on functioning. This search for pathways linking health and behavior represents one of the most promising research directions in behavioral epidemiology research.

Self-care practices that are used by older adults to compensate for declining physical, cognitive, or mental capacities and to help extend overall life activities are described in the chapter by Gordon DeFriese and colleagues. The chapter defines the concept of "self care" and emphasizes its importance as an integral component of the complete spectrum of health care. It also includes research results from the first national survey on self-care behaviors practiced by elderly persons in the United States. For example, preliminary results indicate that the probability of engaging in self-care activities varies with levels of disability, as does the type of self care strategy employed. In a concluding section of the chapter unsolved research and policy issues are explored.

Moving away from an emphasis on mortality, health researchers are now focusing greater attention on the antecedents and consequences of disability in later life. Lois Verbrugge explores the impact of disabilities in late life and the implications of both individual and societal approaches to disability prevention. Presenting the epidemiology of disability, the chapter offers a conceptual scheme that includes predisposing risk factors, interventions, and exacerbators in the disablement process, exploring each from pathology to impairment to functional limitation to disability. Several themes relevant to aging and quality of life are discussed including: (1) disability as a multidimensional concept reflecting the gap between personal capacities and environmental demands, (2) comparisons of life-long and late-life disability, and (3) projections of future levels of disability in an aging society. Complementing the chapter by DeFriese and colleagues, Verbrugge also suggests the value of self-care strategies for slowing down the disablement process.

Part III: Physical Health, Quality of Life, and Aging

The theme in Part III is quality of life and aging in relation to general frailty, as well as specific age-related physical diseases. This section considers a basic assessment issue which often arises, that is, whether quality of life concepts and measurement should assess general health and functioning states, or be adapted to disease-specific conditions. T. Franklin Williams opens the section with a discussion of the importance of retaining or regaining the older person' independence for determining quality of life. The chapter discusses the interplay between intrinsic and extrinsic factors of age-related changes and the potentials for restoring or at least improving independence for those who have lost functions because of disease or lifestyle practices. Specific examples are given to illustrate how the application of rehabilitation principles can improve the functioning and quality of life of older persons with disabling conditions, such as arthritis, stroke, or hip fracture.

In the next chapter, the attention is focused on cancer, a condition that is especially prevalent in old age. With more than half of all cancers occurring in people over age 65, detection and treatment of cancer in older people needs to be more aggressive. Yet, stereotypical assumptions that older people cannot tolerate chemotherapy and radiation therapies paradoxically act to limit the use of aggressive therapies in one of the most "at risk" segments of the population. Barrie Cassileth addresses the impact of new and effective treatments of cancer that have refocused cancer research on rehabilitation, psychosocial status and quality of life. This chapter examines older cancer patients and compares their reactions, problems, coping styles, and age-related psychosocial well-being to those of younger patients. The surprising trend toward better quality of life among older versus younger cancer patients suggests the need for further examination of aging influences on the capacity to cope with chronic diseases and disability.

In the chapter that follows, Peter Vitaliano and colleagues address quality of life issues as they relate to caregivers, who are often the "hidden" patients. Formulating a conceptual model of stress effects on health, they examine how caregiving reactions and responsibilities affect the health and well-being of the caregiver. They use the literature on cardiovascular risk factors in caregivers of people with Alzheimer's disease as a particular example. The effects of two psychological factors, anger and depression, on the presence of cardiovascular risk factors (e.g., reactivity, lipid levels, blood pressure) are examined. Not only are elderly caregivers' risk for cardiovascular problems aggravated by their emotional states, but there is also some suggestion that older people are more vulnerable than younger persons to the health risks of caregiving stressors. Such basic research on older caregivers' vulnerabilities and resources can contribute to the selection of strategies for identifying caregivers at risk and helping them cope with their caregiving responsibilities.

Part IV: Older People and Their Environments

Chapters in Part IV address older people's health and functioning in relation to their social and physical environments. Emphasis in this section is on the significance of support networks and older people's sense of control for successful aging and effective functioning in the community, as well as in institutions. Implicit in the concept of "successful aging" is the ability to maintain mastery over one's environment. Therefore, attention is given to the physical environment and the dynamic interactions between the aging person and environmental demands. Robert Kahn begins the section with a review of the content, causes, and consequences of social supports in terms of their effects on mortality and morbidity. He proposes a theoretical model of social support across the life course and considers strategies for increasing available supports for older people, especially the vulnerable. Kahn addresses the lack of consensus on the definition and measurement of social support, as well as causal mechanisms linking social support and health outcomes. Models, such as those proposed by Kahn, advance the state-of-the-art in research by providing a theoretical framework for specifying components of social supports over the life course.

Margie Lachman, Mauri Ziff, and Avron Spiro discuss another major social science construct that is often related to quality of life, the sense of control. Along with social support, sense of control emerges as one of the most powerful predictors of morbidity and mortality. A developmental framework of beliefs about control in later life is used to interpret correlations between control beliefs and functioning. Using age-related declines in memory as an example, they examine the impact of self-efficacy beliefs on memory aging, as well as specific interventions designed to modify negative control beliefs. This chapter presents the potential benefits of cognitive restructuring techniques for helping older people deal with memory losses. With special training, older people can retain a sense of personal mastery despite age-related deficits. As with the previous chapter by Kahn, the chapter points out the need for greater attention to definitional clarity and conceptually driven assessment methodologies.

Influences of environmental factors on older people's quality of life are addressed in the chapter by Margaret Baltes. The chapter discusses whether certain environments, such as long-term care institutions, hinder the processes necessary for successful adaptation to the imbalance between gains and losses with old age. Institutions that recognize the need to maximize the fit between personal abilities and environmental demands will be most successful in maintaining personal competencies. Baltes stresses the importance of three behavioral processes —selection, compensation, and optimization—for maximizing functioning in the face of declining physical or mental abilities. The implementation of this model would require that care in the typical nursing home be reoriented. Change from institutional care models that inadvertently reinforce dependency to highly individualized approaches that stress independence and autonomy is recommended.

Robin Barr addresses the importance of the physical and technological environment for effective functioning. Barr discusses the need for extending principles of human factors research (the science of matching the physical and technological environment to the intended users) to research on aging. A human factors approach can be applied to understanding and specifying tasks involved in older peoples' accomplishment of activities of everyday living, medication adherence, driving, and paid work. The findings presented in this chapter suggest strategies for reducing task demands and enhancing performance. A review of progress made in human factors and aging research argues for a reorientation within the gerontological research and services community to realize the full potential of this newly emerging discipline.

Part V: Social Structures, Quality of Life, and Aging

Gerontological research has exploded the myth that aged populations are necessarily frail, dependent, and homogeneous. In fact, research has demonstrated tremendous diversity within the aged population. Part V explores the physical, social, and economic needs of the population, noting how these changes depend on the individual's social strata. Matilda White Riley and Karyn Loscocco open the section with a discussion of the gap that has developed between the interdependent processes of aging and changing social structures. They address changes in society by counterposing two ideal types of age structures, an "age-differentiated" type and an "age-integrated" type. Riley and Loscocco also discuss current pressures that are moving modern societies toward an "age-integrated" structure and propose a conceptual model for understanding the complex processes that link aging and structural change. Identifying barriers to change, Riley and Loscocco are nevertheless hopeful about the consequences of current social trends that will facilitate the emergence of more flexible work structures. These trends would result in improved quality of life and productivity of older people who are now spending over one third of their lives in "retirement."

There is considerable literature suggesting that people in different socioeconomic status (SES) strata experience significant differences in mortality, morbidity, and disability as they age. Stephanie Robert and James House discuss the implications of SES on changes in health as people age. Their chapter reviews evidence of SES differences in health over the life course and discusses six theories that attempt to explain why SES differentials in health may diminish in later old age. These include: (1) a data artifacts explanation, (2) the drift hypothesis, (3) a selective survival explanation, (4) an access to health care explanation, (5) a lifestyle behavior and psychosocial factors explanation, and (6) an age stratification explanation. Understanding the mechanisms linking SES to health over the life course requires additional theoretical and methodological attention. This review suggests the involvement of multiple explanations and the need for complex models that examine the effects of multiple and interacting factors.

A focus on specific subgroups within the aged population is important for examining the impacts of socioeconomic status. Toward this goal, the section next focuses on the socioeconomic status of two subgroups: the healthy older American and the poor older American. James Smith begins by discussing the socioeconomic status of *healthy* older people in the United States. This chapter presents three fundamental changes — new findings in research on aging, the emergence of important new data sets for collecting state-of-the-art health and economic information, and the emerging transnational character of aging research. It highlights new research findings that affect older people's ability to age successfully and explores how well new directions in aging research will transfer to other cultural settings. Economic research on transition to retirement, adequate income, and interactions between economic well being and health among the elderly is critical for formulating public policies for aging societies. Moreover, recent research indicating cross-national similarities in the relationships between economic factors and health behaviors of older people suggest a benefit of sharing economic and health data across national boundaries.

Although the economic well-being of older people as a whole has dramatically improved over the past 20 years, Asuman Kiyak and Nancy Hooyman point out that these improvements have not been equally distributed within the population. Minorities are disproportionately found in the ranks of the poor. This chapter reviews the socioeconomic status, health, and psychosocial well-being of older African Americans, Americans of Hispanic descent, Asian Americans, and Native Americans. By viewing poverty as both a determinant and consequence of quality of life, cumulative effects of life-long conditions (low income, limited education and language difficulties, unemployment and underemployment, and so on) are examined. A major issue for further research is the extent to which social and cultural factors can mediate the negative effects of poverty and enhance quality of life among the elderly minority poor. The problems of future cohorts of minority and ethnic elders in terms of quality of life are also examined.

Part VI: Policy Implications

Section VI examines the impact of social, behavioral, and health services research on the aging individual and society. This final section also speculates on how future cohorts of older people will be affected by changes in the social and health care systems. Carroll Estes and Elizabeth Close emphasize the importance of understanding the linkages between social factors and health across the entire life course. Their chapter highlights four societal forces that have shaped public policy and long-term care: the aging of the American population, the biomedicalization of aging, unresolved problems concerning health care access and costs, and the cummulation of dependency in old age. Estes and Close identify specific research that is needed to assist in the design of long-term care policy. This research agenda is attentive to racial, ethnic, gender and social class differences, as well as subsequent policy considerations.

The next chapter, which is authored by Lennart Levi and Donna Cox, examines macrosocietal influences on the health and functioning of older people. Drawing examples from the Swedish experience, they demonstrate how public policies on healthy aging can make a difference in the lives of older people. Levi and Cox argue for comprehensive intersectorial governmental action involving multiple segments of society, and the testing of social experiments based on principles of applied intervention research. Adaptation of the social environment to the abilities and needs of elderly people is seen as the major health promotion strategy for adding years to life, as well as life to years.

Robert Binstock, Dennis Jahnigen, and Stephen Post conclude the section with a look at American health care for older people as it may emerge in the early twenty-first century. Fundamental changes are occurring in health care which, will affect the quality of life for older persons, and more generally, society. The chapter addresses several emergent changes that will affect older people and their health care providers. These include issues related to doctor–patient relations, geriatric acute care, rehabilitation and long-term care, and law and ethics.

Conclusions

Although it is difficult to predict the future, one certainty prevails: the life experiences and expectations of people who reach old age in the early decades of the twenty-first century will be substantially different from those who grew old in earlier decades. Moreover, societal changes that interact with a rapidly aging population underscore the need for a firm conceptualization and measurement of what is meant by quality of life. As new health technologies and social environments improve the life circumstances for older people, the criteria for a "good" quality of life will undoubtedly change. An understanding of the factors that facilitate or impede enriched quality of life throughout the life course and over time is important for identifying those at risk for less than optimal quality of life and for designing appropriate health-promoting interventions. As indicated in this volume, the past decade has seen the emergence of excellent behavioral sciences research on aging and quality of life. Yet, many unanswered research questions remain. As with explorers in the days of Columbus, the charting of new research territories remains a priority.

References

Aging America: Trends and Projections. (1991). Prepared by the U.S. Senate Special Committee on Aging, the American Association of Retired Persons, the Federal Council on the Aging and the U.S. Administration on Aging. Washington, D.C. : U.S. Department of Health & Human Services.

Fries, J. F. (1989). The compression of morbidity: near or far? *The Milbank Quarterly, 67,* 208–232.

Guralnik, J. LaCroix, A.Z., Everett, D.F., Kovar., M.A. (1989, May 26). *Aging in the Eighties: The prevalence of comorbidity and its association with disability.* Number 170. National Center for Health Statistics.

Hing, E. & Bloom B. (1990). National Center for Health Statistics, *Long-term Care For The Functionally Dependent Elderly.* Vital and Health Statistics, Series 13, No. 104. National Center For Health Statistics. Hyattsville, MD: Public Health Service.

Institute of Medicine. (1991). *Extending Life, Enhancing Life.* A National Research Agenda on Aging. Washington, DC: National Academy Press.

Lawton, M.P. (1983). Environment and other determinants of well-being in older people. *The Gerontologist, 23,* 349–357.

Lawton, M.P. (1991). Quality of life: Medical and other. In J.E. Birren, D.E. Deutchman, J. Lubben, & J. Rowe (Eds.). *The concept and measurement of quality of life in the later years.* New York: Academic Press.

Manton, K.G., Corder, L.S. & Stallard, E. (1993a). Estimates of change in chronic disability and institutional incidence and prevalence rates in the U.S. elderly population from the 1982, 1984, and 1989 National Long Term Care Survey. *Journal of Gerontology. 48:* S153–S166.

Manton, K.G., Corder, L.S. & Stallard, E. (1993b). Changes in the use of personal assistance and special equipment 1982–1989: results from the 1982 and 1989 National Long Term Care Survey. *The Gerontologist, 33:* 168–176.

National Center for Health Statistics. (1991). *Health, United States, 1990.* Hyattsville, MD: Public Health Service.

National Center for Health Statistics. (1993). *Health data on older Americans: United States, 1992.* Series 3, No. 27. Hyattsville, MD: Public Health Service.

Omenn, G. S. (Ed.). (1992, February). Health Promotion and Disease Prevention. *Clinics in Geriatric Medicine,* 1–232.

Ory, M G., Abeles, R P., & Lipman, P. D. (1992). *Aging, Health, And Behavior.* Newbury Park; CA: Sage.

Ory, M. G. & Duncker, A.P. (Eds.). (1992). Introduction: The Home Care Challenge. *In-home care for older people: Health and supportive services (pp. 1–8).* Newbury Park, CA: Sage.

Patrick, D. L. & Bergner, M., (1990). Measurement of Health Status in the 1990s. *Annual Review of Public Health, 11,* 165–183.

Riley, M W. & Riley, J. W. (1989). The quality of aging: Strategies for interventions. *Annals of the American Academy of Political and Social Sciences.* *503,* 9–147.

Schneider, E. I., & Brody, J. A.. (1983). Aging, natural death and the compression of morbidity. *New England Journal of Medicine. 303,* 854–855.

Schumacher, M., Olschewski, M. & Schulgen, G. (1991). Assessment of quality of life in clinical trials. *Statistics in Medicine. 10,* 1915–1930.

Shumaker, S. A., Anderson A. T., & Czajkowski S. M. (1990). Psychological Tests and Scales. In B. Spiker, (Ed.). *Quality of life in clinical trials* (pp. 95–113). New York: Raven Press.

Stewart, A. L, & King, A. C. (1991). Evaluating the efficacy of physical activity for influencing quality of life outcomes in older adults. *Annals of Behavioral Medicine, 13,* 108–116.

Stewart, A. L. & Ware, J. E. (1992). *Measuring functioning and well-being.* Durham, NC: Duke University Press.

Suzman, R. M., Willis D. P., & Manton K. G. (1992). *The oldest old.* New York: Oxford University Press.

U.S. Bureau of the Census. (1993).Sixty five plus in America. *Current Population Reports.* Special Issue. P25–1092. Washington, DC: U.S. Government Printing Office.

Verbrugge, L.M. (1990). The iceberg of disability. *The legacy of longevity.* S.M. Stahl (Ed.), Newbury Park, CA: Sage.

World Health Organization. (1946). Definition of health (Preparatory Committee of the International Health Conference). Geneva: Author.

PART I

Background Perspectives

Chapter 1

Historical Perspective on Aging and the Quality of Life*

Robert N. Butler

Recently Christopher Columbus, that great explorer in the dimension of space, was honored for the European discovery of the Western Hemisphere 500 years ago, even though he was actually looking for another. Few in Columbus's time comprehended or appreciated what he had achieved.

Today we are only beginning to comprehend the discoveries and achievements of other great explorers in the dimension of time. Few can now imagine achieving the "Fountain of Youth." Yet, a related revolution in longevity has occurred in the twentieth century, which is a striking social achievement, not a consequence of biological evolution. Nearly 25 years of average life expectancy has been gained in this century in the industrialized world. This is nearly equal to the gain in life expectancy obtained during the preceding 5,000 years of human history. The "Longevity Revolution" came about primarily as a result of progress in economic well-being and public health. The application of the germ theory of disease has produced striking reduc-

---

*Based on "Searching for the Fountain of Youth: 500 Years of Research to Understand Aging," Keynote for *Aging: The Quality of Life Conference*, Washington, DC, February 10–12, 1992.

tions in maternal, childhood, and infant mortality rates that have, in turn, contributed to the Longevity Revolution. Thus, just as Columbus broke through invisibile spatial barriers, thanks to science, courage, and luck, so are we now breaching the barriers of longevity.

The Rise of Science

Columbus's fifteenth century was not an easy century in which to live. Societies and their economies were still suffering the effects of the Black Death. The universities and even the churches were having difficult times. Science, as now conceived, did not exist. Yet, certain key historic events—such as the Italian Renaissance, the invention of the printing press, and the beginning Spanish and Portuguese explorations marking the European age of discovery—were catalysts for modern science.

If Columbus's fifteenth century saw the beginning of worldwide geographic exploration, the following century saw the birth of modern science. The sixteenth century revolution in science began with Copernicus, Paracelsus, and Vesalius, each attacking long-standing dogmas of alleged authorities. Sir Frances Bacon (1561–1626) urged the scientific method and developed *The Great Instauration*, which was a comprehensive plan to reorganize the sciences and restore to humanity mastery over nature, which was conceived to have been lost by the fall of Adam. (Incidentally, he was also the author of *The History of Life and Death with Observations Natural and Experimental for the Prolongation of Life*, a treatise published in 1623 that is relevant to gerontology.)

Despite over four centuries and great scientific advances, it would be wise to admit how little is really known. Indeed, less is known than is commonly thought about the world and its human and other inhabitants in all respects. Little is known about thousands of species, many of which will become extinct before they are studied. Questions that dominate scientific hypotheses, and even questions reformulated with the passage of centuries, are often unanswerable until newer, more appropriate concepts and technology are developed. The fundamentals of energy and motion have yet to be probed successfully, although it is possible that the superconducting supercollider near Geneva, Switzerland will achieve this goal. The fields of aging and longevity science are in their infancies. Most of all, human behavior is only beginning to be understood, and this may be the most dangerous *terra incognito*.

The process of discovery goes on, however, despite the persistence of human ignorance in the world, massive poverty, repetitive family violence, and persistent conflicts among various national, ethnic, and religious groups who have failed the basic test of tolerance and are unable yet to see the human family as a whole.

Science and various intellectual pursuits continue to struggle against great odds. Both public and private patronage remain limited. Public acceptance of scientific inquiries varies and, most recently, has been affected by rising forces of antiintellectual, antitechnological, and antiscientific sentiment. Indeed, some of the sequelae of science, which those of us in science failed to foretell, have contributed to this negativism and should remind us to assess the impact of scientific discovery and application on people and the environment. Witness, for example, industrial development and pollution, or the ethical issues related to end-of-life decisions that have resulted from discoveries in medicine.

Research in human development, from fetal life to old age, is often suspect in the eyes of many. Some people feel threatened by any tinkering with nature, even if the intention is to preserve and extend life, or to alter negative outcomes of behaviors and social conditions. In part, these concerns stem from fears of an extended life consisting of disability, disease, destititution, and dependence in old age. To alleviate this fear, aging research must focus on maintaining the healthy middle years of life—that is, on seeking a life of high quality, not merely an extended life *per se*. Research plans are required that integrate the biology of aging with clinical conditions as well as with the social and behavioral aspects of aging in order to improve the quality of life in aging.

The New Science of Aging

Just as Columbus and other explorers were following in the footsteps of others, often in science, so-called new discoveries are rediscoveries or reformulations of older, even ancient concepts and findings. The basic theories of aging were laid down centuries ago. Theories of aging can be divided into two kinds: Those that consider aging to be essentially inherent, developmental, or programmed and those that consider aging to be a result of random, stochastic, or environmental ("wear and tear") factors. Some theories involve both. The debate over whether aging is normal or a disease process goes back to Aristotle and Cicero. Despite all scientific efforts, the struggle to disentangle aging, health, and disease continues.

Paracelsus, born in 1493, said "a doctor must be a traveller; knowledge is experience." He appeared to understand that there is a difference between questions about how and why people age and how and why people live as long as they do. Furthermore, Paracelsus put scientists on the track of modern pharmacology, and he appreciated as well the healing process of nature.

During the twentieth century, indeed the last 50 years, many scientific advances have propelled research on aging forward. Beyond the genetic, cellular, and biological organismic levels, many advances are being made in the social, behavioral, economic, and methodological arenas that are the focus of this volume. In addition to the study of Alzheimer's disease, research includes basic biology, clinical syndromes that accompany aging and reflect disease–age interactions, as well as social and behavioral factors. Epidemiological and demographic studies help serve policy development as well as the understanding of the origins, risk factors, incidence, and prevalence of disease and disability at various ages.

As noted earlier, the Longevity Revolution took place over the past century, mainly as a result of improvements in public health. Now, the results of what might be called the "Longevity Revolution II" are beginning to be observed. This refers to the maintenance and even restoration of biological systems that extend life expectancy. If one could maintain the integrity of the immune, central nervous, and endocrine systems, it would have important effects on a variety of diseases and disabilities of old age, not just one. A current practical example is estrogen replacement therapy (ERT), which probably helps prevent heart disease as well as osteoporosis, thus holding great potential for improved quality of life. Another example is the remarkable evidence of research in neuroplasticity that offers great hope for both an extended life expectancy and an extended quality of life of the mind. In addition, a "Longevity Revolution III" may lie ahead, if the ability to affect genes concerned with length of life were to be gained. With these advances—and even those already existing—come new frontiers for social and behavioral sciences: How will people and society adapt to an extended healthy old age?

Aging is a capacious subject. Scientific investigations must go far beyond the current emphasis on Alzheimer's disease to understand

and ameliorate a whole range of diseases and disabilities of old age. Studies of the frail elderly—with complex, multiple, interacting acute and chronic psychological and physical conditions—are needed. Research must be expanded in biology, pharmacology, nutrition, as well as in the social and behavioral aspects of aging (such as the impact of retirement, family life, bereavement, sexuality). Similarly, greater attention is needed to health service delivery research and to analytical and empirical ethics research.

The past has seen fruitful collaborations among The National Institutes of Health (NIH), other Federal agencies, academics and the commercial sector. The complexity of aging research in the future will be best met by similar and expanded collaboration across topical areas as well as across organizations. For example, an unexplored area is work history as a constituent element (e.g., risk factors) in the determination of quality of late life. The National Institute on Aging's (NIA) recently launched Retirement History Study will provide improved understanding of the mutual and complex influences of work experiences, health, and wealth on later life. The resulting knowledge should provide practical information that will shape work, retirement, Social Security, and Medicare policies in the twenty-first century.

Increased emphasis on studies of human performance—the maintenance and restoration of various physical and psychological factors that are conducive to the maintenance of productive aging—should be likewise useful. Inasmuch as individuals live longer, perhaps they should work longer. This is based on the simple premise that a productive life is good for the individual and for society. When Social Security was passed into law, the average life expectancy of men was not yet 60 and that of women was about 63. Now just over 50 years later, average life expectancy is over 70 and nearly 80, respectively. Functional status, not chronological age, should be considered as a determinant of retirement. Ways for individuals to remain productive in a *full-participation society* throughout life should be considered. (See Chapter 13.)

Moreover, genetic diseases and lifestyle need to be explored across wide-spread age, racial, ethnic, and social class groups. Epidemiological and longitudinal studies and augmentation of national health promotion and disease prevention programs for older adults are needed. Given this remarkable, multicultural, multiracial, and multiethnic country, a kind of indigenous anthropology can be practiced, while always appreciating individual differences.

A new stage of aging research has been reached. This is a *new ger-*

ontology, which is interventionist in character. Its beginnings can be traced to studies of healthy, community-residing older people. Through these studies first came the revision of ideas, indeed, myths and stereotypes about aging, such as the natural inevitability of senility. A better understanding of the underlying mechanisms of aging such as immune senescence and osteopenia has been reached. Preventive, therapeutic, and rehabilitative interventions, which include social and behavioral strategies such as the famous Widow-to-Widow Program and various biomedical interventions, often borrowing from other fields (such as dietary, exercise, pharmacologic, and endocrine therapy), have been introduced. As genetic therapy is introduced successfully, genetic strategies will become part of this area of research. Finally, personal responsibility to maintain health is being emphasized, and data suggest that a positive, optimistic disposition is associated with longevity, as are the possession of goals and structure in one's life.

Some interventions in gerontology focus on delay of occurrence, a reasonable approach in late life. For example, if the onset of Alzheimer's disease could be delayed by 5 years, the incidence would be reduced by 50%. Some interventions, including growth hormones, may retard aging or restore earlier stages, though much the same can be accomplished by aerobic (target heart rate) exercise and strengthening. An important sidebar to the great contributions of the new interventionist gerontology is the empowerment of older persons themselves. They have become better-informed consumers, who are more conscious of their power and effectiveness not only through the rise of organizations such as the American Association of Retired Persons, but also in the myriad ways in which older persons remain contributory to their families, their communities, and to the nation.

What people seek in addition to longevity is a reasonable quality of life: The retention of their energy, health, and strength (youth), memory (mind), functioning (mobility and independence), and romance (sexuality). This, after all, is what it is ultimately all about—the maintenance of vigorous and healthy citizenry for as long as possible. Oliver Wendell Holmes' poem, "The Deacon's Masterpiece or The Wonderful One Hoss Shay" (1858), is certainly the lodestar for the voyage of discovery in gerontology. Ultimately the goal is not to imagine living for the sake of living, but maintaining a high quality of life up until the final moments.

Of course, there must not only be a vibrant science of aging and longevity, but also helmsmen to maintain the course of the ships of discovery. In the larger scheme of things, science is no longer a small-time cottage industry. Principles and strategies for health research planning to moderate health politics are needed. Social, economic, and political factors influence research agendas and the delivery of services—and, therefore, the health and well-being of older Americans and, ultimately, of all Americans. It is necessary to understand the unity and continuity of life—that the children of today will one day be old. One age group should not be pitted against another. In particular, the Baby Boomers constitute a generation that will be at risk in its old age, with the forthcoming great numbers of older persons constituting 20% of the population in the decade 2020–2030.

"Knowledge is power," and perhaps modern scholarship, scientific knowledge, and databases constitute as much a concentration of power as do the legislative, judicial, and executive branches of government. Knowledge serves business and business people.

Certainly the issues of an aging workforce compel greater corporate attention. But individual philanthropists and foundations still need to take a more serious look at and invest in research on aging and longevity.

Philosophy is needed to guide us in the new world of aging and longevous societies. Aside from the thoughts of Aristotle in the *Rhetoric*, Cicero's majestic essay *De Senectute*, some of Montaigne's essays, notions concerning the stages of life in Shakespeare and Rousseau, Goethe's *Faust*, the thinking of Tolstoy in *The Death of Ivan Illych* and the great novel *Resurrection*, the books of Eli Metchnioff, Marcel Proust's *Remembrance of Things Past*, the five linked plays *Back to Methuselah* by George Bernard Shaw, some of Carl Gustave Jung's writings, and the twentieth century novel by Gabriel Garcia-Marquez *Love in the Time if Cholera*, as well as Western religious and ethical thinking in such works as *Ecclesiastes* and *Job*, surprisingly little in Western literature exists to contribute to a philosophy of the conduct of life in the later years, understanding of aging and/or the prospect of an enriched longevity, or an approach to the inevitable crisis of illness, loss, dying, and death.

Columbus did not get to his destination—Cathay, the East—nor did Ponce de Leon reach the Fountain of Youth. But many interesting discoveries were made along the way. The destination of the Fountain of Youth may never be reached—a questionable pursuit in any case—but there will surely be fun and profit and serendipity along the way. Now, 500 years after Columbus's famous voyage, both past work and new scientific tools offer hope for prolonged, vigorous, and productive life—a reasonable quality of life in older age.

Reference

Holmes, Oliver Wendell (1955). The deacon's masterpiece or the wonderful one hoss shay. *The new perfect anthology of American verse*. The New York: Pocket Books.

Chapter 2

Conceptualizing and Measuring Quality of Life in Older Populations

Anita L. Stewart and Abby C. King

The purpose of this chapter is to provide a framework for defining quality of life that is appropriate and useful for studying quality of life in older adults, to review issues pertaining to defining and measuring quality of life in this population, and to briefly summarize the variety of measures that are available in this area.

Defining Quality of Life

The term "quality of life" is being used widely by clinicians and researchers, but because of the popular meanings that have been attached to it, the term remains a source of some confusion. In the purest sense, the term *quality* implies an evaluation or subjective rating by the individual. These subjective evaluations can be of life in general or of various components of life such as social life, financial situation, or work (Andrews & Withey, 1976; Campbell, Converse, & Rodgers, 1976). Perhaps because such subjective states are difficult to measure, investigators tend to bypass personal evaluations and *in-*

fer quality of life through knowledge of things about persons that are more observable or "objective." For example, we infer that persons in a wheelchair, with certain diseases, with low income, or limitations in physical functioning have a poor overall quality of life. Such inferences are risky, however, when one considers the countless individuals who have difficult "objective" situations but who consider their lives to be meaningful, satisfying, and enjoyable. In short, inferring subjective quality or well-being from external circumstances does not take fully into account the values, needs, and adaptability of individuals to various life circumstances (Flanagan, 1982).

Our tendency to infer quality from other factors reflects a lack of a clear distinction between *actual* quality of life and what might simply be *predictive* of quality of life. In particular, some confusion has occurred over the past decade because the term "quality of life" has been adopted by health researchers and clinicians to refer to a broad array of concepts that previously were referred to as components of health status or functional status. Thus, in addition to internal, subjective evaluations that represent the heart of the quality of life concept, the term now often includes concepts of physical and cognitive functioning, activities limitations, fatigue, pain, and health perceptions, among other things.

Should these health-related concepts be considered as components or predictors of quality of life? Three arguments favor the first alternative. First, some of these health-related concepts could justifiably be considered as part of subjective well-being and hence are closely aligned with the initial definition of quality of life. Second, one of the most common applications of quality of life assessments is to evaluate health care interventions (procedures, therapies). Third, because the term has now been widely and popularly adopted, it would likely be confusing to return to a more "pure" definition (Guyatt, Feeny, & Patrick, 1991).

Domains of Quality of Life

Because health issues are of primary concern to older adults, we recommend a comprehensive definition of quality of life that includes global, subjective ratings of life quality (satisfaction); other internal subjective states such as psychological distress/well-being, pain and discomfort, energy/fatigue, self-esteem, and sense of mastery/control; ability to function cognitively, physically, socially, sexually; ability to perform usual daily activities including self-maintenance and self-care activities; and perceived health. Although different terms may be used for these concepts by different investigators, the domains they represent remain reasonably similar (George & Bearon, 1980; Kane & Kane, 1981; Lawton, 1991; Patrick & Erickson, 1988). There is reasonably broad agreement on the domains that should be included among different investigators. Nevertheless, there is considerable variation within each domain in terms of how it is defined. To define each domain clearly requires defining the *content area* or components of the domain and the *response dimensions*.

Content Areas

The content area pertains to what aspects of the domain are included in the definition. For example, nearly all definitions of physical functioning include walking and climbing stairs. However, some distinguish among various distances walked (across a room, one block, one mile). Some definitions include complex tasks such as shopping and doing laundry and others include only basic physical functions such as getting out of a chair or getting out of bed. Some include discretionary activities such as running and walking long distances. Social functioning has also been defined in a variety of ways. For instance, it can be defined separately for various types of social relationships such as family, friends, or social groups. Functioning in daily activities, sometimes referred to as role functioning, can pertain to functioning in normal activities of daily life such as child care, care of parents, work, housework, or volunteering. As people age, many roles diminish in importance, especially work and child care, and are replaced by other more discretionary activities such as hobbies and recreation. The latter may be the most important to assess for older populations. Psychological well-being is often defined primarily in terms of depression, but other content areas are also important such as anxiety, anger, and positive affect. Within positive affect, happiness has been distinguished from "zest," which pertains to feeling interested and not bored with life (Liang, 1984).

Response Dimensions

Once the content area of each domain is defined, one needs to clarify what it is about each domain and content area that is of interest. For each content area, several types of response dimensions are possible. The majority of response dimensions in available measures of quality of life focus on defining some *level or state* of a behavior or a feeling. For example, for symptoms such as fatigue or pain, one could assess whether or not the symptom has occurred, how often it has occurred, how long the symptom lasts, and its intensity. Similarly, the response dimension for physical functioning could be extent of difficulty in various physical activities, limitations due to health, or limitations due to arthritis. Response dimensions requiring respondents to report only limitations that are attributable to health in general or to specific health problems may be difficult for older persons, especially if they have more than one condition or problem. For self-care activities, one could assess the duration of any limitations, need for help, receipt of help, the use of special equipment, or the extent of difficulty (Wiener, Hanley, Clark, & VanNostrand, 1990). Questions about specific activities that have a discretionary component such as cooking, doing moderate sports, climbing several flights of stairs, or handling finances, may be problematic for respondents who do not engage in these activities. If one offers a "not applicable" or "I don't do this" choice, then decisions regarding how to score these must be made. Some may not engage in the activity because they *cannot* (i.e., are unable) and have thus found alternatives out of necessity. Some may report not doing an activity because they *do not need to* in their environment (e.g., they can always use an elevator and thus never need to climb stairs). In this case, they may or may not be limited in the activity if they did it. People may not do certain activities because of the normative division of labor between men and women in older cohorts. Thus, men may not cook a meal or do shopping and women may not handle finances or do household repair.

An increasing concern is that measures of quality of life incorporate information on the values or preferences of the respondents and not simply reflect levels or states of health, functioning, or well-being. Knowing the value or importance of the different levels or states to the individual facilitates interpreting scores. One way to obtain such information is to ask respondents to *evaluate* their level of functioning or well-being in a particular domain, that is, rate their satisfaction with their level of functioning or well-being, rate the quality of that particular domain, or report how much they are bothered by a symptom. For example, one person may be perfectly satisfied with some functional limitations because he/she is able to do those things that are the most valued, whereas another person may be unsatisfied with the same limitations because they prevent him/her from doing something valued. Similarly, the value or importance of the level of social contact can be ascertained by asking about satisfaction with amount of contact. For symptoms, such as fatigue, one can ask the extent to which the symptom has been bothersome. Evaluative response dimensions are thus more closely related to the pure definition of "quality" than are the state or level response dimentions. If people report being satisfied with an "objectively" low level or state, it could reflect either a relatively low value placed on that domain or an adaptation or adjustment to the level. An example of the importance of evaluative response dimensions is illustrated by a recent study in which Parkinson's patients were asked about their level of functioning and well-being on a variety of domains and then were asked parallel items about the extent to which they were bothered by their problems on each domain. The correlations of the evaluative items (bothersomeness) were much stronger in relation to psychological well-being than were the correlations of the level or state on the domains (Brod, Cohen, & Mendelsohn, 1992).

Finally, some response dimensions are *comparative*, that is, they ask respondents to compare their present state on some domain with either a prior time point (e.g., worse, better, about the same relative to 1 year ago) or with their "usual" level or state (e.g., better or worse than usual). Because older individuals are often viewed as health optimists (Kutner et al., 1992), investigators might ask respondents to rate their health or functioning compared to others their own age. Clearly, each of these types of response dimensions yields different information. Thus, defining the response dimension is an extremely important part of the conceptualization process.

Quality of Life Conceptual Framework

Given the plethora of potential domains, content areas, and response dimensions, it is apparent that no single definition or conceptual framework of quality of life will suit all investigators or studies. Thus, in Table 2.1, we present a framework of *potential* domains, content areas, and response dimensions that could be useful in defining quality of life in aging studies. For each domain of quality of life outlined above, we list various content areas that might be defined. For example, within psychological distress/well-being, we have identified several content areas such as depression, anxiety, anger, and perceived stress. We then present possible response dimensions taken from various available instruments, organized into either level/state or evalua-

TABLE 2.1 Conceptual Framework of Quality of Life

Domain	Potential Content Areas	State/Level	Evaluative
		Potential Response Dimensions	
Physical functioning	Lower body (walking, climbing stairs, getting out of a chair) Upper body (e.g., reaching, carrying) Dexterity Basic movements (e.g., standing, walking short distances, climbing a few stairs) Discretionary movements (e.g., running, walking long distances) Mobility, ability to go places	Amount of difficulty (perceived or observed) Need for help Presence of problem Extent of limitation Able to perform	Satisfaction with level of functioning Extent to which bothered by limitation
Self-maintenance, self-care	Self-care (bathing, dressing, toileting, transferring, grooming, etc.) Instrumental activities (e.g., shopping, errands, cooking, finances, etc.)	Need for help Amount of difficulty (perceived or observed) Extent of limitation Able to perform	Satisfaction with abilities
Usual activities	Work, employment Child care Caregiving (of family, friends) Volunteer, community work Hobbies, recreational activities Work around the house	Unable to do because of health Any limitation because of health Extent of limitation due to health in general or due to physical health or due to emotional problems Extent of limitation due to specific health problem Restricted activity days: (e.g., no. of days unable to perform activity, limited in activity)	Satisfaction with ability to perform activity Satisfaction with amount of activities Quality of leisure time Extent to which bothered by limitations
Social functioning	With friends With groups With neighbors Family Spouse/partner	Amount of social contact Extent of limitation in activities due to health in general, due to physical health, or due to emotional problems Extent of limitations due to specific health problem Amount of social contact Social skills, abilities	Satisfaction with amount of contact Quality of social relationships Extent to which bothered by limitations Satisfaction with social life

TABLE 2.1 Continued

Domain	Potential Content Areas	Potential Response Dimensions		
		State/Level		Evaluative
Sexual functioning, intimacy		Frequency of sexual problems Presence of sexual problems		Satisfaction with sex life Extent bothered by sexual problems Satisfaction with level of intimacy
Psychological well-being and distress (Subjective well-being)	Depression Anxiety Anger, irritability Loneliness Positive affect (e.g., interest in life, happiness, hopefulness/optimism, morale, enjoyment) Perceived stress Distress about health	Amount of time experienced various psychological states Presence of various psychological states Frequency of various psychological states		Satisfaction with psychological states
Cognitive functioning	Memory Confusion Attention Concentration Orientation Judgement Alertness	Frequency of cognitive problems Presence of cognitive problems		Worry about cognitive function Concern about cognitive problems Extent to which bothered by cognitive problems
Pain and discomfort	Pain in general Specific pains (e.g., back pain, angina)	Severity/intensity (on average, at its worst) Extent pain interferes with activities Duration of pain Frequency of pain		Extent to which bothered by pain Ability to tolerate pain Ability to manage pain Distress due to pain
Energy/fatigue	Energy, pep Fatigue, tiredness	Frequency of states of fatigue Amount of time experienced states of energy, fatigue		Extent to which bothered by fatigue Satisfaction with level of energy "Enough" energy to do everything

TABLE 2.1 Continued

Domain	Potential Content Areas	Potential Response Dimensions	
		State/Level	Evaluative
Sleep	Sleep disturbance Daytime sleepiness	Frequency of sleep problems Amount of sleep	Perceived adequacy of sleep
Self-esteem	General esteem Physical self-esteem: (e.g., physical appearance, competence) Social self esteem Intellectual self esteem	Agreement with statements about self	Satisfaction with self
Sense of mastery, control	General control Control over health	Agreement with statements about control	Satisfaction with level of control
Perceived health	Current health Future health Past health Resistance to illness	Ratings of health Agreement with statements about health	Satisfaction with level of health
Life satisfaction	Current life in general Past life in general Components of life:[a] (e.g., social life, life situation)		Satisfaction with life Extent to which needs met Contentment with life

[a]Satisfaction with various components of life such as social life, work life, etc. is sometimes defined by the evaluative response dimension in that category (e.g., satisfaction with social life is the evaluative response dimension for social functioning).

tive dimensions. For instance, three potential response dimensions of social functioning are amount of social contact, satisfaction with amount of contact, and perceived quality of social relationships. The comparative response dimension is omitted from the table because it does not vary by domain or content area.

The table is intended to provide a menu of possibilities of measurement for any one concept. By defining the appropriate concepts and dimensions to be measured for a particular study population and question of interest, the subsequent selection of useful and relevant measures can be made easier. Our goal is to provide a way to think about the conceptualization of quality of life rather than to present an exhaustive review of all possible ways in which it has been defined. Thus, although Table 2.1 is reasonably comprehensive with respect to the most common domains of quality of life, there are numerous definitions that are unrepresented here.

One distinction that has been made in this framework is worth noting, between physical functioning and self-care/self-maintenance activities. Although the latter are often considered as indicators of physical functioning, we distinguish them because the ability to perform complex activities depends on not only the physical abilities involved, but environmental factors and the individual's cognitive abilities. For example, the ability to shop depends on people's physical abilities as well as the distance and nature of transportation to the store.

We acknowledge that the domains are highly interrelated and undoubtedly there is considerable overlap in the information across domains. We leave to others the tasks of addressing which of these domains contain the most unique and independent information, or which are more important to assess. For example, social functioning is confounded with usual daily activities, as many daily activities are social in nature. Nevertheless, some response dimensions of social functioning tap quite different aspects of quality of life than limitations in usual activities. Similarly, sexual functioning and intimacy are closely related to social functioning. We retained this as a unique category, however, because individuals can be functioning well socially yet have little intimacy or sexual contact. Because overall life satisfaction concepts are very broad, they often encompass specific components of this framework, especially psychological distress and well-being.

Determinants of Quality of Life

By defining quality of life somewhat inclusively, what remains is to identify factors that could be considered as *determinants* of quality of life. We consider the major categories of determinants of quality of life to be clinical status, health care, lifestyle, social environment, community environment, and personality, socioeconomic, and demographic characteristics. These categories and sample components of each are summarized in Table 2.2.

An understanding of the many determinants of quality of life can serve many purposes. One is to identify the *most important contributors* to quality of life so that they can be targeted for programs and interventions. Another is to provide a *descriptive context* for understanding how to appropriately measure quality of life within a particular study. For example, knowing the range and level of education, literacy, medical problems, and living situation in a particular study sample can aid selection of an appropriate conceptual and measurement approach, for example whether the focus should be on lower- versus higher-levels of functioning, or what methods of data collection are optimal. Finally, scores on such determinants can become useful *covariates* in studies attempting to explain quality of life outcomes, enabling isolation of the unique influence of the independent variables of primary interest.

Issues in Defining and Measuring Quality of Life in Aging Studies

There are numerous conceptual, methodologic, and measurement issues that pertain to defining and measuring quality of life in older populations. They include the wide variability in quality of life, concerns about the time frame, whether one is interested in states or traits, the order in which questions are asked, method of administration, proxy respondents, data quality, number of response choices, sensitivity of measures to change, tradeoffs between using single summary scores and profiles of scores, and use of utility approaches.

Variability in Quality of Life

In a given older population, one finds a very broad range on virtually all quality of life domains. Whereas most younger populations tend

TABLE 2.2
A Sample of Quality of Life Determinants for Older Adults

Clinical Status	Medical and mental conditions
	Sensory limitations
	Physical impairments
Health Care	Medications
	Procedures, therapies
	Information provided
	Interpersonal style of provider
	Treatment regimens
Social environment	Living arrangement
	Privacy
	Social networks, social support
	Marital status
	Life events
Physical/community environment	Dwelling unit – physical layout
	Resources for seniors
	Safety
	Gathering places for seniors
	Recreational opportunities
	Transportation opportunities
Lifestyle	Exercise
	Diet/nutrition
	Smoking
	Alcohol use
	Spiritual practices
	Participation in activities
	Recreational
	Intellectual
	Social
	Community
	Creative
	Other
Personality characteristics	Ability to cope
	Adaptability to change
	Friendliness
	Attitude toward aging
Socioeconomic factors	Employment status
	Financial status, income
	Occupation
Demographic factors	Age
	Gender
	Education
	Race/ethnicity

to be healthy on average, older populations include many who are doing very well and many who are doing very poorly on any domain measured (Rowe & Kahn, 1987). This presents both advantages and disadvantages in quality of life studies. This large variability is statistically advantageous, providing an increased likelihood of detecting associations among variables. However, it presents a problem when attempting to select a measure that is appropriate for individuals at both ends of the continuum. A measure that will capture the variation at one end (e.g., activities of daily living) will create ceiling effects in the group of individuals at the healthy end of the continuum (all will score perfectly on the scale). If a large proportion of the sample has the highest possible score, change in the positive direction is less likely to be detected. For example, measures of ability to perform self-care and self-maintenance activities (e.g., bathe, cook, shop, eat) in an active, healthy, older population would tend to have ceiling effects. One general approach to this problem is to use two measures —one tapping variation in lower-level activities and another extending into higher-level functions (Guralnik & LaCroix, 1992).

Time Frame

Ratings of subjective well-being may vary depending on the time frame of the questions. For example, results varied depending on whether subjects were asked about their overall well-being over the past day, week, or month with the stability being greatest for the longest time period (Flanagan, 1982). Despite this, because of memory problems, shorter time frames such as one or two weeks may be preferable for older respondents. For measures of functioning, the time frame needs to take into account whether one is concerned with acute situations or fairly long-term, chronic circumstances. For example, a measure of physical functioning that asks about limitations over the past month is more likely to tap those caused by chronic health conditions or impairments. If the time frame focuses on the last two days, the limitations reported may have more to do with acute illness, for example, persons not feeling well may feel limited temporarily in their physical functioning because of fatigue. The latter, acute type of limitation is perhaps more appropriately assessed by asking about "disability days."

States or Traits?

In considering concepts of quality of life as potential outcome measures of interventions, we are assuming that such concepts are changeable or mutable, which remains an open question. Although some of the more health-related components (e.g., pain, fatigue) are surely mutable, some of the more subjective and evaluative components may be more stable. For example, levels of psychological distress and well-being may be somewhat stable (McNeil, Stones, & Kozma, 1986), reflecting the tendency of individuals to adapt to changing circumstances. McNeil and colleagues concluded this based on their evaluation of the consistently small proportion of variance explained by various predictors of subjective well-being and the high stability coefficients in many studies of older adults. Changes in psychological well-being may represent acute responses to difficult situations that stabilize over time. To the extent that this is the case, it would be difficult to expect measures of psychological distress and well-being to change much in response to a medical or other intervention. This issue merits some attention. Global evaluations may tend to be more stable than evaluations of specific aspects of one's life. Thus, global evaluations may be more useful as descriptors or predictors of other concepts rather than as outcomes. Longitudinal studies evaluating quality of life dimensions across the life span are needed to better understand this issue.

Ordering of Questions

The order in which quality of life concepts are asked may affect responses. Making older subjects aware of losses or unhappiness may affect their responses to subsequent questions (Kutner et al., 1992). Kutner and colleagues suggest that the order should proceed from questions with less emotional impact to those with more. They further suggest that when questions may be distressing, explaining the purpose of the questions may be helpful.

Methods of Administration

Selection of an appropriate method that will provide quality data requires an understanding of the advantages and disadvantages of each. Special problems of some subgroups of older populations such as cognitive difficulties or sensory limitations may affect the choices regarding the optimal method. Several methods of administration are available—self-administration, self-report using a personal or telephone interview, subjective ratings by trained observers (including clinicians), and performance-based testing. Performance-based assessments are those in which individuals actually perform specific physical, self-care, or cognitive tasks (e.g., walk a certain distance, put on a shirt, count backwards) and are assigned scores by trained observers.

Each of the different methods of data collection has advantages for different populations. Self-administration is the least expensive and offers respondents the most privacy. However, it can be problematic for those with vision, reading, or language problems. When self-administration is used, extensive follow-up of missing and inconsistent responses may be needed. Personal and telephone interviews may be a viable alternative. Although they are more time-consuming than self-administration, both in terms of staff and respondent burden, the savings of time needed to follow up on missing data and nonreturned self-administered forms may somewhat offset these costs. Although hearing impairments are prevalent in the elderly, only 5% of persons over 65 report having difficulty using a telephone (Dawson, Hendershot, & Fulton, 1987). However, telephone interviews may be more stressful for those with hearing problems (Herzog, Rodgers, & Kulka, 1983). For measures of physical functioning, cognitive functioning, and self-care activities, performance-based measures allow assessment of those who are cognitively impaired and who might be unable to complete a self-reported instrument. Disadvantages include their cost and time, the need for special equipment and special training of examiners, and the fact that they tend to assess individuals outside of their own familiar environment, which may result in atypical scores (Guralnik, Branch, Cummings, & Curb, 1989; Guralnik & LaCroix, 1992). When personal interviews are used, the use of response cards with response choices written out has proven helpful (Kutner et al., 1992).

A practical, cost-effective approach in many studies is to use *mixed modes* of data collection, combining the advantages of different modes (Rodgers & Herzog, 1992). Utilizing mixed-mode approaches requires an understanding of the equivalence of the various methods (e.g., interview vs. self-administration) in terms of data quality (Rodgers & Herzog, 1992). The optimal mixed-mode is one that combines telephone and face-to-face interviews because of their general equivalence (Herzog & Rodgers, 1988). Another option is to begin with self-administration and provide help for those who have difficulty with this response mode. However, less is known about the equivalence of self-administration and personal interview (Herzog & Kulka, 1989).

Proxy Respondents

When older persons are unable to respond for themselves because of cognitive impairment or frailty, a spouse or family member may be asked to respond for them. This approach is essential to obtain a representative sample; it becomes more necessary when the sample is older and more disabled (Magaziner, 1992; Rodgers & Herzog, 1992).

Several factors affect the accuracy of proxy reports, including the relationship of the proxy to the respondent, the amount of time spent with the subject, the nature of the questions, and the health, cognitive, and affective status of the respondent (Epstein, Hall, Tognetti, Son, & Conant, 1989; Magaziner, Simonsick, Kashner, & Hebel, 1988). Magaziner (1992) identifies two key issues concerning proxies: response precision and response bias. If errors in proxy ratings are random, the issue can be handled by increasing the sample size. When the errors are biased, more problems are created. If proxies are being used for all respondents and the study is correlational in nature, the issue is less serious than if proxies are being used for some respondents and/or population estimates are being made.

Results of studies on proxy respondents suggest that some bias is introduced by using proxies; the magnitude and nature of the bias depends on a variety of factors. The nature of the bias appears to be reasonably consistent across studies, with proxies tending to report poorer health and functioning than subjects themselves (Magaziner et al., 1988; Rubenstein, Schairer, Wieland, & Kane, 1984). Most studies focus on the ability of proxies to rate somewhat objective facets of the person's life such as their functioning or behavior. One would anticipate even less agreement with regard to more subjective information such as feelings of well-being.

Data Quality

Because of potential problems with memory, comprehension, vision, hearing, and dexterity in older populations, a number of data quality issues are of particular concern. Data quality problems that can affect reliability and validity include not answering certain questions, responding by guessing to questions that are confusing or ambiguous, tending to agree with questions that are in an agree–disagree format, tending to respond "don't know" rather than committing to a choice, and responding in socially desirable ways (Colsher & Wallace, 1989; Sherbourne & Meredith, 1992). Although these problems are not specific to the collection of quality of life data, methods and measures of quality of life may need to be specially designed to assure optimal data quality.

The extent of occurrence of these problems remains controversial and may depend on the content of the questions being asked (Colsher & Wallace, 1989). Because of these potential problems, it is important for investigators to evaluate the data quality in any study of older adults to assure that measures meet minimal psychometric standards in their sample.

One needs to understand not simply *whether* data quality problems increase with age, but the *magnitude* of the problems, that is, whether they are of sufficient magnitude to seriously affect one's ability to utilize the data. Some studies suggest that although data quality is related to age, the magnitude of the problem is not serious (Colsher & Wallace, 1989). For example, Sherbourne and Meredith (1992) evaluated the reliability of self-administered data on functioning and well-being in various age groups in a sample of 2,304 patients in the Medical Outcomes Study. Of the 18 measures evaluated, reliability tended to diminish with age for eight measures. Nevertheless, the reliability coefficients were high in all groups. The results of this important data-quality study suggest that although some decrements were observed in the older age groups, they were not severe and the data quality remained adequate.

Number of Response Choices

The optimal number of response choices is an issue in general research methodology, but is more controversial in studies of older adults. Some believe that in very old subgroups, dichotomous response choices are best. Hence the popularity of the Geriatric Depression Scale, which consists of statements to which respondents answer yes or no (Yesavage et al., 1983). However, others have found that dichotomous items were disliked by most respondents because they could not respond adequately (Carp, 1989).

In one study of older respondents' preferences for different formats, five-point scales were best liked and had the best distributions (Carp, 1989). In a study of different types of response formats for evaluative items, items with 10 response choices tended to yield the best data quality whereas items with only four response choices yielded the worst in a sample of adults aged 60 and older (Rodgers, Herzog, & Andrews, 1988). Methodological research needs to continue to address these issues.

Sensitivity to Change

When quality of life measures are to be used to monitor change over time, it is essential to know whether the measure selected is known to be sensitive to clinically important changes. Although the methodological issue of sensitivity to change is clearly acknowledged (Deyo & Inui, 1984), there is actually very little systematic knowledge related to the sensitivity of particular measures or instruments. One recent study compared several quality of life measures in terms of their ability to detect a treatment effect in arthritis patients (Bombardier & Raboud, 1991). Methods for evaluating the sensitivity of measures to change are available (Deyo, Diehr, & Patrick, 1991).

Several features of measures contribute to their ability to change over time. First, the measures must be assessing a *mutable characteristic* that is likely to change rather than a more stable trait or characteristic. Second, the measure must have enough scale levels to detect small changes. Some measures, especially single-item measures, may be too coarse to be sensitive to small changes. Third, the *variability* in the measure at the initial assessment must be sufficient that change can be detected (e.g., there should not be strong floor or ceiling effects).

For many available measures, information on their ability to discriminate among groups differing in clinical status is more commonly found than information on change in scores over time on the same individuals. The sensitivity of measures to change may be even more important in studies of older populations than in other groups, because of the controversy over whether dysfunction and diminished well-being can be reversed in older adults.

Single Summary Scores versus Profiles

Although there is consensus that quality of life is a multidimensional concept, there continues to be a demand for a single score that reflects overall quality of life. Sometimes investigators depend on a single summary *item* such as an overall rating of life quality (Campbell et al., 1976). Overall subjective well-being *indexes* that combine information across diverse categories may also fulfill this need (Lawton, 1975; Neugarten, Havighurst, & Tobin, 1961).

The most critical issue in selecting a single summary score is the content of that score—each one contains a different mixture of information. Depending on one's definition of "overall quality of life," as well as the characteristics of the population under study and the goals of the investigation, these various summary indexes and items may or may not be adequate.

There are a number of disadvantages to relying primarily on single summary scores instead of using scores on multiple domains of quality of life. If the summary measure is being used to evaluate an intervention or treatment and if the treatment affects different components or domains in different directions (e.g., reduces pain but increases fatigue), these effects might cancel out in a summary score leaving no overall effect. For example, observed impacts of arthritis on specific physical tasks were underestimated when using an aggregated index (Guccione, Felson, & Anderson, 1990). Second, assuming that patients or health care providers might consider some domains more important than others, it may be important to know the effects of interventions on the various domains in order to make informed decisions. In the above example, a patient can choose to accept or reject a treatment depending on the relative importance of fatigue or pain to that patient. The use of summary scores alone would obscure the information by which to make such choices. Third, different domains of quality of life may be affected at different points in time in a treatment or intervention regimen.

Utility Approaches

Utility approaches to measuring quality of life attempt to derive a single score that summarizes overall quality of life; however, unlike simple summary scores, the score reflects the value or preference for the overall state. Utility scores typically range from 0 to 1, with 0 representing death and 1 perfect health. The values for the various health states are determined either by obtaining normative value preferences (e.g., of a group of judges) or by determining the values of the respondent. For example, the Quality of Well-being (QWB) Index is a utility measure in which normative preference weights are applied to each possible combination of levels of health on four domains of health (Kaplan et al., 1989; Patrick, Bush, & Chen, 1973); death is assigned a zero. Most utility measures assume that death is the worst possible state, an assumption that has been questioned because of the choice of some individuals to commit suicide.

There are several standard scaling methods for obtaining preference or value weights (Mulley, 1989). When information on utility and length of life are combined, the product is often referred to as quality-adjusted life years (QALYS) or well-years (Kaplan & Bush, 1982; Loomes & McKenzie, 1989). Such tools are considered useful for making policy decisions about allocation of scarce resources, where the goal is to maximize collective well-being (Mulley, 1989). Utility approaches may also be useful when the information is being used to facilitate clinical decision making or in studies in which death is a likely outcome, for example, studies of nursing home populations. If death is not incorporated into the quality of life measure, biases in time-series analyses can lead to spurious findings (Kaplan et al., 1989).

Some researchers are enthusiastic about the use of utility measures (Torrance, 1987). Others are more cautious, noting a number of problems and issues regarding how scores are obtained and how they are applied (Guyatt & Jaeschke, 1990; Llewellyn-Thomas et al., 1984; Loomes & McKenzie, 1989; Mulley, 1989; Patrick & Bergner, 1990). Utility measures have also been criticized for emphasizing physical health and containing little information on psychological or social domains (Lawton, 1991).

Specific Measures

There are numerous measures of single domains and instruments of multiple domains available from which to choose. The problem is not a lack of measures, but the necessity to become familiar with the choices and to learn how to select an appropriate measure or set of measures to meet the needs of a particular study. Reviews of many of these are available (George & Bearon, 1980; Kane & Kane, 1981; McDowell & Newell, 1987; Wilkin, Hallam, & Doggett, 1992). Reviews of measures specifically developed for aging studies are also available (Applegate, Blass, & Williams, 1990; Wiener et al., 1990). Quality of life measures are cited but not reviewed in two sources (Spilker, Simpson, & Tilson, 1992; Stewart & King, 1991).

Overall life satisfaction and subjective well-being measures include single-item quality of life measures developed in the national studies of the quality of life of Americans (Andrews & Withey, 1976; Campbell et al., 1976), as well as multi-dimensional overall indexes such as the Life Satisfaction Index (Neugarten et al., 1961), and the Philadelphia Geriatric Center Morale Scale (Lawton, 1975; Liang & Bollen, 1983).

Several key *multidimensional instruments* are available, each providing a set of multi-item measures of a variety of domains that are appropriate for older populations. These include the Sickness Impact Profile (Bergner, Bobbitt, Pollard, Martin, & Gilson, 1976), the Medical Outcomes Study (MOS) Functioning and Well-being Profile (Stewart et al., 1992), the SF-36, which is based on the MOS measures (Ware & Sherbourne, 1992), the 20-item MOS short form (Stewart, Hays, & Ware, 1988), the Functional Status Questionnaire (Jette et al., 1986), the Duke UNC Health Profile (Parkerson et al., 1981), the Older Americans Resources and Services (OARS) Multidimensional Functional Assessment Questionnaire (MFAQ) (George & Fillenbaum, 1985), the Multilevel Assessment Instrument (Lawton, Moss, Fulcomer, & Kleban, 1982), the Health Assessment Questionnaire (Ramey, Raynauld, & Fries, 1992), and the Rand Health Insurance Experiment measures (Brook et al., 1979). The Quality of Well-being Scale (QWB) assesses multiple domains but summarizes them into a single score (Kaplan, Bush, & Berry, 1976).

Some of the more commonly used *measures of specific domains* that have been developed *especially for older adults* and that are not part of the above multidimensional instruments include the Katz Activities of Daily Living Index (ADL) (Katz, 1983), Instrumental Activities of Daily Living (IADL) scale (Lawton & Brody, 1969), the Geriatric Depression Scale (Yesavage et al., 1983), and the Mini Mental State (Folstein, Folstein, & McHugh, 1975).

Finally, measures of several *specific domains* that have been used widely in populations of *all ages* include the McGill Pain Index (Melzack, 1975), the Psychological General Well-being Index (Dupuy, 1984), the Center for Epidemiologic Studies (CES–D) Depression scale (Radloff, 1977), the Cohen Perceived Stress scale (Cohen, Kamarck, & Mermelstein, 1983), the Profile of Mood States (McNair, Lorr, & Doppleman, 1981), the Taylor Manifest Anxiety Scale (Bendig, 1956), the Spielberger State-Trait Anxiety Inventory (Spielberger, Gorsuch, & Lushene, 1970), and the Rosenberg Self-Esteem Scale (Rosenberg, 1965).

Selecting an Appropriate Quality of Life Assessment Approach

It is tempting to simply select a standard quality of life instrument that has been widely used. Doing so can save the time of reviewing numerous measures and selecting those that are appropriate. Further, it allows comparability to existing data sets. The instrument may have been subjected to psychometric testing, although this should by no means be assumed. There also may be applications of the instrument in a variety of populations and settings, thus improving the likelihood that it might be useful in yet more settings. However, such an instrument may not adequately focus on areas of special importance to the study, may not have measures that are sufficiently responsive to change in an area in which change is anticipated, and may include concepts that are not important to a study and thus "waste" time and money.

To be sure of adequately addressing the needs of any particular study, a more systematic approach for selecting measures should be taken. Unfortunately, there are only a few guidelines for doing so (Bergner & Rothman, 1987; Ware, Brook, Davies, & Lohr, 1981). We agree with those suggesting a modular approach (Aaronson, Bullinger, & Ahmedzai, 1988). In this approach, a standard instrument is selected that best addresses the concepts of interest and additional measures are included to supplement it—measures that focus on concepts that are missed or inadequately assessed with the standard instrument.

The selection of appropriate measures of the concepts of interest depends on a variety of factors such as the purpose of the study, the setting, and the nature of the population. If the purpose of measurement is descriptive or to identify individuals in need of care or services, the type of approach may differ from a situation in which measures are being used as dependent variables by which to evaluate an intervention. For example, the Katz Activities of Daily Living scale and the OARS were specifically developed to identify needs for various services. Descriptive studies may need to include a broad range of concepts to fully describe the population on a variety of domains.

In studies in which the quality of life measures are to be used as outcomes of an intervention, it is important to first specify a conceptual framework. That is, one needs to first identify the *concepts* that are relevant to that intervention and population before proceeding to select the *measures* of those concepts that are appropriate. Studies evaluating specific interventions need to focus more closely on the problems of that particular population and the likely benefits of the intervention. One approach is to compile a list of candidate measures of each of the concepts identified as relevant and then compare them on their psychometric adequacy, including sensitivity to change in similar situations. Another is to identify those domains that are of most importance to the population being studied. For example, Avery and colleagues (1976) had consensus panels rank order outcomes for patients with each of eight diseases in terms of prevalence and likelihood of improvement with optimal medical care. Rank scores such as these could be used to select measures in order of importance. Another strategy is to select a set of measures that are the most independent of one another, for example by examining correlations among the various domains. A similar process for identifying subjective well-being measures to evaluate educational programs for older adults has been described (Okun, Stock, & Covey, 1982).

For especially important concepts, it might be helpful to include more than one measure of the concept in order to increase the chances of detecting possible effects. For example, in a trial intended to improve shortness of breath, no improvement was observed using a clinical measure of forced expiratory volume (FEV), but improvement was observed using a functionally-based indicator of the effects of shortness of breath (Mahler, Matthay, Snyder, Wells, & Loke, 1985).

Conclusion

Although there has been a growing emphasis on health-related quality of life as a useful discriminator among different population segments, an important predictor of health and health behaviors, and a potentially significant outcome of health-related intervention programs in older adults, the field remains plagued by a number of measurement-related issues and difficulties. The time is ripe for concerted efforts on the part of all researchers interested in quality of life concepts to begin or broaden the systematic collection of the reliability and validity data required to better determine which of the growing number of quality of life instruments perform adequately under which sets of circumstances. In addition, continued efforts to identify those content areas and response dimensions that likely will provide the best discrimination among populations and the greatest sensitivity to change are essential to enable the field to guide future health policy and resources. This is not merely an academic exercise, but an undertaking of potentially far-reaching consequences that requires the continued attention of scientists and policymakers alike.

Acknowledgment

The preparation of this chapter was supported by grants from the National Institute on Aging awarded to Dr. Stewart (AG09931) and Dr. King (AG00440).

References

Aaronson, N. K., Bullinger, M., & Ahmedzai, S. (1988). A modular approach to quality of life in cancer clinical trials. *Rec Results Cancer Results, 101,* 231–249.

Andrews, F. M., & Withey, S. B. (1976). *Social indicators of well-being.* New York: Plenum.

Applegate, W. B., Blass, J. P., & Williams, T. F. (1990). Instruments for the functional assessment of older patients. *New England Journal of Medicine, 322,* 1207–1214.

Avery, A. D., Lelah, T., Solomon, N. E., Harris, L. J., Brook, R. H., Greenfield, S., Ware, J. E., & Avery, C. H. (1976). *Quality of medical care assessment using outcome measures: Eight disease-specific applications (R-2021/2-HEW).* Santa Monica CA: Rand Corporation.

Bendig, A. W. (1956). The development of a short form of the Manifest Anxiety Scale. *Journal of Consulting Psychology, 20,* 384.

Bergner, M., Bobbitt, R. A., Pollard, W. E., Martin, P., & Gilson, B. S. (1976). The Sickness Impact Profile: Validation of a health status measure. *Medical Care, 14,* 57–67.

Bergner, M., & Rothman, M. L. (1987). Health status measures: An overview and guide for selection. *American Review of Public Health, 8,* 191–210.

Bombardier, C., & Raboud, J. (1991). A comparison of health-related quality-of-life measures for rheumatoid arthritis research. *Controlled Clinical Trials, 12,* 243S–256S.

Brod, M., Cohen, F., & Mendelsohn, G. (1992). Stress and coping in Parkinson's disease. *The Gerontologist, 32,*189.

Brook, R. H., Ware, J. E., Davies–Avery, A., Stewart, A. L., Donald, C. A., Rogers, W. H., Williams, K. N., & Johnston, S. A. (1979). Overview of adult health status measures fielded in Rand's Health Insurance Study. *Medical Care, 17 (Supplement).*

Campbell, A., Converse, P., & Rodgers, W. (1976). *The quality of American life.* New York: Russell Sage Foundation.

Carp, F. M. (1989). Maximizing data quality in community studies of older people. In M. P. Lawton & A. R. Herzog (Eds.), *Special research methods for gerontology* (pp. 93–122). Amityville NY: Baywood Publishing Company.

Cohen, S., Kamarck, T., & Mermelstein, R. (1983). A global measure of perceived stress. *Journal of Health and Social Behavior, 24,* 385–396.

Colsher, P. L., & Wallace, R. B. (1989). Data quality and age: health and psychobehavioral correlates of item nonresponse and inconsistent responses. *Journal of Gerontology, 44,* P45–52.

Dawson, D., Hendershot, G., & Fulton, J. (1987). NCHS advance data. Vital and health statistics of the NCHS, Number 133, June 10, 1987.

Deyo, R. A., Diehr, P., & Patrick, D. L. (1991). Reproducibility and responsiveness of health status measures. *Controlled Clinical Trials, 12*(Suppl.) 142S–158S.

Deyo, R. A., & Inui, T. S. (1984). Toward clinical applications of health status measures: Sensitivity of scales to clinically important changes. *Health Services Research, 19,* 276–289.

Dupuy, H. J. (1984). The Psychological General Well-Being (PGWB) Index. In N. K. Wenger, M. E. Mattson, C. D. Furberg, & J. Elinson (Eds.), *Assessment of quality of life in clinical trials of cardiovascular therapies.* New York: LeJacq.

Epstein, A. M., Hall, J. A., Tognetti, J., Son, L. H., & Conant, L., Jr. (1989). Using proxies to evaluate quality of life: Can they provide valid information about patients' health status and satisfaction with medical care? *Medical Care, 27 Suppl.,* S91–98.

Flanagan, J. C. (1982). Measurement of quality of life: Current state of the art. *Archives of Physical Medicine and Rehabilitation, 63,* 56–59.

Folstein, M. F., Folstein, S. E., & McHugh, P. R. (1975). Mini-mental state: A practical method for grading the ccognitive state of patients for the clinician. *Journal of Psychiatric Research, 12,* 189–198.

George, L. K., & Bearon, L. B. (1980). *Quality of life in older persons: Meaning and Measurement.* New York: Human Sciences Press.

George, L. K., & Fillenbaum, G. G. (1985). OARS methodology: A decade of experience in geriatric assessment. *Journal of the American Geriatrics Society, 33,* 607–615.

Guccione, A. A., Felson, D. T., & Anderson, J. J. (1990). Defining arthritis and measuring functional status in elders: Methodological issues in the study of disease and physical disability. *American Journal of Public Health, 80,* 945–949.

Guralnik, J. M., Branch, L. G., Cummings, S. R., & Curb, J. D. (1989). Physical performance measures in aging research. *Journal of Gerontology, 44,* M141–146.

Guralnik, J. M., & LaCroix, A. Z. (1992). Assessing physical function in older populations. In R. B. Wallace & R. F. Woolson (Eds.), *The epidemiologic study of the elderly* (pp. 159–181). New York: Oxford University Press.

Guyatt, G., Feeny, D., & Patrick, D. (1991). Issues in quality-of-life measurement in clinical trials. *Controlled Clinical Trials, 12,* 81S–90S.

Guyatt, G. H., & Jaeschke, R. (1990). Measurements in clinical trials: Choosing the appropriate approach. In B. Spilker (Ed.), *Quality of life assessments in clinical trials* (pp. 37–46). New York: Raven, Ltd, Press.

Herzog, A. R., & Kulka, R. A. (1989). Telephone and mail surveys with older populations: A methodological overview. In M. P. Lawton & A. R. Herzog (Eds.), *Special research methods for gerontology* (pp. 63–89). Amityvill, NY: Baywood.

Herzog, A. R., & Rodgers, W. L. (1988). Interviewing older adults: Mode comparison using data from a face-to-face survey and a telephone resurvey. *Public Opinion Quarterly, 52*, 84–99.

Herzog, A. R., Rodgers, W. L., & Kulka, R. A. (1983). Interviewing older adults: A comparison of telephone and face-to-face modalities. *Public Opinion Quarterly, 47*, 405–418.

Jette, A. M., Davies, A. R., Cleary, P. D., Callans, D.R., Rubenstein, L.V., Fink, A., Kosecoff, J., Young, R.T., Brook, R.H., & Delbanco, T.L. (1986). The Functional Status Questionnaire. *Journal of General Internal Medicine, 1*, 143–149.

Kane, R. A., & Kane, R. L. (1981). *Assessing the elderly: a practical guide to measurement*. Lexington MA: Lexington Books.

Kaplan, R.M., Anderson, J.P., Wu, A. W., Mathews, C., Kozin, F., & Orenstein, D. (1989). The Quality of Well-Being Scale: Applications in AIDS, cystic fibrosis, and arthritis. *Medical Care, 27 Suppl.*, S27-S43.

Kaplan, R. M., & Bush, J. W. (1982). Health-related quality of life measurement for evaluation research and policy analysis. *Health Psychology, 1*, 61–80.

Kaplan, R. M., Bush, J. W., & Berry, C. C. (1976). Health status: Types of validity and the index of well-being. *Health Services Research, 11*, 478–507.

Katz, S. (1983). Assessing self-maintenance: Activities of daily living, mobility, and instrumental activities of daily living. *Journal of the American Geriatrics Society, 31*, 721–727.

Kutner, N. G., Ory, M. G., Baker, D. I., Schechtman, K. B., Hornbrook, M. C., & Mulrow, C. D. (1992). Measuring the quality of life of the elderly in health promotion intervention clinical trials. *Public Health Reports, 107*, 530–539.

Lawton, M. P. (1975). The Philadelphia Geriatric Center Morale Scale: A revision. *Journal of Gerontology, 30*, 85–89.

Lawton, M. P. (1991). A multidimensional view of quality of life in frail elders. In J. E. Birren, J. E. Lubben, J. C. Rowe, & D. E. Deutchman (Eds.), *The concept and measurement of quality of life in the frail elderly* (pp. 3–27). San Diego: Academic Press, Inc.

Lawton, M. P., & Brody, E. M. (1969). Assessment of older people: Self-maintaining and instrumental activities of daily living. *The Gerontologist, 9*, 179–186.

Lawton, M. P., Moss, M., Fulcomer, M., & Kleban, M. H. (1982). A research and service oriented Multilevel Assessment Instrument. *Journal of Gerontology, 37*, 91–99.

Liang, J. (1984). Dimensions of the Life Satisfaction Index A: A structural formulation. *Journal of Gerontology, 39*, 613–622.

Liang, J., & Bollen, K. A. (1983). The structure of the Philadelphia Geriatric Center Morale Scale: A reinterpretation. *Journal of Gerontology, 30*, 77–84.

Llewellyn-Thomas, H., Sutherland, H. J., Tibshirani, R., Ciampi, A., Till, J. E., & Boyd, N. F. (1984). Describing health states: Methodologic issues in obtaining values for health states. *Medical Care, 22*, 543–552.

Loomes, G., & McKenzie, L. (1989). The use of QALYs in health care decision making. *Social Science and Medicine, 28*, 299–308.

Magaziner, J. (1992). The use of proxy respondents in health studies of the aged. In R. B. Wallace & R. F. Woolson (Eds.), *The epidemiologic study of the elderly* (pp. 120–129). New York: Oxford University Press.

Magaziner, J., Simonsick, E. M., Kashner, T. M., & Hebel, J. R. (1988). Patient-proxy response comparability on measures of patient health and functional status. *Journal of Clinical Epidemiology, 41*, 1065–1074.

Mahler, D. A., Matthay, R. A., Snyder, P. E., Wells, C. K., & Loke, J. (1985). Sustained-release theophylline reduces dyspnea in nonreversible obstructive airway disease. *American Review of Respiratory Disease 131*, 22–25.

McDowell, I. Y., & Newell, C. (1987). *Measuring health: A guide to rating scales and questionnaires.* New York: Oxford University Press.

McNair, D. M., Lorr, M., & Doppleman, L. F. (1981). *EITS manual for the profile of mood states.* San Diego CA: Educational and Industrial Testing Service.

McNeil, J. K., Stones, M. J., & Kozma, A. (1986). Subjective well-being in later life: Some issues concerning measurement and prediction. *Social Indicators Research, 18*, 35–70.

Melzack, R. (1975). The McGill Pain Questionnaire: Major properties and scoring methods. *Pain, 1*, 277–299.

Mulley, A. G. (1989). Assessing patients' utilities: Can the ends justify the means? *Medical Care, 27*, S269–S281.

Neugarten, B. L., Havighurst, R. J., & Tobin, S. S. (1961). The measurement of life satisfaction. *Journal of Gerontology, 16*, 134–143.

Okun, M. A., Stock, W. A., & Covey, R. E. (1982). Assessing the effects of older adult education on subjective well-being. *Educational Gerontology, 8*, 523–536.

Parkerson, G. R., Gehlbach, S. H., Wagner, E. H., James, S.A., Clapp, N.E., &

Muhlbaier, L.H. (1981). The Duke–UNC Health Profile: An adult health status instrument for primary care. *Medical Care, 19,* 806–828.

Patrick, D. L., & Bergner, M. (1990). Measurement of health status in the 1990s. *Annual Review of Public Health, 11,* 165–183.

Patrick, D. L., Bush, J. W., & Chen, M. M. (1973). Methods for measuring levels of well-being for a health status index. *Health Services Research, 8,* 228–245.

Patrick, D. L., & Erickson, P. (1988). What constitutes quality of life? Concepts and dimensions. *Clinical Nutrition, 7,* 53–63.

Radloff, L. S. (1977). The CES–D scale: A self-report depression scale for research in the general population. *Applied Psychological Measurement, 1,* 385–401.

Ramey, D. R., Raynauld, J. P., & Fries, J. F. (1992). The Health Assessment Questionnaire 1992: Status and review. *Arthritis Care and Research, 5,* 119–129.

Rodgers, W. L., & Herzog, A. R. (1992). Collecting data about the oldest old: Problems and procedures. In R. M. Suzman, D. P. Willis, & K. G. Manton (Eds.), *The oldest old* (pp. 135–156). New York: Oxford University Press.

Rodgers, W. L., Herzog, A. R., & Andrews, F. M. (1988). Interviewing older adults: Validity of self-reports of satisfaction. *Psychology and Aging, 3,* 264–272.

Rosenberg, M. (1965). *Society and the Adolescent Self-Image.* Princeton NJ: Princeton University Press.

Rowe, J. W., & Kahn, R. L. (1987). Human aging: Usual and successful. *Science, 237,* 143–149.

Rubenstein, L. Z., Schairer, C., Wieland, G. D., & Kane, R. (1984). Systematic biases in functional status assessment of elderly adults: Effects of different data sources. *Journal of Gerontology, 39,* 686–691.

Sherbourne, C. D., & Meredith, L. S. (1992). Quality of self-report data: A comparison of older and younger chronically ill patients. *Journal of Gerontology, 47,* S204–S211.

Spielberger, C. D., Gorsuch, R. L., & Lushene, R. E. (1970). *Manual for the State-Trait Anxiety Inventory.* Palo Alto CA: Consulting Psychologists Press.

Spilker, B., Simpson, R. L., Jr., & Tilson, H. H. (1992). Quality of Life Bibliography and Indexes: 1991 update. *Journal of Clinical Research and Pharmacoepidemiology, 6,* 205–266.

Stewart, A. L., Hays, R. D., & Ware, J. E., Jr. (1988). The MOS Short-form General Health Survey: Reliability and validity in a patient population. *Medical Care, 26,* 724–735.

Stewart, A. L., & King, A. C. (1991). Evaluating the efficacy of physical activity for influencing quality of life outcomes in older adults. *Annals of Behavioral Medicine, 13,* 108–116.

Stewart, A. L., Sherbourne, C. D., Hays, R. D., Wells, K. B., Nelson, E. C., Kamberg, C. J., Rogers, W. H., Berry, S. D., & Ware, J. E., Jr. (1992). Summary and discussion of MOS measures. In A. L. Stewart & J. E. Ware Jr. (Eds.), *Measuring Functioning and Well-Being: The Medical Outcomes Study Approach.* Durham NC: Duke University Press.

Torrance, G. W. (1987). Utility approach to measuring health-related quality of life. *Journal of Chronic Diseases, 40,* 593–600.

Ware, J. E., & Sherbourne, C. D. (1992). The MOS 36–item Short-Form Health Survey (SF–36): I. Conceptual framework and item selection. *Medical Care, 30,* 473–483.

Ware, J. E., Jr., Brook, R. H., Davies, A. R., & Lohr, K. (1981). Choosing measures of health status for individuals in general populations. *American Journal of Public Health, 71,* 620–625.

Wiener, J. M., Hanley, R. J., Clark, R., & VanNostrand, J. F. (1990). Measuring the activities of daily living: Comparisons across national surveys. *Journal of Gerontology, 45,* S229–237.

Wilkin, D., Hallam, L., & Doggett, M. A. (1992). *Measures of need and outcome for primary health care.* Oxford: Oxford University Press.

Yesavage, J. A., Brink, T. L., Rose, T. L., Lum, O., Wuang, V., Adey, M. B., & Leirer, V. O. (1983). Development and validation of a geriatric depression screening scale: A preliminary report. *Journal of Psychiatric Research, 39,* 37–49.

PART II

Life Style and Quality of Life

Chapter 3

Behavioral and Social Factors in Healthy Aging

George A. Kaplan and William J. Strawbridge

Healthy Aging

Two counter-currents characterize discussions of aging. On the one hand, living to an advanced age while retaining independence and vigor is desirable. On the other hand, many believe that aging is inevitably characterized by increased disease, dependence, and dementia. Although neither view is without supportive evidence, recent developments in the biology, physiology, and epidemiology of aging are providing increasing support for the more optimistic of these positions. Emphasis on the ability to maintain health and function in old age, versus inevitable declines, is based on observations of substantial heterogeneity in health and functioning at all ages (Rowe & Kahn, 1987), the impact of behavioral, social, and psychological factors on the health of the elderly (Kaplan & Haan, 1989), and the positive impact of interventions (Buchner & Wagner, 1992; Buchner et al., 1992).

Emerging from this growing body of evidence is the concept of healthy aging. Although many agree that healthy aging constitutes an important focus, its definition is unclear. Healthy aging could be defined as "in a normal condition." However, this raises the important issue of separating the impact of disease from the aging process, with normal being used in the sense of "usual" (Rowe & Kahn, 1987).

Healthy aging could also be defined as being disease and dysfunction free. This use comes close to that of "successful aging" as used by Rowe and Kahn (1987) and others (Roos & Havens, 1991). Although this concept of healthy aging may be very informative for understanding basic mechanisms and modulators of aging, the high burden of disease and disability among the elderly means that it will apply to a relatively small, elite portion of the population. Furthermore, as our abilities to diagnose pathophysiological processes noninvasively and to measure physiological and performance dysfunction increases, a smaller and smaller portion of the population will be classified as healthy agers, thereby limiting the public health significance of this definition. Finally, healthy can also be defined as "good" or "sound." This is either a moralistic use of the term that mainly reflects the user's value system or represents a nonnormativistic view of health and disease based on biological absolutism (Caplan, 1990).

An Alternative Definition of Healthy Aging

We believe that a more productive view of healthy aging builds on the idea of prevention and emphasizes all three types—primary, secondary, and tertiary. It uses the term healthy aging to refer not just to those who are free of disease and dysfunction, but also to those in whom the progression of disease or dysfunction has been slowed or reversed, and to those in whom the consequences of disease or dysfunction have been reduced. Thus, it refers to successful aging that is contextual. Understanding the heterogeneity in outcomes at these three stages, and the primary, secondary, and tertiary efforts to improve outcomes for all, becomes the goal of the researcher and practitioner. We recognize that this concept of healthy aging is far from viewing healthy aging as referring to those with high levels of health and functioning. We propose it as an alternative that could lead to a potentially more productive focus on improving the health and quality of life of all older persons, regardless of whether they are in some pristine state of "optimal" health, are in the early stages of a degenerative disease, or are frail and cognitively impaired. Efforts to understand the heterogeneity in health and quality of life at these very different stages may lead to a fuller understanding of aging itself, as well as interventions that can benefit the majority of older persons. As will be seen later, there is much evidence to support such an approach.

The Behavioral and Social Determinants of Healthy Aging

There is abundant evidence that the entire natural history of health and functioning in the elderly bears the imprint of behavioral and social processes (Kaplan, 1992b; Kaplan & Haan, 1989). Adoption, maintenance, and elimination of major risk factors for the leading causes of morbidity and mortality are heavily determined by behavioral and social factors. This is not to deny the impact of genetic or biological factors, but only to emphasize the critical involvement of behavioral and social processes. In the case of genetic factors, the behavioral and social environment provides the context that determines the expression of these factors. Even more importantly, behavioral and social factors may dynamically interact with biological processes to determine the health of the elderly. Finally, the heterogeneity of aging, with variation by time, place, and social structure argues for the importance of behavioral and social modifications of the aging process (Riley & Riley, 1989).

Behavioral and Social Factors in Longevity

Although increased longevity is not to be confused with healthy aging, most agree that increased longevity and the elimination of premature (early) mortality are desirable. An extensive literature now exists indicating that behavioral factors are strongly associated with risk of death. Although a number of behavioral factors have been implicated as risk factors for mortality, the strongest evidence is found for smoking and physical activity.

Smoking

Although there are some conflicting studies (e.g., Branch and Jette, 1984) the predominant pattern is higher risk of death among older smokers (Barrett-Connor, Suarez, Khaw, Criqui, & Wingard, 1984; Feldman, Makuc, Kleinman, & Cornoni-Huntley, 1989; Kaplan, Roberts, Camacho, & Coyne, 1987; LaCroix et al., 1991; USDHHS, 1990). In addition, the risk for those older persons who formerly smoked is generally less than for current smokers. In the Alameda County Study, quitting smoking was associated with decreased risk of death over the subsequent nine years (Kaplan & Haan, 1989). Although those who continued smoking had a 76% higher risk of death than those who discontinued smoking previously, those who quit during the first 9-year period had only a 33% higher risk. These results persisted even when there was statistical adjustment for prevalent health conditions at baseline and incident conditions that occurred during the period in which the smoking pattern was assessed. A beneficial effect of quitting smoking on all-cause mortality was also found in analyses of the nonsurgical control group in the Coronary Artery Surgery Study (Hermanson et al., 1988). In this study of patients with angiographically documented coronary artery disease, survival was better for those who had quit smoking in the year before the beginning of the study and who continued to not smoke throughout follow-up compared to those who continued to smoke. There was no indication of a weakening effect of cessation with increasing age.

Physical Activity

Low levels of physical activity have been shown to be associated with increased risk of death. Alameda County Study participants who were 70 or more years old and who reported no leisure-time physical activity were at 37% increased risk of death compared to those who reported some leisure-time physical activity (Kaplan et al., 1987). Interestingly, the increased risk associated with inactivity did not vary substantially by age. Follow-up data from NHANES II also indicated increased risk associated with a sedentary life style (Foley et al., 1990) as did low levels of physical activity for both older men and women involved in health screening at the Cooper Clinic (Blair et al., 1989). Changes in level of leisure-time physical activity also appear to be related to changes in risk of death. In the Alameda County Study, participants were asked on two occasions 9 years apart about the frequency and strenuousness of their leisure-time physical activity (Kaplan & Haan, 1989). Those who increased their level of activity showed a decreased risk of death and those who decreased their level of activity showed an increased risk of death compared to those who remained at the same level. This relationship persisted even when the analyses were restricted to those who were healthy at baseline and there was statistical adjustment for incident chronic conditions, alcohol consumption, changes in weight, smoking, and other variables. Similarly, Paffenbarger et al. (1993) found that older men who began moderately vigorous sports activities had lower mortality rates over an 8-year period than did those who remained less active.

Social Risk Factors

Seeman, Kaplan, Knudsen, Cohen, and Guralnick (1987) found that low social network participation was associated with a 69% increased risk of death over 17 years in a group that was 70 years of age or older. Similar results were found for men, but not women, in a population-based study in Sweden (Orth-Gomer & Johnson, 1987). In another Swedish study of persons 60 years old, low levels of activities outside the home and social activities were associated with increased risk of death over a 9-year follow-up period (Welin, Larsson, Svardsudd, Tibblin, & Tibblin, 1992). Using data from the Longitudinal Study on Aging, Steinbach (1992) found that low level of participation in social activities and low frequency of visits with friends and neighbors were associated with increased risk of death. There is some evidence that social participation may have a stronger relationship with mortality for those recovering from illness than in preventing new disease. Vogt and colleagues (1992) found that the relationship between social participation and mortality over a 15-year follow-up was stronger for persons with incident Ischemic Heart Disease (IHD), cancer, and stroke than for those free of illness at baseline.

Blazer (1979) found that low availability of social attachments and low perceived support were both associated with a doubling of 2.5 year risk of death in those 65–93 years of age. Using more extensive measures of both social networks and support, a recent study of men born in Malmö, Sweden found that measures of social anchorage, adequacy of social participation, and availability of social support were all associated with risk of death (Falk, Hanson, Isacsson, & Ostergren, 1992). Although there have been no population-based interventions on social support or social networks, Kaplan and Haan's (1989) analyses indicated that increases in social network participation were prospectively associated with decreased risk of death, and vice versa.

Socioeconomic level has also been found to be associated with risk of death in the elderly. In analyses based on the almost 50,000 persons 75 years of age or older in the Cancer Prevention Study-I (Lew & Garfinkel, 1990), there was a clear relationship between education and risk of death. In almost all age/sex strata, those with less than a high school education had the highest mortality rates. Branch and Ku

(1989) found that poverty status was an important predictor of mortality risk in the Massachusetts Health Care Panel Study of those 65 years of age or older. For all age/sex strata except men who were 80 years or older, those at the poverty level had increased rates of death.

Questions about Increases in Longevity Lead to a Focus on Functional Ability

Thus, there is substantial evidence suggesting that behavioral and social factors are related to longevity in older persons, and nascent findings suggesting that alteration in behavioral and social factors might decrease mortality rates. These observations, coupled with the large decline in mortality risk and resultant increases in life expectancy at older ages, are reasons for optimism. But the impression they create could be misleading. Extending longevity in no way guarantees that the added years of life are spent in good health with high quality of life. This issue is at the heart of discussions of compression of morbidity, (Fries, 1989) and active life expectancy (Katz et al., 1983). In fact, some evidence suggests that these added years of life have been accompanied by increased prevalence of disabling chronic disease (Kaplan, 1991). The unanswered questions concerning the meaning of increased life expectancy at older ages for quality of life have turned attention to studies of functional status among the elderly, including physical, cognitive, social, and psychological functioning. In the discussion that follows, we will focus on physical functioning because it is an important factor in the ability to live independently, provides an important substrate for other domains of function, and appears to be modifiable in both the fit and frail elderly (Buchner & Wagner, 1992; Buchner et al., 1992).

What are the Determinants of Problems in Physical Functioning?

Chronic and Acute Disease

Table 3.1 summarizes evidence indicating that some of the strongest determinants of physical functioning are related to chronic conditions and acute events such as falls. Such results suggest opportunities for preventing declines in physical functioning. To the extent that chronic

TABLE 3.1
Chronic and Acute Conditions Associated with Physical Functioning:
Prospective Studies

Study	Population	Results (RR = Relative Risk)
Harris et al. (1989)	LSOA, 2-year follow-up Age 80+ at baseline	Among those physically able at baseline, arthritis (RR 1.9) and cardiovascular disease (RR 2.1) were associated with subsequent functional impairment
Guralnik & Kaplan (1989)	Alameda County Study, 19-year follow-up Age 65–89 at follow-up	Hypertension (RR 4.3), back pain (RR 2.0), and arthritis (RR 2.8) were associated with subsequent poorer physical functioning
Keil et al. (1989)	Charleston Heart Study, 25-year follow-up Age 60+ at follow-up	Cardiovascular disease (RR 1.6 to 2.6) and elevated systolic blood pressure (RR 1.4 to 2.3) were associated with subsequent difficulties in physical functioning
Lammi et al. (1989)	Finnish cohorts in Seven Countries Study, 10–25 year follow-up Age 65+ at follo-wup	Low vital capacity, intermittent claudication, cerebrovascular disease, coronary heart disease, and emphysema were associated with subsequent lower physical functioning
Mor et al. (1989)	LSOA, 2-year follow-up Age 70–74 at baseline	Diabetes (RR 1.6) was associated with subsequent functional decline
Pinsky et al. (1987)	Framingham Heart Study, 21-year follow-up Age 56+ at follow-up	Ventricular rate in initially healthy males was associated with subsequent functional decline
Kaplan (1992a)	Alameda County Study, 9-year follow-up Age 59+ at follow-up	8 conditions and symptoms (RR 1.8 to 6.8) were associated with subsequent incidence of mobility/self care problems
Guralnik et al. (1993)	EPESE cohorts, 4-year follow-up Age 65+ at baseline	Incident myocardial infarction (RR 1.7 to 2.3), cancer (RR 1.2 to 2.6), stroke (RR 2.2 to 3.0), and hip fracture (RR 1.9 to 4.4) were associated with subsequent loss of mobility
Kaplan et al. (1992)	Alameda County Study, 6-year follow-up Age 65+ at baseline	Incident hip fracture, fall, stroke, and myocardial infarction were associated with subsequent decline in physical functioning

and acute conditions can be prevented or delayed, there will be higher levels of physical functioning. Although the evidence is impressive, considerably more detailed studies still need to be done (such as the Women's Aging Study being carried out with National Institute on Aging support at Johns Hopkins University) before it is possible to pinpoint the exact mechanisms by which chronic and acute disease influence functioning and quality of life.

Behavioral and Social Factors

Although chronic and acute disease are important determinants of physical functioning, behavioral and social factors also have a role. Table 3.2 summarizes results from studies that have prospectively examined the impact of smoking and physical activity on subsequent levels of functioning in older populations. These studies should be seen as preliminary as they do not firmly establish the temporal ordering of the incident conditions and changes in functioning. In addition, it is possible that the incident chronic conditions are more severe in those who smoke or who are sedentary. Measures of disease severity will be necessary to clarify this issue. Nevertheless, the evidence is consistent with the hypothesis that levels of smoking and physical activity are important predictors of later declines in physical functioning. It is, of course, biologically plausible that smoking and low levels of physical activity will lead to compromised physiological functioning, without manifest disease, which will then lead to poorer physical functioning.

A variety of social factors have also been implicated in the natural history of physical functioning. For example, low socioeconomic level has been prospectively associated with poorer functioning in many studies (Camacho, Strawbridge, Cohen, & Kaplan, 1993, Branch & Ku, 1989; Clark & Maddox, 1992; Guralnik & Kaplan, 1989; Guralnik et al., 1993; Harris, Kovar, Suzman, Kleinman, & Feldman, 1989; Kaplan, 1992a; Kaplan, Strawbridge, Camacho, & Cohen, 1993b; Keil et al., 1989; Lammi et al., 1989; Maddox & Clark, 1992; Mor et al., 1989; Pinsky et al., 1987; Rogers, Rogers, & Belanger, 1992). Although there is abundant evidence that socioeconomic factors are associated with increased risk of poor physical functioning, it is not possible to specify the pathways that account for this association. For example, because socioeconomic level is associated with a wide variety of diseases (Haan, Kaplan, & Syme, 1989) it is possible that the association with function simply reflects increased incidence and prevalence

TABLE 3.2
Association between Smoking and Physical Activity and Physical Functioning: Prospective Studies

Study	Population	Results
Guralnik & Kaplan (1989)	Alameda County Study, 19-year follow-up Age 65+ at follow-up	Current smokers twice as likely to have low/moderate function compared to past/never smokers
Mor et al. (1989)	LSOA, 2-year follow-up Age 70–74 at baseline	Reports of no regular exercise in men and not walking one mile in women associated with decline in physical functioning
Pinsky et al. (1987)	Framingham Heart Study, 21-year follow-up Age 56+ at follow-up	Smoking in males associated with decline in function in healthy subset
Branch (1985)	Massachusetts Health Care Panel Study, 5-year follow-up Age 65+ at baseline	Smoking associated with incident disability
Kaplan (1992a)	Alameda County Study, 9-year follow-up Age 59+ at follow-up	Smoking and low leisure-time physical activity associated with incident mobility and self-care problems
Kaplan et al. (1993)	Alameda County Study, 6-year follow-up Age 65+ at baseline	Smoking and low physical activity associated with declines in physical functioning
Camacho et al. (1993)	Alameda County Study, 19-year follow-up Age 80+ at follow-up	Cumulative effect of low level of physical activity over previous 19 years on physical function

of disease. Although several studies have attempted to statistically adjust for underlying disease, most have used self-reported acute and chronic conditions that may not be sensitive enough. The consistency of the finding of an association between socioeconomic level and poorer functioning argues for focused research aimed at understanding this relationship.

There is also some evidence that marital status and levels of social networks or social support are prospectively associated with poorer physical functioning. For example, being unmarried was associated with poorer functioning in Mor et al.'s (1989) analysis of the Longitudinal Study of Aging cohort. In a 6-year follow-up of persons 65 years old or older, Kaplan et al. (1993) found that being unmarried and having a low level of social network participation were both associated with greater declines in functioning. Camacho et al. (1993) found a cumulative effect of social isolation such that persistent social isolation over the preceding 19 years was associated with lower levels of physical functioning in those who reached at least 80 years of age. Although we do not fully understand the pathways accounting for the impact of social factors on physical functioning, the literature is consistent enough to suggest that socioeconomic level, marital status, social network participation, and social support may be important predictors of physical functioning.

Do Behavioral and Social Factors Modify the Impact of Disease on Functioning?

Compression of morbidity is a highly desirable goal, yet there is little evidence supporting movement in that direction. Given the low probability of ever eliminating all disease among the elderly—leading to people dying "healthy"—and the burden of disability associated with acute and chronic diseases among the elderly, it is reasonable to ask if behavioral and social factors might reduce the impact of disease on disability. There are, unfortunately, very few studies that have examined these issues with respect to physical functioning, although there are some studies that have looked at behavioral and social factors as modifiers of mortality risk after acute or chronic events (Berkman, Leo-Summers, & Horwitz 1992; Ruberman, Weinblatt, Goldberg, & Chaudhary, 1984; Williams et al., 1992). So far the evidence is relatively consistent. The notion of behavioral and social modifiers of disease-related problems in functioning is not unreasonable because it is likely that physical function is determined by an interacting set of physiologic, behavioral, cognitive, psychological, and environmental factors. Evidence supporting an ameliorative role for behavioral and social factors is summarized in Table 3.3

What are the Environmental Factors Supportive of Healthy Aging?

The evidence reviewed so far has focused primarily on the role of factors in the individual that predict healthy aging. Although the evi-

TABLE 3.3
Behavioral and Social Modifiers of Disease-Related Problems in Physical Functioning

Study	Population	Results
Cummings et al. (1988)	Hip fracture patients 6-month follow-up Age 60+ at baseline	Greater number of social supports associated with increased ability to walk unaided
Verbrugge et al. (1991)	Supplement on Aging Self-reported arthritis Age 55+ at interview	Being married, higher education, and non-black status associated with higher levels of functioning
Nickel & Chirikos (1990)	Cohort of patients hospitalized for coronary care, 6 month–9 year follow-up Mean age 74 (males) and 59 (females) at baseline	Among those who survived to 8–9 year follow-up, greater disability associated with lower income; for women being unmarried associated with less disability
Kaplan (1992a)	Alameda County Study, 9-year follow-up Age 59–89 at follow-up	Among those with incident heart trouble, stroke, or arthritis, smoking and inadequate income associated with twice the risk of incident mobility problem
Magaziner et al. (1990)	Hip fracture patients, one-year follow-up Age 65+ at baseline	Greater contact with social network at 2 months associated with better walking ability, less physical dependence and less instrumental dependence at 1 year
Marottoli et al. (1992)	New Haven EPESE cohort, 6-week and 6-month follow-up of hip fracture patients Age 65+ at baseline	Higher levels of physical functioning pre-fracture associated with higher physical function post–fracture
Kaplan et al. (unpublished)	Alameda County Study, 6-year follow-up Age 65+ at baseline	In those with incident stroke, prior low income and low physical activity associated with greater decline in physical functioning

dence suggests that modification of these factors holds promise in promoting our expanded concept of healthy aging, there are important factors outside the individual that need to be considered.

The Healthcare Environment

Much more attention needs to be paid to the influence of access to and provision of health care services to the elderly, including preventive, rehabilitative, and case management services (Ory & Bond, 1989). It is likely that if we can prevent or delay the onset of chronic and acute diseases and their sequelae in the later years, we will be able to prevent the progressive declines in functioning that interfere with healthy aging. Evidence suggests that rehabilitative services and possibly interventions that increase exercise capacity and strength might have a substantial impact on the postponement of frailty (Buchner & Wagner, 1992). Unfortunately, these services are limited in availability and are seldom reimbursed by second-party payers.

The Social Environment

We have reviewed several studies which suggest that social support, social networks, education, socioeconomic level, and other socioenvironmental factors are associated with level of disability both in the presence and absence of diagnosed disease. The evidence with respect to recovery of function post-hip fracture is particularly consistent (Cummings et al., 1988; Magaziner, Simonsick, Kashner, Hebel, & Kenzora, 1990). Several Swedish studies also illustrate the impact of socioenvironmental interventions on functioning for older persons. Arnetz and colleagues (1983, 1987) conducted an intervention in a senior citizen apartment building, with two floors randomly assigned to control and intervention status. The intervention consisted of a "social activation" program directed at increasing social activity and independence, and the impact of this intervention was evaluated at 3 and 6 months. Positive changes associated with the intervention included increased social activity, independence, and resistance to control, increased height, and increased anabolic and decreased catabolic hormones indicating decreased stress. In another study, elderly female pensioners who rated themselves as lonely and were awaiting placement in housing units were assigned to group meetings with peers or a waiting list (Andersson, 1984). At a 6-month follow-up, the participants in the peer group meetings were less lonely, had greater self-confidence, and lower blood pressure. Finally, Lökk, Theorell, Arnetz, and Eneroth (1991) conducted a trial with adult day care patients, most of whom suffered from cerebrovascular disease. The intervention engaged patients in small group activities, including discussing the goals and progress of rehabilitation and going on outings, and encouraged them to contact each other outside the facility. At 24 weeks, those in the intervention group scored higher on a number of psychological scales, showed greater improvement in physical functioning, and showed decreases in plasma prolactin, possibly indicating lower stress. Thus, interventions aimed at modifying the social context of aging could significantly promote healthy aging. These studies indicate that relatively simple interventions, focused on social support and autonomy, can help to promote "healthy aging," even in patients requiring adult day care.

The Physical Environment

The role of the physical environment in promoting healthy aging is relatively unstudied. Some current interventions are directed at reducing hazards in home environments that lead to falls (Stevens, Hornbrook, Wingfield, Hollis, & Greenlick, 1991). But even broader interventions might be necessary. The evidence we have reviewed suggests that higher levels of physical activity promote "healthy aging," and it is reasonable to ask if there are environmental barriers that interfere with physical activity. One possible barrier is traffic. If older persons cannot cross streets, they might restrict their walking. Based on walking speeds from the Established Populations for the Epidemiologic Study of the Elderly (EPESE) studies (J. Guralnik, personal communication) we have illustrated in Figure 3.1 how far older persons might get across the street in front of the authors' office. Assuming a 2-second delay in beginning to cross after the light turns green, males and females who are 65+ years of age would get only three quarters of the way across the street before the light turns red. An 80+ year old woman would get less than half way. It seems reasonable to believe that environmental factors like these impede activity among the elderly.

Unanswered Questions

We have contended that an expanded view of healthy aging is required, one that considers the importance of primary, secondary, and tertiary prevention. Although the small amount of evidence available supports such a perspective, considerably more work needs to be done to meet the conceptual and methodologic challenges posed by

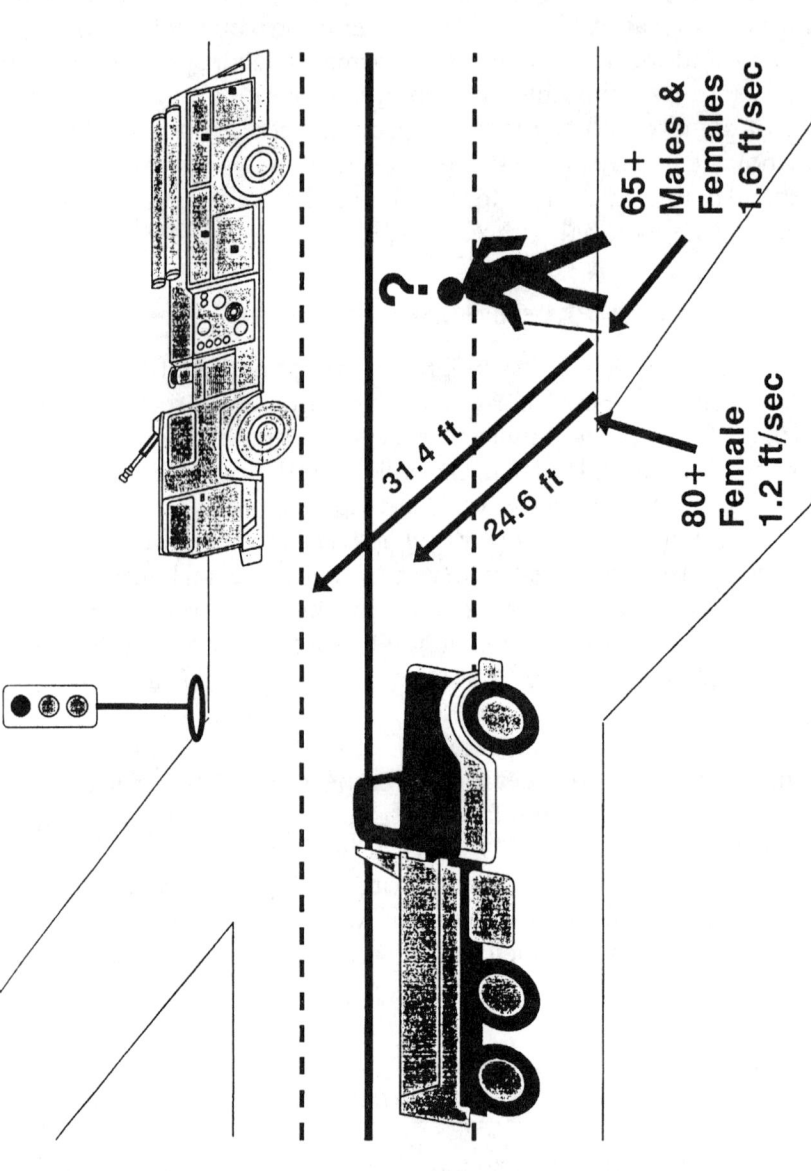

FIGURE 3.1 Schematic illustration of problems encountered by the elderly when crossing intersections. Arrows indicate distances covered by indicated groups before light turns red. Walking speeds taken from National Institute on Aging Established Populations for the Epidemiologic Study of the Elderly (J. Guralnik, personal communication).

this view. In this chapter we restricted our discussion to physical functioning. It is clear that a full view of healthy aging will need to consider the full spectrum of domains of functioning (Roos & Havens, 1991). Such consideration will lead to new definitions of active life expectancy that involve domains beyond physical functioning, and that, consistent with a conceptualization of healthy aging, are applicable throughout the disease spectrum.

We also need to know the mix of short- and long-term determinants of healthy aging. That is, the respective contribution of long-term, lifetime exposures and more proximal exposures that are amenable to modification in later life. The preliminary evidence with respect to smoking suggests that smoking cessation at older ages reduces mortality risk, but we do not know if it also improves functioning. In general we recommend that existing longitudinal studies that have data covering decades before reaching the older years be exploited to investigate this issue. An initial approach to this was taken by Camacho et al. (1993) who examined the cumulative effects of behavioral, social, and psychological factors on physical functioning in those who had reached 80 years of age or more. Over the previous two decades, higher functioning was related to the consistency of the patterns of physical activity, moderate alcohol use, moderate weight for height, and absence of depression. There was also suggestive evidence of a cumulative effect of social isolation.

Finally, we must recognize that any adequate approach to healthy aging will have to accept the recursive, interdependence of health status, physical, social, cognitive, and psychological functioning (Kaplan, 1992b). Figure 3.2 presents the pattern of interrelationships found in the Alameda County Study. High levels of depressive symptoms are associated with declines in physical activity (Kaplan, Lazarus, Cohen, & Leu, 1991) and increased risk of social isolation (G. Kaplan et al., unpublished data). Low levels of physical activity are associated with increased risk of incident depression (Camacho, Roberts, Lazarus, Kaplan, & Cohen, 1991), and increased social isolation (G. Kaplan et al., unpublished data). At the same time, social isolation is associated with declines in physical activity (Kaplan et al., 1991), and increased risk of depression (Kaplan et al., 1987). Although this web of causation leads to analytic difficulties, it is a reality that needs to be addressed in approaches to healthy aging.

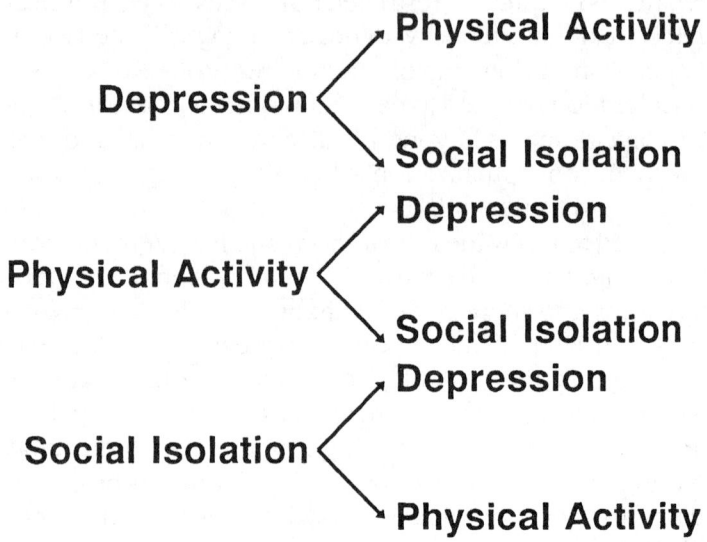

FIGURE 3.2 The recursive interplay of behavioral, social, and psychological factors. Based on prospective data from the Alameda County Study.

Conclusion

Although we may hope for the outcomes portrayed in Figure 3.3, it is a view of aging whose time has not yet come for the bulk of the population. An expanded view of healthy aging that recognizes the possibility of increasing health, functioning, and quality of life at all stages of the health–disease continuum creates exciting possibilities for primary, secondary, and tertiary prevention and leads to the following conclusions:

- Age is not destiny. There is substantial variation in health and functioning between individuals of the same age.
- Behavioral and social factors are associated both with mortality and with the level of health and functioning among those who survive to older ages.
- Disease is not destiny. Behavioral and social factors may modify the impact of acute and chronic disease on functioning.

BEHAVIORAL AND SOCIAL FACTORS IN HEALTHY AGING • 73

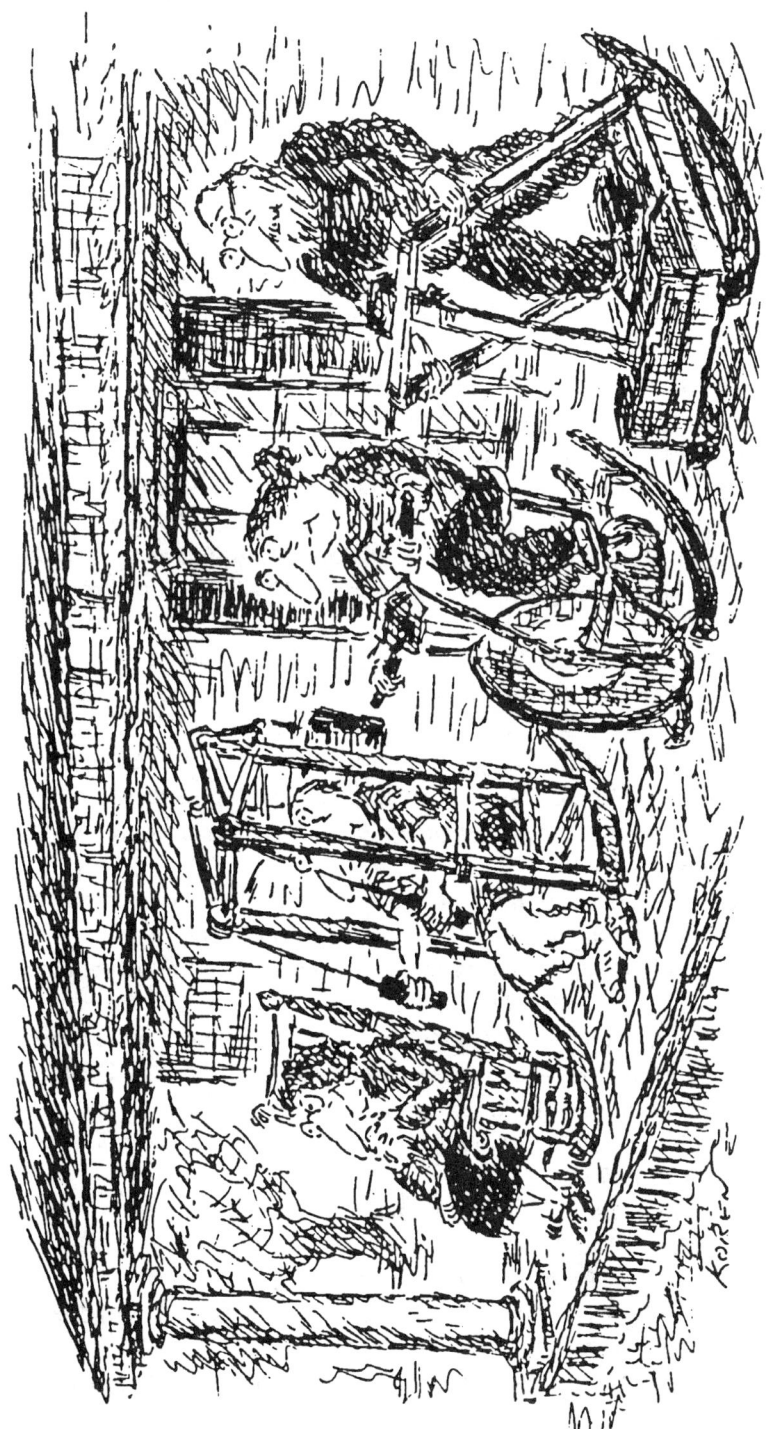

FIGURE 3.3 Some people's view of healthy aging. Copyright © 1991 by the New York Times Company. Printed by permission.

- Such a perspective leads to increasing optimism about the possibilities for increasing the levels of healthy aging in the population, thereby adding "life to years."

References

Andersson, L. (1984). *Aging and loneliness: An interventional study of a group of elderly women.* Stockholm: Karolinska Institute.

Arnetz, B., & Theorell, T. (1987). Long-term effects of a social rehabilitation programme for elderly people: Physiological predictors and mortality data. *Clinical Rehabilitation, 1,* 225–229.

Arnetz, B., Theorell, T., Levi, L., Kallner, A., & Eneroth, P. (1983). An experimental study of social isolation of elderly people—Psychoendocrine and metabolic effects. *Psychosomatic Medicine, 45,* 395–405.

Barrett-Connor, E., Suarez, L., Khaw, K., Criqui, M., & Wingard, D. (1984). Ischemic heart disease risk factors after age 50. *Journal of Chronic Diseases, 37,* 903–908.

Berkman, L., Leo-Summers, L., & Horwitz, R. (1992). Emotional support and survival after myocardial infarction: A prospective, population-based study of the elderly. *Annals of Internal Medicine, 117,* 1003–1009.

Blair, S., Kohl, H. I., Paffenbarger, R., Clark, D., Cooper, K., & Gibbons, L. (1989). Physical fitness and all-cause mortality: A prospective study of healthy men and women. *Journal of the American Medical Association, 262,* 2395–2401.

Blazer, D. (1979). Social support and mortality in an elderly community population. *American Journal of Epidemiology, 115,* 684–694.

Branch, L. (1985). Health practices and incident disability among the elderly. *American Journal of Public Health, 75,* 1436–1439.

Branch, L., & Jette, A. (1984). Personal health practices and mortality among the elderly. *American Journal of Public Health, 74,* 1126–1129.

Branch, L., & Ku, L. (1989). Transition probabilities to dependency, institutionalization, and death among the elderly over a decade. *Journal of Aging and Health, 1,* 370–408.

Buchner, D., Beresford, S., Larson, E., LaCroix, A., & Wagner, E. (1992). Effects of physical activity on health status in older adults. II. Intervention studies. *Annual Review of Public Health, 13,* 469–488.

Buchner, D., & Wagner, E. (1992). Preventing frail health. *Clinics in Geriatric Medicine, 8,* 1–17.

Camacho, T. C., Roberts, R. E., Lazarus, N. B., Kaplan, G. A., & Cohen, R. D.

(1991). Physical activity and depression: Evidence from the Alameda County Study. *American Journal of Epidemiology, 134,* 220–231.
Camacho, T. C., Strawbridge, W. J., Cohen, R. D., & Kaplan, G A.. (1993). Functional ability in the oldest old: Cumulative impact of risk factors from the preceding two decades. *Journal of Aging and Health, 5.* 439–454.
Caplan, A. (1990). Can philosophy cure what ails the medical model? In R. Berg & J. Cassells, (Eds.) *The second fifty years: Promoting health and preventing disability* (pp. 291–310). Washington, DC: National Academy Press.
Clark, D., & Maddox, G. (1992). Racial and social correlates of age-related changes in functioning. *Journals of Gerontology, 47,* S222–S232.
Cummings, S., Phillips, S., Wheat, M., Black, D., Goosby, E., Wlodarczyk, D., Trafton, P., Jergesen, H., Winograd, C., & Hulley, S. (1988). Recovery of function after hip fracture. The role of social supports. *Journal of the American Geriatrics Society, 36,* 801–806.
Falk, A., Hanson, B., Isacsson, S., & Ostergren, P. (1992). Job strain and mortality in elderly men: Social network, support, and influence as buffers. *American Journal of Public Health, 82,* 1136–1139.
Feldman, J., Makuc, D., Kleinman, J., & Cornoni-Huntley, J. (1989). National trends in educational differentials in mortality. *American Journal of Epidemiology, 129,* 919–933.
Foley, D., Branch, L., Madans, J., Brock, D., Guralnik, J., & Williams, T. (1990). Physical function. In J. Cornoni-Huntley, R. Huntley, & J. Feldman (Eds.), *Health status and well-being of the elderly: National Health and Nutrition Examination Survey—I. Epidemiologic follow-up study* (pp. 221–236). New York: Oxford University Press.
Fries, J. (1989). The compression of morbidity:Near or far? *Milbank Quarterly, 67,* 208–232.
Guralnik, J. M., & Kaplan, G. A. (1989). Predictors of healthy aging: Prospective evidence from the Alameda County Study. *American Journal of Public Health, 79,* 703–708.
Guralnik, J. M., LaCroix, A. Z., Abbott, R. D., Berkman, L. F., Satterfield, S., Evans, D. A., & Wallace, R. B. (1993). Maintaining mobility in late life. I. Demographic characteristics and chronic conditions. *American Journal of Epidemiology, 137,* 845–857.
Haan, M. N., Kaplan, G. A., & Syme, S. L. (1989). Socioeconomic status and health: Old observations and new thoughts. In J. P. Bunker, D. S. Gomby, & B. H. Kehrer (Eds.), *Pathways to health: The role of social factors* (pp. 76–135). Menlo Park, CA: Henry J. Kaiser Family Foundation.

Harris, T., Kovar, M., Suzman, R., Kleinman, J., & Feldman, J. (1989). Longitudinal study of physical ability in the oldest-old. *American Journal of Public Health, 79*, 698–702.

Hermanson, B., Omenn, G., Kronmal, R., Gersh, B., Participants in the Coronary Artery Surgery Study, et al. (1988). Beneficial six-year outcome of smoking cessation in older men and women with coronary artery disease: results from the CASS Registry. *New England Journal of Medicine, 319*, 1365–1369.

Kaplan, G. A. (1991). Epidemiologic observations on the compression of morbidity: Evidence from the Alameda County Study. *Journal of Aging and Health, 3*, 155–171.

Kaplan, G. A. (1992a). Health and aging in the Alameda County Study. In K. W. Schaie, D. Blazer, & J. S. House (Eds), *Aging, health behaviors, and health outcomes* (pp. 69–88). Hillsdale: Lawrence Erlbaum Associates.

Kaplan, G. A. (1992b). Maintenance of functioning in the elderly. *Annals of Epidemiology, 2*, 823–834.

Kaplan, G. A., & Haan, M. N. (1989). Is there a role for prevention among the elderly? Epidemiological evidence from the Alameda County Study. In M. Ory, & K. Bond (Eds.), *Aging and health care: Social science and policy perspectives (pp. 27–51)*. London: Routledge.

Kaplan, G. A., Lazarus, N. B., Cohen, R. D., & Leu, D. J. (1991). Psychosocial factors in the natural history of physical activity. *American Journal of Preventive Medicine, 7*, 12–17.

Kaplan, G. A., Roberts, R. E., Camacho, T. C., & Coyne, J. C. (1987). Psychosocial predictors of depression: Prospective evidence from the Human Population Laboratory Studies. *American Journal of Epidemiology, 125*, 206–220.

Kaplan, G. A., Strawbridge, W. J., Camacho, T., & Cohen, R. D. (1993). Factors associated with change in physical functioning in the elderly: A six-year prospective study. *Journal of Aging and Health, 5*, 140–153.

Katz, S., Branch, L., Branson, M., Papsidero, J., Beck, J., & Greer, O. (1983). Active life expectancy. *New England Journal of Medicine, 309*, 1218–1224.

Keil, J., Gazes, P., Sutherland, S., Rust, P., Branch, L., & Tyroler, H. (1989). Predictors of physical disability in elderly blacks and whites of the Charleston Heart Study. *Journal of Clinical Epidemiology, 42*, 521–529.

LaCroix, A., Lang, J., Scherr, P., Wallace, R., Cornoni-Huntley, J., Berkman, L., Curb, J., Evans, D., & Hennekens, C. (1991). Smoking and mortality among older men and women in three communities. *New England Journal of Medicine, 324*, 1619–1625.

Lammi, U., Kivela, S., Nissinen, A., Punsar, S., Puska, P., & Karvonen, M.

(1989). Predictors of disability in elderly Finnish men—A longitudinal study. *Journal of Clinical Epidemiology, 42,* 1215–1225.

Lew, E., & Garfinkel, L. (1990). Mortality at ages 75 and older in the Cancer Prevention Study (CPS–I). *CA: A Cancer Journal for Clinicians, 40,* 210–224.

Lökk, J., Theorell, T., Arnetz, B., & Eneroth, P. (1991). Physiological concomitants of an "autonomous day programme" in geriatric day care. *Scandinavian Journal of Rehabilitation Medicine, 23,* 41–46.

Maddox, G., & Clark, D. (1992). Trajectories of functional impairment in later life. *Journal of Health and Social Behavior, 33,* 114–125.

Magaziner, J., Simonsick, E., Kashner, T., Hebel, J., & Kenzora, J. (1990). Predictors of functional recovery one year following hospital discharge for hip fracture: A prospective study. *Journal of Gerontology, 45,* M101–107.

Marottoli, R., Berkman, L., & Cooney, L. (1992). Decline in physical function following hip fracture. *Journal of the American Geriatrics Society, 40,* 861–866.

Mor, V., Murphy, J., Masterson-Allen, S., Willey, C., Razmpour, A., Jackson, M., Greer, D., & Katz, S. (1989). Risk of functional decline among well elders. *Journal of Clinical Epidemiology, 42,* 895–904.

Nickel, J., & Chirikos, T. (1990). Functional disability of elderly patients with long-term coronary heart disease: A sex-stratified analysis. *Journal of Gerontology, 45,* S60–S68.

Orth-Gomer, K., & Johnson, J. (1987). Social network interaction and mortality: A six year follow-up study of a random sample of the Swedish population. *Journal of Chronic Diseases, 40,* 949–958.

Ory, M., & Bond, K. (Eds.). (1989). Health care for an aging society. *Aging and health care: Social science and policy perspectives.* London: Routledge.

Paffenbarger, R. Jr., Hyde, R., Wing, A., Lee, I., Jung, D., & Kampert, J. (1993). The association of changes in physical-activity level and other lifestyle characteristics with mortality among men. *New England Journal of Medicine, 328,* 538–545.

Pinsky, J., Leaverton, P., & Stokes III, J. (1987). Predictors of good function: The Framingham Study. *Journal of Chronic Diseases, 40 (Suppl. 1),* 15S–67S.

Riley, M.W., & Riley, J. W., Jr. (Eds.). (1989). The quality of aging: Strategies for interventions. *Annals of the American Academy of Political and Social Science, 503,* 9–147.

Rogers, R., Rogers, A., & Belanger, A. (1992) Disability-free life among the elderly in the United States. *Journal of Aging and Health, 4,* 19–42.

Roos, N., & Havens, B. (1991). Predictors of successful aging: A twelve-year study of Manitoba elderly. *American Journal of Public Health, 81,* 63–68.

Rowe, J., & Kahn, R. (1987). Human aging: Usual and successful. *Science, 237,* 143–149.

Ruberman, W., Weinblatt, E., Goldberg, J., & Chaudhary, B. (1984). Psychosocial influences on mortality after myocardial infarction. *New England Journal of Medicine, 311,* 552–559.

Seeman, T. E., Kaplan, G. A., Knudsen, L., Cohen, R., & Guralnik, J. (1987). Social network ties and mortality among the elderly in the Alameda County Study. *American Journal of Epidemiology, 126,* 714–723.

Steinbach, U. (1992). Social networks, institutionalization, and mortality among elderly people in the United States. *Journals of Gerontology, 47,* S183–S190.

Stevens, V., Hornbrook, M., Wingfield, D., Hollis, J., & Greenlick, M. (1991). Recruitment and intervention for a falls prevention project: The study of accidental falls in the elderly. In R. Weindruch, E. Hadley, & M. Ory (Eds.), *Reducing frailty and falls in older persons* (pp. 277–292). Springfield, IL: Charles C Thomas.

U.S. Department of Health and Human Services. (1990). *The health benefits of smoking cessation.* Rockville, MD: USDHHS, Public Health Service, Centers for Disease Control, Office on Smoking and Health.

Verbrugge, L., Gates, D., & Ike, R. (1991). Risk factors for disability among U.S. adults with arthritis. *Journal of Clinical Epidemiology, 44,* 167–182.

Vogt, T., Mullooly, J., Ernst, D., Pope, C., & Hollis, J. (1992). Social networks as predictors of ischemic heart disease, cancer, stroke, and hypertension: Incidence, survival and mortality. *Journal of Clinical Epidemiology, 45,* 659–666.

Welin, L., Larsson, B., Svardsudd, K., Tibblin, B., & Tibblin, G. (1992). Social network and activities in relation to mortality from cardiovascular diseases, cancer, and all causes: A 12 year follow up of the study of men born in 1913 and 1923. *Journal of Epidemiology and Community Health, 46,* 127–132.

Williams, R., Barefoot, J., Califf, R., et al. (1992). Prognostic importance of social and economic resources among medically treated patients with angiographically documented coronary heart disease. *Journal of the American Medical Association, 267,* 520–524.

Chapter 4

Disability in Late Life

Lois M. Verbrugge

For most adults, the time between the onset of chronic morbidity and death is long, measured in years and decades. Discomfort and limitations become everyday matters—perpetual for some people, episodic for others. In the long run, symptoms and dysfunctions tend to increase, and correspondingly, so do professional and personal efforts to slow the progress of medical conditions, blunt symptoms, and restore function. Many such interventions are successful so that people return to work, play tennis again, readily get out for movies and shopping, feel hopeful about the future, and stow away the medical paraphernalia they no longer need.

"Disability" refers to the impact that chronic conditions have on people's ability to act in necessary, expected, and personally desired ways in their society. Chronic conditions are progressive diseases and sensory or structural abnormalities; their onset is usually in middle or older ages. Examples are arthritis, ischemic heart disease, hypertension without heart disease, Alzheimer's disease or other dementia, emphysema, bunions, persistent hemorrhoids, hearing loss, vision loss, and chronic low back pain. Our attention is on long-term, but not necessarily static, consequences of those conditions on functioning.

Available statistics on disability give a brief, narrow picture of the disability experience. They focus on abilities to perform basic personal care, household management, and work activities. They query a person's intrinsic ability, that is, without another person's or mechanical assistance; "naked before the world." And, they measure abilities for a given point in time. Listening to older persons, we realize the disability experience is far deeper and elongated: First, disability penetrates many valued domains of life besides those mentioned; hobbies, socializing, recreation, and sleep can be greatly affected by a chronic health problem. Second, people evaluate their disability by how well they are achieving goals *with* current assistance, not without it; actual disability is on their minds, not the hypothetical notion of intrinsic disability. Third, disability changes over time depending on disease status and the efficacy of interventions; it is not a static phenomenon and it is not a unidirectional (downhill) one. Finally, as the disability experience stretches over months and years, it develops history; people can recount worst times, best times, and the overall trajectory of their functioning. This personal history greatly affects how someone deals with disability now; for example, the motivation to try a new therapy or find still another physician, feelings of weariness about today and interest in tomorrow.

The limited content in surveys is due, in part, to financial limits. Nevertheless, intellectual limits can and should be avoided in survey design and analysis. Presuming that the included questions constitute the "all" of disability, or the only important aspects of it, is not faithful to reality. By contrast, recognizing the full scope of disability and then carefully choosing items for some of it, with stated reasons for the "some," *is* faithful.

This chapter covers five topics of direct relevance to aging and quality of life: (1) the epidemiology and prevention of disability, (2) current prevalence and dynamics of disability in the U.S. population, (3) the importance of viewing disability as a gap between personal capability and environmental demand, (4) comparisons of life-long and late-life disability, and (5) future prospects for chronic morbidity and disability in our population. Because chronic conditions and their long-term consequences constitute the usual health situation in mid- and late life, I omit from discussion acute conditions (whose rates decline with age) and associated short-term disability. A bibliography with references for further reading is appended; text references are included.

Epidemiology of Disability

A classic aim of epidemiology is to understand the etiology of disease; that is, to trace the natural history of diseases and to identify their causative agents in the population. The "epidemiology of disability" employs the perspective and techniques of epidemiology for a different purpose: to describe trajectories of disablement, and to identify factors that propel or slow its pace and alter its course. Diseases now are predictors that help explain the outcome, rather than themselves the outcome to be explained. "Disablement" denotes dynamics, the process by which pathology affects functioning of specific body systems and the whole person.

Conceptual Framework for the Disablement Process

In recent decades, various conceptual schemes have been developed to think through the disablement process. Here, I describe one that is being widely accepted, elaborated, and put to use in science and public health policy. It originates in work by the sociologist Saad Nagi (1965, 1991) and has gained visibility recently through its acceptance by an Institute of Medicine panel (Pope & Tarlov, 1991). The scheme has a main pathway of impact from Pathology to Impairment to Functional Limitation to Disability. Briefly defined, Pathology is biochemical and physiological abnormalities that, if detected, become medically labeled (e.g., arthritis, schizophrenia, diabetes). The term Pathology includes diseases, injuries with long sequelae, and congenital/developmental abnormalities. Impairment refers to dysfunctions in specific body systems, measurable by clinical signs, clinical tests, or symptoms. Functional Limitation is restriction in doing basic physical and mental actions such as grasping, walking, speaking intelligibly, a reading regular print. These actions are fundamental building blocks for complex activities such as bathing, housecleaning, driving a car, hiking in the woods, and gardening. Disability is difficulty in performing complex activities because of a long-term physical or mental condition. The pace and direction of the disability process are affected by biological, behavioral, and environmental factors (together called risk factors in the Institute of Medicine scheme). In addition, the disability process affects a person's sense of well-being and overall quality of life.

This general scheme has been elaborated by Verbrugge and Jette (1994) in a manner suitable for clinical and epidemiological research. The scheme is shown in Figure 4.1. Measurement issues for each concept are discussed, and factors that affect the pace and direction of the

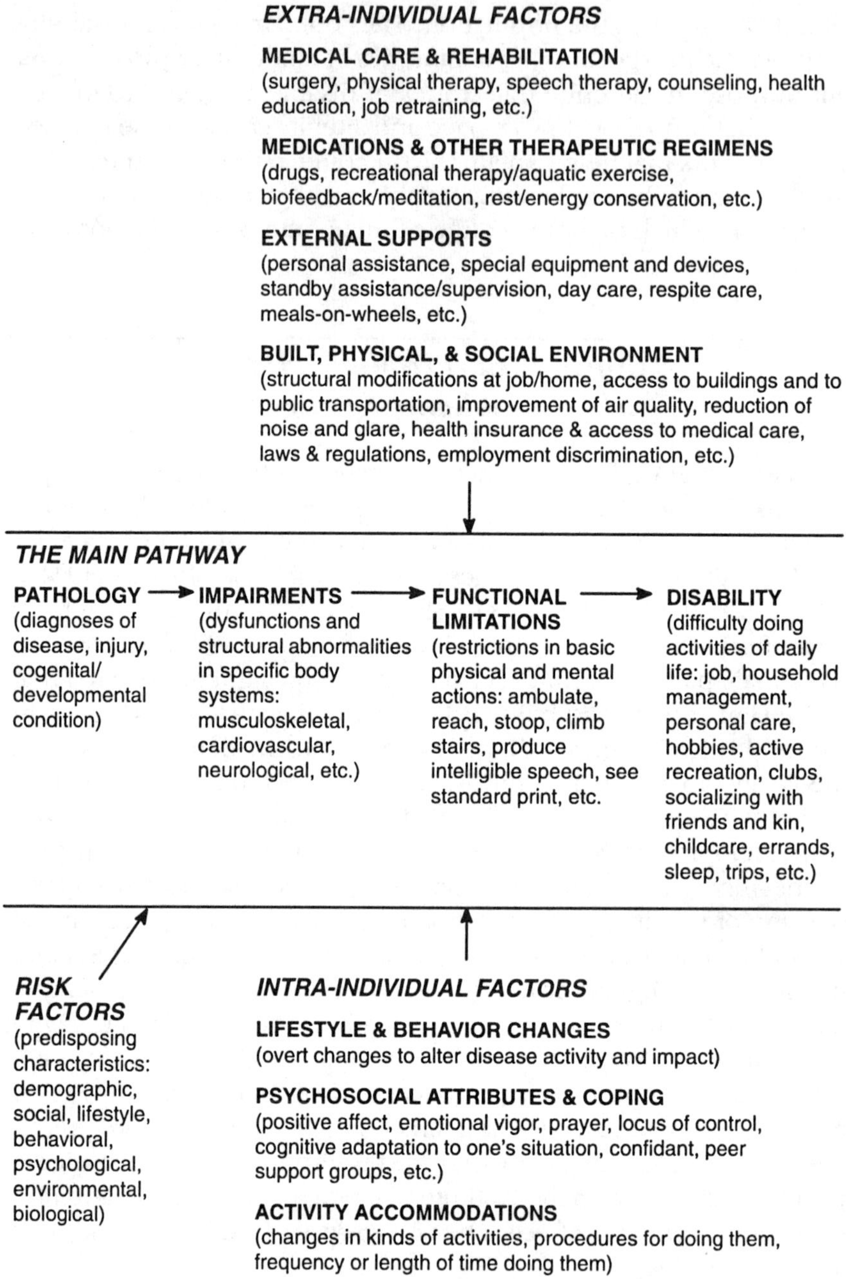

EXTRA-INDIVIDUAL FACTORS

MEDICAL CARE & REHABILITATION
(surgery, physical therapy, speech therapy, counseling, health education, job retraining, etc.)

MEDICATIONS & OTHER THERAPEUTIC REGIMENS
(drugs, recreational therapy/aquatic exercise, biofeedback/meditation, rest/energy conservation, etc.)

EXTERNAL SUPPORTS
(personal assistance, special equipment and devices, standby assistance/supervision, day care, respite care, meals-on-wheels, etc.)

BUILT, PHYSICAL, & SOCIAL ENVIRONMENT
(structural modifications at job/home, access to buildings and to public transportation, improvement of air quality, reduction of noise and glare, health insurance & access to medical care, laws & regulations, employment discrimination, etc.)

↓

THE MAIN PATHWAY

PATHOLOGY →	IMPAIRMENTS →	FUNCTIONAL LIMITATIONS →	DISABILITY
(diagnoses of disease, injury, cogenital/ developmental condition)	(dysfunctions and structural abnormalities in specific body systems: musculoskeletal, cardiovascular, neurological, etc.)	(restrictions in basic physical and mental actions: ambulate, reach, stoop, climb stairs, produce intelligible speech, see standard print, etc.	(difficulty doing activities of daily life: job, household management, personal care, hobbies, active recreation, clubs, socializing with friends and kin, childcare, errands, sleep, trips, etc.)

↑   ↑

RISK FACTORS
(predisposing characteristics: demographic, social, lifestyle, behavioral, psychological, environmental, biological)

INTRA-INDIVIDUAL FACTORS

LIFESTYLE & BEHAVIOR CHANGES
(overt changes to alter disease activity and impact)

PSYCHOSOCIAL ATTRIBUTES & COPING
(positive affect, emotional vigor, prayer, locus of control, cognitive adaptation to one's situation, confidant, peer support groups, etc.)

ACTIVITY ACCOMMODATIONS
(changes in kinds of activities, procedures for doing them, frequency or length of time doing them)

FIGURE 4.1 A model of disablement process.

SOURCE: Verbrugge & Jette (1994).

disablement process are distinguished: namely, predisposing risk factors, interventions to slow the disability process, and exacerbators that propel it. *Risk factors are* longstanding or permanent features of an individual that exist at or before the outset of the disablement process; for example, gender, age, socioeconomic status, personality style, lifetime smoking behavior. (Our definition is more restricted and traditional than in the Institute of Medicine report.) *Interventions* are introduced during the disablement process in a deliberate effort to avoid, retard, or reverse outcomes (impairments, functional limitations, disability). They serve as buffers. Examples are physical and occupational therapy, therapeutic drugs, surgery, professional counseling, personal assistance, special equipment and devices, psychological coping, peer support groups, lifestyle changes, modifications of the built environment, changes in roles and regular activities. Interventions are numerous, changeable, and often multiple (co-existing). The timing of their effects may be immediate, delayed, or cumulative. All of this makes estimating the effects of specific interventions problematic in observational research. But interventions cannot be ignored in surveys, as they are a commonplace and influential aspect of the disability experience. *Exacerbators* are unwished-for intrusions in the disablement process. They occur when interventions go badly awry, or when people adopt behaviors to relieve stress or discomfort, but that have unfortunate effects on health and disability. Still more pernicious are exacerbators that simply exist in longstanding social custom and expectation; examples are architectural barriers, inflexible work hours, and social prejudice against people who do not look or act "right." Persons with disabilities confront many for-granted aspects of society that inhibit them from doing things they can and wish to do; that is the essence of "handicap." To undo these fixed features often requires public laws because societal mind and manners are slow to change on their own.

Disability precedes and influences outcomes of dire or global nature. Empirical research shows that the more disabled an individual is, the more likely hospitalization, institutionalization, and death are in a prospective period such as a year. Disability also has a powerful effect on happiness, life satisfaction, and other global well-being indicators. In our conceptual scheme, these big outcomes stand to the right of Disability (see Fig. 3 in Verbrugge & Jette, 1994).

Finally, we note what conceptual schemes accomplish, and what they do not. A conceptual scheme delineates and distinguishes key features, provides names, and lays out basic causal trajectories. It is

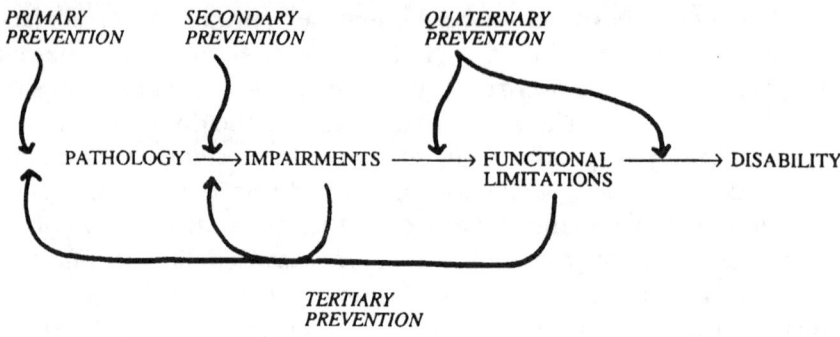

FIGURE 4.2 Prevention strategies.

not a formal scientific model, replete with specific hypotheses, stated rationales, and operational indicators. Good conceptual schemes gain wide acceptance in a field, provide general guidance for research designs, and ultimately enhance the pooling of research results from separately-conducted studies.

Prevention of Disability

"Prevention of disability" is becoming a popular term that signals programmatic and clinical interest in disability. It is actually contained in the epidemiological concept of *"tertiary prevention"*; namely, interventions to reduce disease impacts (Last, 1988). Examples of disability prevention are drugs to diminish my mother's arthritis pain so that she can write letters more easily; a sturdy cane so that my 96-year old sweetheart can walk through and enjoy his desert garden; long prayers to the Lord by my frail aunt so that she can accept the narrowing of her activities and quietness of her days.

The classic triumverate of prevention strategies also includes primary prevention (efforts to avert onset of pathology) and secondary prevention (early detection and management of pathology). In a conceptual scheme for disablement, *primary prevention* acts at the far left side before Pathology (Figure 4.2). *Secondary prevention* acts ahead of and on Impairment, by detecting abnormalities and trying to slow their progress or even eliminate (cure) them. *Tertiary prevention* encompasses everything to the right of Impairment; it includes efforts to avert onset of secondary conditions, to maintain and restore function, and to sustain life by heroic care. Its broad sweep reflects the relative disinterest in functioning among medical professionals for most of the twentieth century, when the typology was created and promulgated. A current, attractive proposal is to use "tertiary prevention" just for disease-related efforts (secondary conditions and heroic care) and to use *"quaternary prevention"* for function-related efforts.

Disability Prevalence and Dynamics

Disability is inherently multifaceted. First, it can occur in *any activity*, whether it is obligatory, committed, or discretionary. Obligatory activities are personal care (activities of daily living or ADLs, necessary for the body's survival), some household management activities (instrumental activities of daily living or IALs, necessary for independent living), and sleep. Committed activities are job, keeping house (when it constitutes one's main work; includes at-home and shopping/errand activities), and childcare/eldercare. Discretionary activities are the vast array of leisure-time pursuits; examples are hobbies, active sports, attending religious services, socializing with friends and relatives. Second, disability can range in *severity* from slight ("a little") difficulty performing an activity to complete inability ("unable") to do it.

The obvious consequence of this variety is that disability can be measured in many ways, by many indicators, with many cutpoints. There is no single rate and no single count of persons with disabilities in the population. This has frustrated politicians and journalists who demand simplicity for their deliberations and reports. At best, public officials and other statistics users are frustrated by disability data; at worst, they distrust and discredit them.

Variety is easier for scientists to accept, but it can tax their serenity at some points, too. First, different surveys asking about the same activity have generated quite different rates, indicating that context and wording of disability questions is very important. Second, the personal standards and external requirements for performing an activity vary across people—a good deal for their favorite hobbies, and far less but certainly not absent for dressing and eating. So, reports of difficulty are not measured against a fixed, uniform level of demand that applies to everybody. Further, an individual's roles and standards change over time. In short, levels of demand have both interindividual variation at a given time and intraindividual variation over time.

This truth is usually left unstated because it proves to be disconcerting, suggesting that disability statistics are squishy and soft, without a firm foundation. Third, panel studies show that substantial percentages of people who are disabled at an initial point are not disabled at a later one. Much of that recovery of function is real, but just how much is due to random or systematic measurement error? The same question arises for losses of function: How many people whose answers change from "no difficulty" to "difficulty" really made that transition?

In sum, it is best to accept, rather than ignore, the fact that disability is multidimensional, genuinely subjective, relative to one's own standards, and changeable over time. This becomes the complex content for scientific measurement and understanding. It can also spur scientists to conduct methodological work that improves the quality of disability statistics by extirpating bias, artifact, and unreliability.

Immersed in the variety, scientists must also appreciate public officials' need for standard, global indicators of disability. The current notion of "active life expectancy" (ALE) aptly fulfills that need. It condenses age-specific disability prevalence rates (and if available, incidence rates) into a single figure, stating the number of years a person can expect to live free of disability. Subtracting that from life expectancy (the number of years a person can expect to be alive) gives an estimate of disabled years. Recent statistics show that U.S. males have an active life expectancy of 60 years; this is 84% of their whole lifetime (Pope & Tarlov, 1991). U.S. females can expect 64 years of disability-free life; but this constitutes slightly less (82%) of their lifetime. Considering just older persons, U.S. men who reach age 65 expect 9 of their remaining 15 years to be active, or 60%. Women that age anticipate more active years (11) but also more disabled ones (8); the percentage of active years ends up just less (58%) than men's. In most statistical series, women's rates of disability exceed men's. But women's disability is more often mild or moderate, whereas men's is more often severe. This changes at advanced ages; elderly women have more severe disabilities.

The attractiveness of ALE is immense for health planners and others who need compact statistics to garner funds and compel public attention. Officials of localities, states, and other nations welcome the notion and ask how it can be measured for their population. Scientists could answer readily if there were a single global indicator of disability and a single appropriate statistical technique for ALE; once again, variety poses a problem! Currently, there is active work by health statisticians and demographers to craft a few compact comprehensive in-

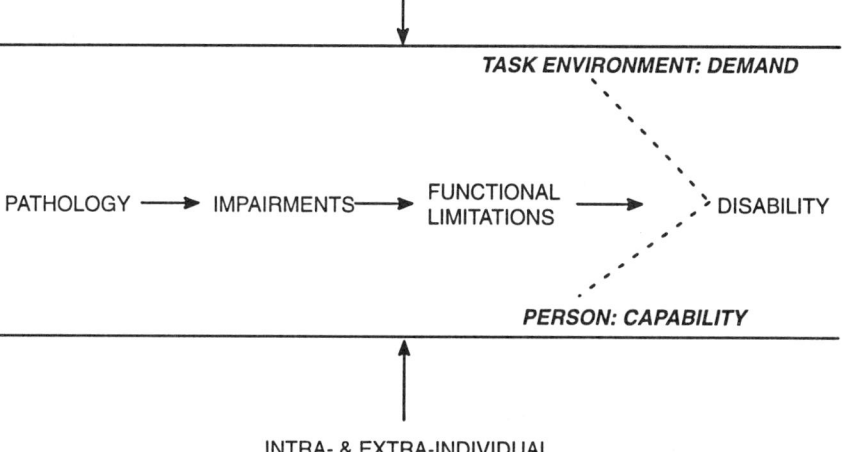

SOURCE; Verbrugge & Jette (1994).

FIGURE 4.3 Disability as a gap between capability and demand.

dicators about disability and to develop calculation approaches for disability prevalence and incidence data.

Disability as a Gap

So far, the discussion implies that disability is a personal feature, in the same way as age or occupation is. In truth, disability is not inherent in a person. Instead, it denotes a relationship between a person and his/her environment (Figure 4.3). Disability occurs for a given activity when there is a gap between personal capability and the activity's physical and mental demand. Disability can be alleviated on either side—by increasing capability or by reducing demand. Strategies to *increase capability* are medical care and rehabilitation, medications and other therapeutic regimens, and lifestyle and behavior changes to reduce key risk factors. Strategies to *reduce demand* are modifications of the built, physical, and social environment, activity accommodations (changes in roles and time management), external supports (personal assistance or supervision, special equipment), and psychosocial coping.

Medical care and public health programs focus on interventions to improve or maintain capability, that act on a person's physical or mental interior. This person-centered approach ignores the importance and malleability of demand. In real life, changes in demand are a common feature of the disablement process, and they can reduce disability swiftly and greatly.

Changes in demand are common; some are private and invisible, others public and visible. Consider the *private* ways: People modify their regular activities to reduce the physical and mental demands posed. For example, my mother goes shopping less often and plans those ventures carefully so she is not on her feet for more than a couple of hours. And, from one year to the next, my father planted more small evergreens in his flower garden so the zone of flowers narrowed and was manageable as his asthma and anemia advanced. My mother and father did not announce these changes; they just gradually adjusted their behavior to match their stamina. Similarly, psychosocial coping is usually private (prayer, acceptance, laughter, reading humorous or inspirational books), or shared with intimates (peer support group). Consider the *public* ways: Opting for human or equipment assistance can alleviate disability. But there are costs, both financial and personal (changes in self-identity and social appearance). At more distance from a person's own physical periphery, modifications can be made in the built, physical, and social environments at home, jobsites, and the broader public arena. For example, my uncle moved to a house without stairs; employers buy special furniture for staff with chronic back pain; cities offer special bus services for mobility-limited persons; laws prohibit employment discrimination for disability. Environmental changes cost money, and they require planning and goodwill. Accomplishing them in broad societal venues can take a great deal of time and uncover deep resistance from those whose pockets will be touched.

Why does the person-centered perspective exist and persist? There are three reasons. First, medicine contemplates the person in his or her whole—or more usually his or her parts—and asks: what is wrong in here?, what can be done to make things right in this body or mind?

The medical viewpoint has a very pervasive influence on health research, including the research done by social scientists. Second, surveys are the standard technique for obtaining information about health and disability. Methods are well-developed for samples and interviews of individuals, and this inevitably steers scientific questions to be framed from that perspective. Third, even if the importance of demand is recognized, scientists are uncertain how to measure it in a compact manner. It is appropriate to query respondents about capabilities (these are indeed their own) and difficulties doing activities (the perceived gap). But it is much harder—even unreasonable, maybe impossible—to ask them about environmental features that pose high or excessive demand. Can people perceive environmental barriers, talk about unmet needs, envision technical and social solutions for their disabilities? A key issue on the scientific agenda is to devise ways to measure demand, especially "unfair demand" (the essence of handicap).

In sum, intellectual limitations can be removed easily, given enough motivation and illumination. Research that has a person-centered approach will and should continue, but the importance and fundamental veracity of seeing disability as a relationship, not a personal characteristic, can be kept firmly in mind while doing it. Methodological limitations can also be removed, given enough scientific time and energy.

Life-long and Late-life Disability

The terms "life-long" and "late-life" designate when a serious chronic condition and its impact on functioning enter life. That timing, or onset, makes a great difference in the nature of the disability experience.

The usual causes of life-long disability are congenital conditions and developmental conditions or severe injury in childhood or youth. Disability is often profound, pervasive, essentially static, and (for injuries) rapid in onset. By contrast, the usual causes of late-life disability are chronic diseases that cross clinical thresholds in mid- or late life and declines in sensory function or structural integrity not directly related to disease. Disability tends to be mild or moderate, initially restricted to a few domains but expanding over time, dynamic with fluctuations to and fro, and slow in evolution.

There are many differences in the disablement process for the two groups. Life-long disabled persons do not enjoy the expansion of skills and activities in adulthood or the total diversity of lifetime experiences, as do their nondisabled peers. For many, the issue of activity accommodation by substituting or dropping activities is effectively moot; the struggle is always to expand what one does in daily life. Capabilities are very restricted and usually fixed (not easily or at all remediable). Demand looms large for virtually any activity. In this situation, attention focuses on external supports (human assistance and special equipment) and on environmental and social access. High quality and reasonable expense for equipment and human services are paramount concerns. Achieving personal control after years of dependency is a courageous goal; it is the central theme of the independent living movement. Access to buildings, vehicles, and jobs is demanded as a basic social right. For very good reasons, a constant plaint of life-long disabled persons is "Change the milieu, not me!"

By contrast, late-life disability is a gradual process, and people devote attention to restoring the capabilities they once enjoyed and recall very well. Their diverse experiences and adaptations to other troubles over a lifetime serve as resources when activity accommodations need to be made. External supports come into daily life gradually, and problems of access are frustrating but seldom defeating. The disability process involves gradual adjustment and a good deal of personal choice. At far points—when capabilities are greatly reduced by disease, external supports are present and critical, and mobility is greatly diminished—late-life disability comes closest to looking like life-long disability. But the sentiment is never the same. The difference between a young disabled adult who yearns to experience life's delights and an elderly disabled person who has done so is indubitably vast.

For all the differences, it is still true that the same overall conceptual scheme—from Pathology to Disability, with risk factors, interventions, and exacerbators—is suitable for both groups. The relative importance and dynamics of the conceptual pieces vary greatly, but not the pieces themselves. This has real-world political and technological implications. There is a fundamental intersection for young and old persons with disabilities: their wish to do more things in life or to do things with greater ease. The older persons have the power of numbers; the younger persons have the power of established advocacy groups. It is hard to persuade older persons to join "the disability movement"; many do not think of themselves as disabled (or, as contemporary language dictates, "a person with a disability"). Older persons have quieter clout. Their personal demands in physicians' offices and in print gradually prompt broad-based political concern, inspire clinical and epidemiological research, and motivate design engineers. Further, as survival of life-long disabled persons increases, more of them will join the older population; their savvy and spirit will undoubtedly influence how their peers with more moderate disabilities voice needs and complaints. In years ahead, life-long and late-life disabled persons will recognize their intersections and exploit them for political and technological benefit for people of all ages.

Future Prospects

What changes in population morbidity, disability, and mortality can we expect in coming decades? *Population aging* will propel upward the numbers of ill and disabled persons and the crude rates of morbidity and disability in the population. That is a certainty; it is important from a health services standpoint but not especially from a scientific one. The important scientific questions concern *age-specific rates*: For example, a half century hence, will elderly persons be more likely to have heart disease than their age-peers today?; among those who do, will they be less disabled by it?; and will they live longer with the disease?

What happens will depend on the relative advances in primary, secondary, tertiary, and quaternary prevention. First, consider great strides in *primary prevention*: If science identifies key risk factors for the most prominent fatal conditions and figures out how to diminish those risks for people's lifetimes, then incidence and prevalence rates will fall for morbidity, disability, and mortality. There will be a "clean sweep" of improvement. If risk factors for key nonfatal conditions are also elucidated, there will be further improvements in morbidity and disability. Next, consider *secondary prevention*: The issue is further development of diagnostic procedures and of therapies that slow disease progression, followed by widespread use of these procedures and therapies in clinical practice. Earlier diagnosis and more efficacious therapy mean that people have milder cases of diseases. They avoid death longer (lower case fatality), but then have a disease for more years and a larger fraction of their lives. Ill people who would otherwise have died in an earlier decade now remain in the population for awhile. In sum, the likely result of secondary prevention is rising rates of morbidity and disability, with a shift toward mildness for both, and declining rates of mortality. This scenario of "longer life but worsening health" can disappoint public health officials, who count success only when rates drop. Yet advances in secondary prevention *are* success; their impact on population health may be counterintuitive but it should be welcomed and applauded. *Tertiary prevention* protects ill/disabled individuals from serious complications such as new health problems due to deconditioning, death from global frailty, and iatrogenic problems from long-term therapy. Successes tend to be hard-won; the complications may be delayed but ultimately eventuate. Compared to secondary prevention, relatively few people are affected and their morbidity/disability status and mortality risks are not altered much. The consequences on population rates due to tertiary prevention are tiny—small upward pushes in age-specific morbidity and disability, and small downward pushes in mortality. Finally, *quaternary prevention* ignores etiology and focuses on function. Advances can occur in a multitude of ways: design of assistive devices, laws that require public transportation for mobility-limited persons, inclusion of home health services in public insurance programs, development of peer support groups for persons with arthritis, home exercise programs for postsurgery patients, and so on. Industry, medicine, and government units can all engage in the development and dissemination of tertiary prevention. Changes like these, when numerous and widespread, can reduce population disability greatly, both its prevalence and average severity. Morbidity rates are unaffected. Mortality rates are likely to drop somewhat as people are more functional and fit at any given age.

These are pure scenarios. In any given decade, advances in all four kinds of prevention occur, with greater or lesser proportions of each. Their impacts are simultaneous, and it may be difficult to untangle their relative importance no matter how fine the empirical data are.

Large-scale phenomena like morbidity, disability, and mortality rates are slow to change (except in catastrophic situations). Thus, describing and understanding trends in the past half century is usually the best guide for speculations about the next one. Researchers have been studying trends in age-specific prevalence of chronic conditions, prevalence of work disability, activity limitation, and dependency (use of personal or equipment assistance), and rates of mortality. Studies indicate rising rates of population *morbidity and disability* in the 1960s and 1970s, but whether those trends continued in the 1980s is unclear (the answer varies for different indicators) (Crimmins, 1993; Manton, Corder, & Stallard, 1993; Verbrugge, 1989a). *Mortality* has taken a different course: Rates were static in mid-century; to everyone's surprise they began to fall in the late

1960s, particularly sharply at oldest ages; the decline continued through the 1980s. This whole set of trends is consistent with a scenario of secondary prevention as the preeminent (though not exclusive) force. It is well-recognized that contemporary medicine's strength indeed lies in early diagnosis and management of chronic disease, particularly fatal diseases, far more than in primary, tertiary, or quaternary prevention.

Secondary prevention is likely to continue as a key focus of medical development and clinical care. For some time, then, we should expect to see rising age-specific morbidity and disability prevalences (but shifts toward milder forms of both) joined with falling mortality. There is an important caution for this future: If biomedical research and medical therapies remain focused on fatal diseases, with relative inattention to nonfatal conditions, we will slowly see a redistribution of health problems within individuals' lives—with ever-growing prominence of nonfatal ones, the conditions that bother and disable but do not kill. Already the leading kinds of conditions for middle-aged and older persons, they will become still more so.

One attractive and widely discussed future scenario deserves comment. The "compression of morbidity" is a specific version of primary prevention. It posits that most people might never acquire chronic diseases and will ultimately die from multisystem physiological frailty. On average, only a small fraction of life will be spent ill and disabled before death. The central premise for the scenario is that improvements in morbidity and disability rates will outpace mortality reductions. (This contains many specific assumptions: that morbidity, disability, and mortality rates all fall, that primary prevention for numerous diseases happens, and that mortality rates bump up against some limit to human life expectancy.) Whether this scenario is a genuine possibility for human populations is not certain, but it definitely will not happen soon.

Reasoned speculation is important in science as a guide to hypothesis development and data collection. But empirical evidence is the essential commodity we want. We must continue current statistical series and establish new ones that allow us to describe changes in morbidity and disability. Explaining those changes and determining the relative importance of the four prevention scenarios will be very difficult, but we must try.

Conclusion

The Quincentennial has prompted some thoughts about the nature of our work as scientists, and I shall conclude with them.

Science is but one way of knowing. There are others: religion, love, poetry, intuition, meditation. Science is but one way of asking questions and obtaining answers. There are others: exploration, invention, consultation with seers, the wisdom of experience.

Science as a craft and profession rises and falls in eminence across history. A central way of knowing in the twentieth century, it was not always so, and may not be so in the future. In Christopher Columbus' time, adventurers and tinkerers contributed greatly to knowledge; not scientists. In the future, visionaries or redeemers may be more trusted for knowledge. Our way of knowing is characterized by empirical data, a combination of inductive and deductive reasoning, documentation of procedures and results, and the canon of replication. The best protection of science for the future is twofold: first, ethical and fastidious performance of our craft and, second, stewardship of what we study—the earth, its inhabitants, and the cosmos beyond.

We are scientists for noble reasons. Awed and curious by things around us, we stop to ask a question or two, have a hunch or idea, and ultimately commit ourselves to finding answers by particular (namely, scientific) procedures. The best reward is learning something that no one has ever known before. (I credit that statement to a woman scientist whose name, sadly, I have forgotten.) The delight is telling what we learned to others and, if we are very lucky, having something we learned become fundamental and enduring. We are also scientists for private and often unacknowledged reasons. Some of us answer personal questions about life's meaning and human relationships through science. Or we find order and control in the lab that offsets the chaos of personal life.

As a curious creature of this century, I became a scientist because I had fun answering questions in science projects as a teenager, because my college affair with mathematics waned, and because I deeply admired a physicist (my father, Frank Verbrugge, 1913–1985) and a geologist (the antarctic explorer and scientist, Laurence McKinley Gould, b.1896). The topics I have studied vary a good deal, but they have sequential ties and all pertain to the life and death of men and women. They are also connected by three steady convictions: that science must remain faithful to real-world experiences; that results must be conveyed in understandable language; and that the gift of survey respondents' time and information must be returned by scientists in the public media.

I study disability because it is a nondramatic commonplace experience of older persons' days and years. I study arthritis because it is nonfatal, is the leading chronic condition for middle-aged and older persons, and is the most often-cited reason for disability in mid and late life. Biomedical and epidemiological research has focused on the dramatic and dire during the twentieth century. Fatal diseases and death have held center-stage. Nonfatal diseases and disability deserve scientific and public health attention that is commensurate with their importance in people's lives. This will happen if scientists and older people insist on it enough.

Acnowledgements

The author thanks Laurence Z. Rubenstein for suggesting the term "quaternary prevention."

References

Adams, P. F., & Benson, V. (1991). Current estimates from the National Health Interview Survey, 1990. *Vital and Health Statistics, 10.* (181), DHHS Publ. No. (PHS)92–1509. Hyattsville, MD: National Center for Health Statistics.

Berg, R. L., & Cassells, J. S. (Eds.). (1990). *The second fifty years. Promoting health and preventing disability.* Washington, DC: National Academy Press.

Branch, L. G., Guralnik, J. M., Foley, D. J., Kohout, F. J., Wetle, T. T., Ostfeld, A., & Katz, S. (1991). Active life expectancy for 10,000 Caucasian men and women in three communities. *Journal of Gerontology: Medical Sciences, 46,* M145–150.

Chirikos, T. N. (1986). Accounting for the historical rise in work-disability prevalence. *The Milbank Quarterly, 64,* 271–301.

Corbin, J. M., & Strauss, A. (1988). *Unending work and care. Managing chronic illness at home.* San Francisco: Jossey-Bass.

Crimmins, E. M. (1993). Trends in health of the U.S. population: 1957–1989. In J. Simon (Ed.), *The state of humanity.* Basil: Blackwell Pub.

Crimmins, E. M., & Ingegneri, D. G. (1992). Trends in health among the

American population. In Anna M. Schieber & Sylvester J. Schieber (Eds.), *Demography and retirement: The 21st Century* (pp. 259-278). Westport CT: Greenwood Publishing Group Inc.

Crimmins, E. M., Saito, Y., & Ingegneri, D. (1989). Changes in life expectancy and disability-free life expectancy in the United States. *Population and Development Review, 15,* 235-267.

Fox, D. M., & Willis, D. P. (Eds.). Disability policy: Restoring socioeconomic independence. *The Milbank Quarterly, 67,* Suppl. 2, Parts 1 & 2.

Fries, J. F. (1983). The compression of morbidity. *Milbank Memorial Fund Quarterly, 61,* 397-419.

Fries, J. F. (1989). The compression of morbidity: Near or far? *The Milbank Quarterly, 67,* 208-232.

Haan, M. N., Rice, D. P., Satariano, W. A., & Selby J. V. (Eds.). (1991). Living longer and doing worse? Present and future trends in the health of the elderly. *Journal of Aging and Health, 3* (2).

House, J. S., Kessler, R. C., Herzog A. R, Mero, R., Kinney, A.,& Breslow, M. (1990). Age, socioeconomic status, and health. *The Milbank Quarterly, 68,* 383-411.

Kaplan, R. M., Anderson, J. P., & Wingard, D. L. (1991). Gender differences in health-related quality of life. *Health Psychology, 10,* 86-93.

Katz, S. (Ed.). (1987). The Portugal Conference: Measuring quality of life and functional status in clinical and epidemiological research. *Journal of Chronic Diseases, 40* (6).

LaPlante, M. P. (1991). Disability risks of chronic illnesses and impairments. *Disability Statistics Report,* No. 2. Washington, DC: National Institute on Disability and Rehabilitation Research, U.S. Department of Education.

Last, J. M. (1988). *A dictionary of epidemiology,* 2nd edition. New York: Oxford University Press.

Lawton, M. P. (1982). Competence, environmental press, and the adaptation of older people. In M. P. Lawton, P. G. Windley, & T. O. Byerts, (Eds.), *Aging and the Environment: Theoretical approaches* (pp. 33-59). New York: Springer Publishing Co.

Lawton, M. P. (1983). Environment and other determinants of well-being in older people. *The Gerontologist, 23,* 349-357.

Maddox, G. L., & Clark, D. O. (1992). Trajectories of functional impairment in later life. *Journal of Health and Social Behavior, 33,* 114-125.

Manton, K. G. (1982). Changing concepts of morbidity and mortality in the elderly population. *Milbank Memorial Fund Quarterly, 60,* 183-244.

Manton, K. G. (1988). A longitudinal study of functional change and mortality in the United States. *Journal of Gerontology: Social Sciences, 43,* S153-161.

Manton, K. G., Corder, L. S., & Stallard, E. (1993). Estimates of change in chronic disability and institutional incidence and prevalence rates in the U.S., elderly population from the 1982, 1984, and 1989 National Long Term Care Survey. *Journal of Gerontology: Social Sciences, 48*, S153-166.

McKinlay, J. B., McKinlay, S. M., & Beaglehole, R. (1989). A review of the evidence concerning the impact of medical measures on recent mortality and morbidity in the United States. *International Journal of Health Services, 19*, 181-208.

Nagi, S. Z. (1965). Some conceptual issues in disability and rehabilitation. In M. B. Sussman (Ed.), *Sociology and rehabilitation* (pp. 100-113). Washington, DC: American Sociological Association.

Nagi, S. Z. 1991. Disability concepts revisited: Implications for prevention. In A. M. Pope, & A. R. Tarlov (Eds.), *Disability in America: Toward a national agenda for prevention* (pp. 309-327). Washington, DC: National Academy Press.

Olshansky, S. J., & Ault, A. B. (1986). The fourth stage of the epidemiologic transition: The age of delayed degenerative diseases. *The Milbank Quarterly, 64*, 355-391.

Omran, A. R. (1971). The epidemiologic transition: A theory of the epidemiology of population change. *Milbank Memorial Fund Quarterly, 49*, 509-538.

Pope, A. M., & Tarlov, A. R. (Eds.). (1991). *Disability in America: Toward a national agenda for prevention.* Washington, DC: National Academy Press.

Riley, J. C. (1989). *Sickness, recovery and death: A history and forecast of ill health.* London: MacMillan.

Rogers, R. G., Rogers, A., & Belanger, A. (1989). Active life among the elderly in the United States: Multistate life-table estimates and population projections. *The Milbank Quarterly, 67*, 370-411.

Rothenberg, R. B., & Koplan, J. P. (1990). Chronic disease in the 1990s. In J. E. Fielding, L. B. Lave, & L. Breslow (Eds.), *Annual Review of Public Health,* Volume 11 (pp. 267-296). Palo Alto, CA: Annual Reviews Inc.

Stahl, S. M. (Ed.). (1990). *The legacy of longevity: Health and health care in later life.* Newbury Park, CA: Sage.

Verbrugge, L. M. (1984). Longer life but worsening health: Trends in health and mortality of middle-aged and older persons. *Milbank Memorial Fund Quarterly, 62*, 475-519.

Verbrugge, L. M. (1989a). Recent, present, and future health of American adults. In L. Breslow, J. E. Fielding, & L. B. Lave (Eds.), *Annual Review of Public Health,* Volume 10 (pp. 333-361). Palo Alto, CA: Annual Reviews Inc.

Verbrugge, L. M. (1989b). Gender, aging, and health. In K. S. Markides (Ed.), *Aging and health: Perspectives on gender, race, ethnicity, and class* (pp. 23-78). Newbury Park, CA: Sage.

Verbrugge, L. M. (1990). The iceberg of disability. In S. M. Stahl (Ed.), *The legacy of longevity: Health and health care in later life* (pp. 55-75). Newbury Park, CA: Sage.

Verbrugge, L. M. (1991). Physical and social disability in adults. In H. Hibbard, P. A., Nutting, & M. E. Grady (Eds.), *Primary care research: Theory and methods* (pp. 31-57). Conference Proceedings. AHCPR Publ. No. 91-0011. Rockville, MD: Agency for Health Care Policy and Research, U.S. Dept. of Health and Human Services.

Verbrugge, L. M., & Jette, A. M. (1994). The disablement process. *Social Science and Medicine, 38,* 1-14.

Verbrugge, L. M., Lepkowski, J. M., & Imanaka, Y. (1989). Comorbidity and its impact on disability. *The Milbank Quarterly, 67,* 450-484.

West, J. (Ed.). (1991). *The Americans with Disabilities Act. From policy to practice.* New York: Milbank Memorial Fund.

Chapter 5
Self-Care and Quality of Life in Old Age

Gordon H. DeFriese, Thomas R. Konrad, Alison Woomert, Jean E. Kincade Norburn, and Shulamit Bernard

It was not so very long ago, in the 1970s to be specific, that the concept of *self-care* was seen by many American health care professionals as a polemical concept intended to suggest the *counter-medical* message of various groups who advocated a stronger and more central role for patients in clinical decision making. The nihilism, which unfortunately became associated with the writings of some of the most widely known authors on the subject, suggested to many health care professionals that self-care (and the associated term *self-help*) expressed a separatism between formal and informal sources of assistance in time of sickness or need, and preferential reliance on the latter whenever possible. Some formal, and certainly many professional, providers of care felt they were relegated through the concept and practice of self-care to a secondary (i.e., less desirable) status, suggesting the necessity for a posture of submissiveness, acquiescence, and subordinate role to the client/patient. On the other hand, many authors within the self-care field of the 1970s saw self-care as a form of lay education for personal health functioning that could empower and protect the individual from the sometimes negative consequences of the professionalization and medicalization of health in modern societies (Barofsky, 1978; Butler, Gertman, Oberlander, 1979; Levin, 1976a; Levin, 1976b.) Self-care was defined so as to include the active participation and collaborative partnership between patient and health care provider, thus relieving the formal care provider of total responsibility for medical care decisions that affected their patients' lives.

Yet, as strange as it would have seemed a decade earlier, by the end of the decade of the 1980s the concept of self-care had achieved a clear acceptance within the formal literature and practice of medical care in this country (Hickey, 1988; Vickery, Golaszewski, & Wright, 1988;) and in Europe (Dean, 1986). By 1980, there was a huge formal literature on self-care ranging over a wide array of disciplines (Woomert, Bond, McFarland, & Graham, 1982), and between 1984 and 1989 the medical literature was enlarged by more than 400 bibliographic references that described the application of self-care approaches to disease management and the maintenance of functional health status for a wide variety of health conditions. Findings from studies of self-care educational programs throughout the United States showed that most programs offered instruction to lay persons for performing skills considered by health care professionals to be relevant to health, easily taught, and of relatively low risk when performed by lay persons (DeFriese, Woomert, Guild, Steckler, & Konrad 1989; Wilkinson, Darby, & Mant, 1987). In 1983 self-care became an official entry in *Index Medicus*, an official publication of the National Library of Medicine, indicating the legitimacy associated with the concept in American health care and clinical medicine.

This chapter discusses the conceptualization, role, and importance of self-care as part of a national strategy emphasizing the social and behavioral aspects of *healthy aging*. It highlights the research of the past several years, which has furthered understanding of the place of self-care education and practice in American health care. This chapter also projects some of the potential benefits that may arise from increased self-care research and practice among older adults in the decades ahead as policymakers attempt to assure a higher quality of life for those who live to experience old age in America.

Conceptualizing Self-Care

Self-care has tended to be defined broadly so as to encompass all activities a lay person undertakes to maintain or promote personal health, as well as those activities (requiring specific skills) for the detection, prevention, and treatment of common health problems and conditions (Haug, Akiyama, Trybon, Sonoda, & Syklo, 1991). Some have even defined the decision to do nothing in response to illness symptoms as self-care (Dean, 1986; Stoller, Foster & Portugal, 1993). The definition promulgated by a work group convened over a decade ago by the World Health Organization (WHO) has proven to be a useful starting point for a discussion of the term self-care. Accordingly,

> *Self-care in health refers to the activities individuals, families and communities undertake with the intention of enhancing health, preventing disease, limiting illness, and restoring health. These activities are derived from knowledge and skills from the pool of both professional and lay experience. They are undertaken by lay people on their own behalf, either separately or in participative collaboration with professionals (World Health Organization, 1983)*

There are several significant points to emphasize about this definition. First, it presupposes that self-care is *intentional,* with the aim of making a positive contribution to health through actions whose purpose is to *prevent disease, limit illness, and restore health*. But there is more. It is a positive step toward the *enhancement of existing states of "health."* Second, these activities or strategies depend on (or are derived from) *technical knowledge and skills*, which may be different from the knowledge and skills available to health professionals. Such knowledge may have a basis in "folk medicine" rather than mainstream medicine. Usually, however, the self-care knowledge of the lay public is a less extensive or less current version of the technical information used by health care professionals. Finally, the WHO definition refers to lay and professional "participative collaboration." That is, it is presumed that professionals would see in self-care and in lay persons' values and perspectives something useful to the purposes of both diagnosis and therapy, as well as to the maintenance of optimum levels of health. Likewise, patients and their families will recognize the value of professional skills and experience in dealing with health and illness conditions.

Dimensions of Self-Care

The "Self-care Assessment of Community-Based Elderly Study" conducted at the University of North Carolina at Chapel Hill, with support from the National Institute on Aging (NIA), defined three general domains of self-care that flowed from the WHO definition. These domains were (1) healthy lifestyle practices that enhance health, reduce established health risk factors, or prevent disease; (2) medical self-care practices for diagnosing and treating commonly occurring acute conditions, and for seeking health information; and (3) self-care practices related to basic, mobility and instrumental activities of daily living, often in response to enduring and recurrent health problems (e.g., chronic conditions and psychosocial behavioral conditions). Although the first two domains, health lifestyle and medical self-care activities, are important for an overall view of self-care in healthy aging processes, the third domain of self-care for functional limitations and chronic conditions merits particular attention for some segments of the older population.

This chapter focuses on the third domain of self-care among older adults and the narrower range of purposive activities in which older persons compensate for declining physical, cognitive, or mental functioning, which can detract from their quality of life. This study conceptualized three dimensions of self-care in response to functional limitations and chronic conditions: (1) acquisitions and use of special *equipment* and *assistive technology*, such as a hearing aid or cane (Centers for Disease Control, 1992; DeWitt, 1991), to accomplish activities of daily living; (2) physical changes in one's living *environment*, such as installing grab bars in the bathroom, which enhance the opportunity for independent functioning or mobility; and (3) behavioral adjustments in everyday activities (e.g., avoiding stairs) to overcome or circumvent specific physical or cognitive impairments. Although the study sought information about activities intended to promote healthy lifestyles and medical self-care, this chapter gives primary emphasis to these three activity types representing the multidimensional assessment of self-care practice, each requiring quite different skills pertinent to distinct aspects of daily functional routines and focused on the achievement of qualitatively different goals.

Contexts of Self-Care

The increasing incidence of health and functional difficulties of older persons is not essentially a result of advancing age. Commonly observed declines in functional and health status do parallel advances in age, but the susceptibilities and frailties associated with aging are

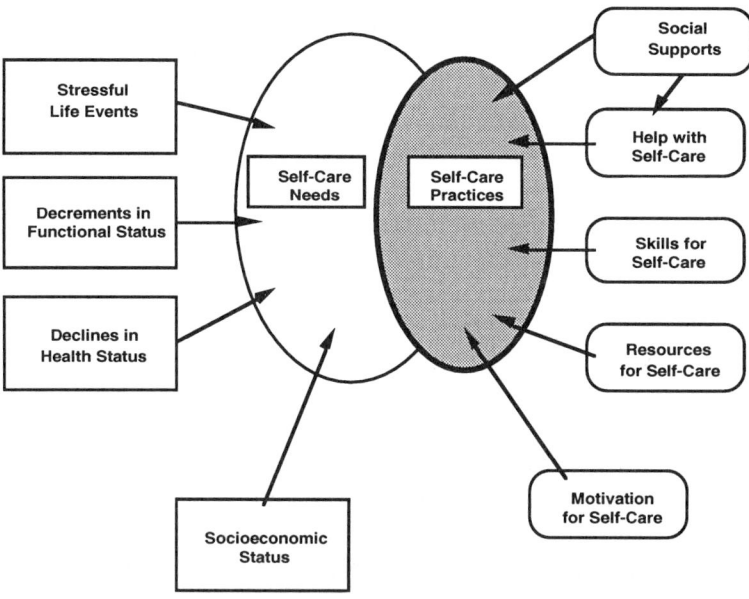

FIGURE 5.1 Self-care and its contexts.

mediated by other statuses of older people, such as gender, ethnicity, social class, and community of residence (particularly urban vs. rural environments). Advancing age is but one factor contributing to the need for adaptation among older people. Self-care, like other responses to conditions of health and illness, occurs in a sociocultural context in which opportunities are of varying availability and where personal decisions are made.

Our definition of self-care *behavior* is directed to activities individuals engage in for themselves and members of primary social groups, such as families or local neighborhoods; one facet of self-care refers to activities individuals and groups undertake in order to deal with the gap that may exist between personal levels of *susceptibility* and available sources and types of *support* (Konrad, Norburn, Woomert, Bernard, & DeFriese, 1991). A corollary of this focus is that the actions of health care professionals and of health care systems and formal organizations enter into the picture only by way of background, supplying a context within which self-care is performed by individuals and primary social groups.

Figure 5.1 portrays two aspects of self-care by discriminating between self-care requirements or needs and self-care practices or behavior. At the center of the diagram, these two aspects are represented by partially overlapping fields, which suggest that at any given time some self-care requirements are unmet, whereas other self-care behaviors are being performed, but not in response to specifically identifiable or immediately apparent care requirements.

A schematic representation of self-care and the contexts in which it occurs can be seen in Figure 5.1. On the left-hand side of the diagram various life contingencies are represented, some of which are associated with aging, which affect what kind of, and how much, self-care is required for an individual to function successfully. Such contingencies include declines in health status, decrements in functional status, and events that induce stress. In a similar fashion, on the right-hand side of the diagram other contextual factors are displayed that affect whether and how individuals respond to the challenges represented by self-care requirements. These behavioral changes are affected not only by the availability of external forces in a person's immediate social field, such as general levels of social support and specific help received from others, but also by internal resources such as motivation, skills, and knowledge mobilized to meet these challenges.

Effective and efficient self-care performance can be represented by maximal overlap of these two regions such that available personal resources are being employed to meet care requirements and the number of inappropriate or "surplus" activities (i.e., strategies employed for which no needs are evident) are at a minimum.

Deficient conditions are represented graphically by the combination of a large circle, reflecting care requirements, and a relatively small or ill-positioned circle, reflecting self-care activities. Such a combination suggests extensive self-care requirements in the face of strategies that are either of limited strength or magnitude, or inappropriately deployed by the individual.

Self-care, therefore, reflects a capacity and an intention to adapt to a wide spectrum of limiting influences on human social life of consequence to health status. Self-care behavior takes place in the context of attempts to maintain control of life and to do so with competence, autonomy, and self-reliance. It denotes a wider spectrum of behaviors than those merely aimed at "filling a gap" in one's ecology of social life; self-care includes the deliberate effort of lay persons to balance a variety of personal risks and resources in the achievement of specific goals and objectives in everyday experience. In the study of self-care *behavior*, and the *capacities* this behavior both requires and represents, our focus is on those activities through which individuals mobilize personal and social resources proactively to sustain and enhance the quality and length of their own and each others' lives (Konrad et al., 1991). The concept of self-care, the behaviors to which it refers, and the context in which it occurs, may represent an important practical response to the declinations in physical and cognitive functioning so often assumed to accompany the aging process. Beyond this fact, however, is the possibility that the promotion of self-care programs that emphasize a positive value on enhancing healthy lifestyle and vigilant and self-reliant responses to acute illness can add "life to years."

Figure 5.1 clearly oversimplifies the inherently complex reality of individual members of a heterogeneous and changing population of older persons. The need for self-care will vary a great deal among older adult populations, and individuals differ in the specific self-care skills exercised when the need arises. Further, over time, each individual is in a dynamic situation in which emerging challenges are met by countervailing responses. Although the trend for the population as it ages is one of decline, for any given individual at any particular stage no irreversible series of steps along this path is inevitable. In each individual the character and magnitude of need can expand or contract quite rapidly depending on the factors previously identified. Similarly, the magnitude and scope of resources applied can also expand or contract either in reaction to or in anticipation of a change in health and/or functional status. Finally, there is the possibility that more recent cohorts of older persons, shaped by different experiences and possessing different expectations from their predecessors, will move into the first decade of the twenty-first century in a new technological and normative environment. They may exhibit a strikingly different pattern of care needs and enact a different scale and scope of self-care capacities and behaviors than did people of similar ages in previous decades. These highly variable conditions affecting the quality of life in older persons during the late stages of life give rise to an almost unlimited range of policy scenarios—from the most optimistic to the most pessimistic. Hence, it is imperative that aging policy researchers search out whatever evidence is available to suggest the extent to which self-care may be useful in diminishing the need for health care and in enhancing functional health status and quality of life.

Importance of Self-Care to the Future Health Status of Older Populations

Recent gerio-demographic research (Lakata, 1985; Manton, Corder, & Stallard, 1993a) has begun to question the inevitable linkage of increasing age and decreasing functional capacity. Many previous studies suffered from design flaws that led to the observation of a direct link between advancing age and functional limitations in samples of older adults that represented the entire population of persons in these age categories. Because there is a tendency for the prevalence of chronic disease to increase with age, these studies masked the causal connection between the association of chronic disease with functional decrements. This explained the increasing prevalence of functional limitations as a result of increasing age, and not the result of the increasing prevalence of chronic illness among the populations studied. It is now becoming widely accepted that there are wide variations in the prevalence of chronic conditions among older adults and that there is likewise a high degree of variation in the prevalence (and duration) of functional limitations as well (Manton, Corder, & Stallard, 1993b). Rather than a long-term trajectory of decreasing functional capacity as aging occurs, individual patterns of aging and quality of life are highly variable and are often characterized by very rapid and short periods of functional decline prior to death (Manton, 1989). Chronic conditions do not lead to easily predictable patterns of behavior or functional capacity in all persons of advancing age; rather, the functional capacities of older adults may be altered through a variety of targeted interventions. Moreover, functional capacity among older adult populations is best evaluated on an individual rather than a collective basis.

Self-care, health maintenance, and lifestyle variations within these age groups assure the heterogeneity of functional status among the elderly population, even among the oldest age groups. Moreover, the heterogeneity of this age group is likely to include individuals with a wide range of educational and lifestyle characteristics who *age* into these older groups. The shifting pattern of gender roles, work roles, and the nature and extent of kinship and family care among widely dispersed families with complex patterns of divorce and remarriage only complicate the picture. Manton (1989) has pointed out that there is now evidence that, under some conditions, physiological processes may lead to reversal of functional declinations through regeneration of physiological capacities.

The demographic aging of the U.S. population is likely, no matter what interventions are introduced, to lead to large increases in the number of disabled elderly in this country over the next two or three decades. Manton (1989), using data from the National Long-Term Care Survey, identifies a number of ADL and IADL limitations that remain unmet for sizable numbers of older adults. The domains in which most improvements seem possible are those in which physical equipment and changes in the *built environment* are associated with specific functional limitations. In his discussion of problems remaining in this area of research, Manton points out that little data are available to assess the extent of unmet need for assistance to those with disabling conditions. Further, it is difficult to "characterize the dimensions of the problem, and to monitor the efficacy of different interventions." Data have not been collected "to identify major cohort differences or accurately assess whether active or healthy life expectancy has increased or decreased as life expectancy at later ages increases. This is a serious hindrance to the development of effective policies to meet the problems of a rapidly aging population" (Manton, 1989 p. 55).

There is controversy about whether declining rates of mortality among the elderly population has led, or will lead, to increasing years of dependency and inadequate health. The "compression of morbidity" thesis advanced by Fries (1983) presents the view that, as mortality has been compressed into the later years of the life cycle, morbidity has been compressed (or delayed) as well. Fries has argued that chronic, debilitating diseases will decrease in prevalence and their effects will be felt only at the very end of life. Analyses by Manton and his colleagues (1993a) based on three waves of the National Long-Term Care Survey demonstrate that increased survivorship in the older age groups has been accompanied by decreased rates of incidence for functional limitations. Absolute needs for long-term care are likely to increase because of increased survival of the oldest–old, the age group with the largest number of persons with disabilities. Although the decline in age-specific incidence of disability was real, over the 1980s it did not wholly compensate for the aging of the population, but it did have some impact. Manton estimated that the number of chronically disabled elderly persons in the population during the period 1982 to 1989 would have been 353,000 greater than it actually was if the rates of disability had not declined.

Verbrugge, Lepkowski, and Imanaka (1989:464) used data from the 1984 Supplement on Aging (SOA) to the National Health Interview Survey to examine the extent to which comorbidities among the elderly population affect social and physical disability. They raise the question of whether and to what extent the total number of accumulated diseases and impairments, or particular conditions and combinations of them, influence physical and social functioning. There is an important question here of whether certain diseases act independently, or synergistically, to propel disability. Their focus is on disability, not on disease. The items in the SOA used by Verbrugge and her colleagues deal with *difficulty* of activities of daily living (ADL) and instrumental activities of daily living (IADL) performance, not *dependence* among community-dwelling populations. This research followed from previous work by Verbrugge and Ascione (1987) in which it was found that acute and chronic conditions lead to quite different patterns of behavioral response. Whereas with acute health care conditions people tend to respond more immediately and in relation to specific symptoms, chronic conditions lead to the development of more organized *strategies* of response, which hinge on the availability of resources and the pattern of roles and attitudes characterizing an individual's illness response over a lifetime. These strategies are then employed when chronic symptoms are experienced.

The overall picture from the research by Verbrugge et al. (1989) is a profile of low levels of disability among the community-dwelling older adult population. Most older people (85%) have no difficulty in walking due to a health problem, but other types of mobility limitations and declines in strength are common. Almost half of the population 55 years of age and older have one or more functional limitations, and 17.3% have five or more limitations. The prevalence of chronic conditions tends to be the major determinant of disability in the older age groups. These tend to be conditions with either (1) high prevalence and low (or only moderate) impact on disability, or (2) low prevalence and high impact. As Verbrugge et al. (1989 p. 477) have explained:

> *(A)rthritis is the leading chronic condition for middle-aged and older persons, but it has modest impact compared to CVD, osteoporosis, and fracture of hip, all much less common. This disjunction between prevalence and impact means that the aggregate level of disability in the community-dwelling population has very diverse sources, to which the sheer frequency of some diseases and the high impact of others both contribute.*

One of the important features of the Verbrugge et al., paper is the recognition of the important "buffering" effect of self-care in modifying the potential transition from chronic condition to physical disability, or modifying the transition from *physical* disability to *social* disability. They conclude that:

> (h)ealth problems are the main driver of disability, and socio-demographic characteristics have only small additional effects. Initial age effects almost vanish when morbidity is controlled; thus, a person's age is not nearly so important in determining the level and extent of disability as what chronic problems she/he has. Women continue to have slightly higher disability levels than men, and nonwhites higher disability than whites, even when morbidity is controlled. (Verbrugge et al., 1989, p. 477)

Their research has begun to lay the groundwork for better understanding of what combinations of conditions among certain population groups pose the greatest risk and potential burden of care. Such findings have much to contribute to future aging policy, and may provide new information on the role of self-care in altering these seemingly inevitable outcomes. As the number of people with chronic conditions continues to rise (some with multiplicative effects), self-care will become even more important to program development for older adults.

New Research on Self-Care Among Elderly Populations

Over the past several years, the Cecil G. Sheps Center for Health Services Research of the University of North Carolina at Chapel Hill (UNC-CH) designed and implemented a new national survey of self-care practices among a national probability sample of persons over age 65. The study selected a nationally representative sample of older adults with equal numbers of participants in each of three age-gender categories: 65-74, 75-84, and 85 and older. In-person interviews, averaging just over an hour in length, were conducted with 3,485 community-dwelling persons (or their proxies) in 1990. Currently, the data from that survey are being analyzed.

The focus of this study goes a bit beyond the place where Manton, Verbrugge, and others have left off with respect to the potential role of social and demographic factors in the modification of age and disease factors in the determination of levels of disability and dependency among the nation's elderly population.

Analyses from the UNC-CH study data indicate that the activities of daily living for which specific functional limitations are pertinent are best conceptualized and measured according to a three-dimensional structure. The study, therefore, distinguishes among: basic activities of daily living (BADL), instrumental activities of daily living (IADL), and mobility activities of daily living (MADL).

The results show that older persons are far more likely to make behavioral modifications in their daily routines in order to compensate for functional limitations than they are to acquire and use special equipment and devices or to make changes in their built environments. More than 75% of older adults have made some form of behavioral adaptation with regard to basic or mobility activities of daily living during the year before the survey. This includes activities such as avoiding bending or stooping and doing things less often or more slowly (Norburn et al., 1993). About 42% of this national sample reported using special equipment, whereas almost one-third had altered their built environment.

It was found that the relationship between the severity of disability in these three dimensions and the probability of engaging in self-care practices is not linear. In general, the probability of engaging in self-care activities varies with levels of disability, as does the type of strategy employed. People with slight functional impairments tend to change their behavior whereas those with moderate levels of impairment rely more on special equipment.

Although older people with specific functional limitations are more likely to engage in self-care practices when compared with persons with no disability, data from the UNC-CH study indicate that a large proportion of older adults practice self-care *in the absence of disabilities*. It is unclear whether or not this represents an instance of "preclinical disability" (Fried, Herdman, Kinn, Rubin, & Turano, 1991), whereby older persons "anticipate" the problems associated with activity limitations as they grow older, and begin self-care strategies in advance of the actual experience of these problems.

Older adults who receive help from others are also more likely to engage in self-care practices. This suggests that practicing self-care and receiving help from another person with activities of daily living are not substitutes for one another; rather, they are supplementary. Although age, race, gender, education, and occupational prestige do not consistently relate to the likelihood of engaging in self-care among persons with at least some disability, those who live in rural areas, and those who live alone are more likely than urban dwellers or those living with another person to engage in some form of self-care behavior.

One of the most interesting findings thus far from the UNC-CH study concerns the extent to which older adults are engaged in the provision of assistance to others. A large proportion of older adults, even those with some self-reported ADL functional limitation, report that they regularly provide social support and assistance to another person (e.g., by helping with the performance of specific ADL activities (35.1%), providing child care (15.7%), doing volunteer work in community agencies (19.7%), and/or listening or providing advice to others (39.7%)). This raises an exciting set of issues related to the complementarity of social support among elders and its relationship to caregiver burden and the costs of health and social care for older adults. As Manton et al. (1993a) have pointed out, lower societal rates of informal care anticipated due to increased female labor force participation and smaller family size may be partly offset by increases in the proportion on nondisabled elderly persons. The help actually extended to other older adults by persons in these age categories may offset other costs associated with care and services needed by this population. Furthermore, volunteer work and child care provided by older adults may offset some health care costs associated with other nonelderly population groups.

Indications of the Responsiveness of Older Adults to Self-Care and Health Promotion Educational Program Interventions

Despite increasing evidence that individuals living in the community are never too old to benefit from health promotion and disease prevention programs (Berg and Cassels, 1990; Riley and Bond, 1983), problems in implementing such programs remain. Conventional wisdom holds that older adults are unpredictable, perhaps even unreliable, attenders of organized programs for imparting health information or changing lifestyles/behaviors. They may attend when the activity coincides with another activity (e.g., group meals) that they may already attend on a regular basis and in which they find some social enjoyment. Yet, they do not attend with regularity any activity that causes them undue perceived inconvenience or danger (e.g., walking in a "bad" neighborhood at night, crossing busy streets, or driving a car at night).

Recent research has found that older persons who participated in a health promotion program differed systematically both from those who declined participation in a health promotion program and from those who initially committed to participate but failed to follow through (Dodge, Clark, Janz, Liong, & Schork, 1993). Decliners generally reported that they did so out of lack of interest in the content of the program (even though their physicians believed that the program might be of some benefit to them). On the other hand, the noncompliers failed to attend scheduled group sessions for a variety of easily understandable reasons: self-reported physical limitations, transportation problems, and conflicting personal or social commitments. In another study it was found that specific practical steps, including the provision of free transportation, scheduling activities during "off-peak" daylight hours, and making use of other older persons in recruitment and staffing (Stevens et al., 1992), could stimulate participation. Assuming that effective self-care education programs can be designed and fielded, two challenges remain: (1) identifying those individuals objectively at risk of high self-care needs and/or low self-care responses, reaching them, and convincing them of the benefit of participating in such programs; and (2) implementing these programs in attractive and supportive barrier-free contexts, preferably staffed by personnel with whom older persons can readily identify. Credibly designed and effectively-marketed self-care education programs can foster the interest of older persons. But the actual implementation of these programs must anticipate and work around real and perceived barriers in order to sustain the ongoing participation of older persons over a relatively long period of time. Increased responsiveness of older adults to such programs seems to presuppose a more attractive program design.

Substitutability of self-care for formal health care is likely to occur. The older population, particularly those with significant functional limitations who live independently, have proven to be very inventive in their attempt to find ways of managing despite their limitations and in assisting their spouses and other older persons within the household in coping with similar challenges and impairments. The greatest worry of many older persons is that they might have to face the necessity of being dependent on anyone, particularly a formal health or social service provider.

The real problem faced in this area is in developing a precise measurement strategy for ascertaining the extent to which intentional actions occur in response to concrete symptoms and problems in everyday personal life. Substantial progress has been made in measuring, both in physical terms and through verbal questions in survey research, the presence or absence of physical limitations (even though much more work needs to be done). Despite the considerable progress in the development of measures of the self-care actions people take for themselves to deal with these limitations and the extent to which they are still dependent on the help they get from others, much work remains to further develop and refine such measures and research strategies appropriate for older adults (Ory, 1988).

Conclusions

There are several *unsolved problems* in this area of research and policy development. There is as yet no clear way of taking self-care into account in the allocation of health care resources to defined populations, such as older adults. Further, because self-care by its very nature functions outside of a commodity-based service economy, it is difficult to estimate the volume, the need, or the economic value of self-care. Nonetheless, the extent to which self-care has reduced the need for, or substituted for, informal caregiving or formal health care services has yet to be estimated. Finally, in addition to these policy questions, certain technical questions also remain. The primary one is the delineation of essential or necessary skills for adequate self-care and the appropriate processes of continuing/remedial education necessary to offset skill "decay" and obsolescence.

There is a considerable volume of needed research if self-care is to achieve its potential as a meaningful component of health care in this country:

- Valid and reliable measurement tools and research strategies relevant to self-care and health promotion in the older adult population must be developed and refined. Furthermore, these must take the heterogeneity of the older adult population into account.
- How and to what extent does substitution of self-care for informal and formal care occur? Is this a gradual process, or does it occur as a result of the sudden onset of a health or family crisis?
- To what extent does self-care extend and/or make more effective formal health care? Can self-care be better fostered through cer-

tain types of programs (e.g., Social health maintenance organizations, senior centers, etc.)?
- To what extent do those who engage in self-care practice extend their knowledge and experience in helping others?
- To what extent is self-care practice modified by the availability of social support?

Promising research that provides hope for improving quality of life for older adults will include:

- Studies, like the work by Stoller et al., (1993), in which health diaries were used to uncover ways in which self-care meshes with the broad spectrum of health and illness behavior, therefore enabling older adults to self-manage symptoms as they occur and thus to avoid the aspects of formal care use so disruptive of one's pattern and quality of life.
- Studies that investigate trends in self-care practices among older adults over time.
- Studies that investigate the skill demands of an expanded scope of self-care practice among older adults that might be met by formal or informal programs offering learning or skill-enhancement training for this population.

Self-care can be viewed as both a capacity for the performance of the essential activities of daily living and as a protection against the disability prevalent in old age. The challenge is to find appropriate and effective strategies, programs, and policies to facilitate health improvement and maximize health and functional independence of the older adult population in the United States. With further research and programmatic implementation, the next decade presages a coming of age for self-care, both as a practical strategy for individuals and families and as a vital adjunct for health and social policies aimed at preventing, delaying, and reversing the onset of declinations in health and functional status among older persons.

Aknowledgments

Research described in the paper was partially supported by a cooperative agreement No. AG-07929-03 with the National Institute on Aging of the NIH and the Division of Nursing of the Bureau of Health Professions, Health Resources and Services Administration.

References

Barofsky, I. (1978) Compliance, adherence and the therapeutic alliance: Steps in the development of self-care. *Social Science and Medicine*, 12, 369-376.

Berg, R. L., Cassells, J. S.(1990). *The second fifty years: Promoting health and preventing disability*. Washington, D.C.: National Academy Press.

Butler, R. N., Gertman, J.S., Oberlander, D. L., & Schindler, L. (1979), Self-care, self-help and the elderly. *International Journal of Aging and Human Development*, 10, 95-119. (1992, September 16).

Centers for Disease Control. *Advance data: Assistive technology devices and home accessibility features: Prevalence, payment, need and trends*. National Center for Health Statistics, U.S. Public Health Service. Number 217.

Dean, K. (1986). Lay care in illness. *Social Science and Medicine*, 22, 275-284.

DeFriese, G. H., Woomert A, & Guild, P. A., Steckler, A. B., Konrad, T. R. (1989). From activated patient to pacified activist: a study of the self-care movement in the United States. *Social Science and Medicine*, 29, 195-204.

DeWitt, J. C., (1991). The role of technology in removing barriers. *Milbank Quarterly*, 69, (Suppl. 1-2): 332.

Dodge, J. A., Clark, N. M., Janz, N. K., Liang, J. & Schork, MA. (1993). Nonparticipation of older adults in a heart disease self-management project: Factors influencing involvement. *Research on Aging*. 15, 220-237.

Fried, L. P., Herdman, S. J.H., Kuhn, K. E., Rubin, G., Turano, K. (1991). Preclinical disability: Hypotheses about the bottom of the iceberg. *Journal of Aging and Health*, 3, 285-300.

Fries, J. F., (1983). Aging, natural death, and the compression of morbidity. *New England Journal of Medicine*, 303, 130-135.

Haug, M. R., Akiyama, H. Tryban, G., Sonoda, K., & Sykle, M. (1988). Self-care: Japan and the U.S. compared. *Social Science and Medicine*, 33, 1011-1022.

Hickey, T. (1988). Self-care behavior of older adults. *Family and Community Health*, 11, 23-32.

Konrad, T. R., Norburn, .JK, Woomert, A., Bernard, S., & DeFriese, G. H. (1991). *Rural-urban differences and similarities in self-care performance among non-institutionalized elderly persons: Findings of a national survey*. Roundtable on Aging in Rural Environments, Gerontological Socicty of America, San Francisco, November 22, 1991.

Lakatta, E. G., (1985). *Health, disease, and cardiovascular aging. In America's aging: Health in an older society.* Institute of Medicine, National Research Council, National Academy of Sciences (pp. 73–104). Washington DC: National Academy Press.

Levin, L. S., (1976a). The layperson as the primary health care practitioner. *Public Health Reports, 91,* 206–210.

Levin, L. S., (1976b). Self-care: An international perspective. *Social Policy, 7,* 70–75.

Manton, K. G., (1989). Epidemiological, demographic, and social correlates of disability among the elderly. *Milbank Quarterly, 67 Suppl. 2,* 13–58.

Manton, K. G., Corder, L. S., & Stallard E. (1983a). Estimates of change in chronic disability and institutional incidence and prevalence rates in the US elderly population from the 1982, 1984, and 1989 National Long Term Care Survey. *Journal of Gerontology, 48,* S153–S166.

Manton, K.G., Corder, L.S, & Stallard E. (1993b). Changes in the use of personal assistance and special equipment from 1982 to 1989: Results from the 1982 and 1989 NLTCS. *The Gerontologist, 33,* 168–176.

Norburn, J. E, Bernard, S.L, Konrad, T. R., Woomert, A., DeFriese, & G. H., Kalsbeek, W. D., & Koch, G. G. (1993). *Self-care and assistance from others in coping with functional status limitations among a national sample of older adults.* Unpublished data. Cecil G. Sheps Center for Health Services Research, University of North Carolina at Chapel Hill.

Ory, M. G., (1988). Considerations in the development of age-sensitive indicators for assessing health promotion. *Health Promotion 3,* 139-150.

Riley, M. W., Bond, K. (1983). Beyond ageism: Postponing the onset of disability. In M. W. Riley, B. B. Hess, & K. Bond. (Eeds.), *Aging in society: Selected reviews of recent research.* (pp. 243-252). Hillsdale, NJ: Lawrence Erlbaum Associates,

Stevens, V. J., Hornbrook, M. C., Wingfield, D. J., Hollis, J. F, Greenlick, M. R., & Ory, M. G., (1992). Design and implementation of a falls prevention intervention for community-dwelling older persons. *Behavior, Health, and Aging,* 257–73.

Stoller, E. P., Forster, L. E., & Portugal, S. (1993). Self-care responses to symptoms by older persons: a health diary study of illness behavior. *Medical Care, 31,* 24–42.

Verbrugge, L. M., & Ascione, F. J. (1987). Exploring the iceberg: common symptoms and how people care for them. *Medical Care, 25,* 539–569.

Verbrugge, L. M., Lepkowski, J. M. & Imanaka, Y. (1989). Comorbidity and its impact on disability. *Milbank Quarterly, 67,* 450–484.

Vickery, D. M., Golaszewski, T. J., Wright, E. C., Kalmer, H. (1988). The effect of self-care interventions on the use of medical service within a Medicare population. *Medical Care, 26,* 580–588.

Wilkinson, I. F., Darby, D. N., Mant, A., (1987). Self-care and self-medication: an evaluation of individuals' health care decisions. *Medical Care, 25,* 965–978.

Woomert, A., Bond, B. A. McFarland, M. E., & Graham, R. M., (1982). *Self-care: an annotated bibliography.* Atlanta: Centers for Disease Control.

World Health Organization. (1983). Health education in self-care: possibilities and limitations. Report of a scientific consultation. Geneva: November, 21-25 1983.

PART III

Physical Health, Quality of Life, and Aging

Chapter 6
Rehabilitation in Old Age

T. Franklin Williams

Achieving and maintaining maximum functional independence and autonomy is clearly one of the essential and major components of a meaningful quality of life for anyone at any age. This is especially so for older people who are more likely to have disabling conditions that cause loss of independence. Equally important is the still-too-prevalent, erroneous perception held by people in general, and health professionals as well, that old age is a time of inevitable decline in function. This perception very often results in accomplishments that are less than optimal in restoring and maintaining maximum functional capabilities in older people.

Fortunately, the understanding and appreciation of a rehabilitative, restorative philosophy and goal as being at the heart of and fundamental to all geriatric health care is becoming more widely recognized and included in geriatric teaching and practice (Brummel-Smith, 1990; Williams, 1984, 1987, 1990). After addressing elements of knowledge and understanding of aging itself as well as rehabilitative potentials and approaches, this chapter will provide examples of how these principles have been and can be applied to enhance the quality of life in several of the common disabling conditions affecting older people. Additionally, issues will be identified calling for further research and development.

It is always important to keep in mind that the restoration and maintenance of maximum possible functioning and autonomy is a necessary, but not the only essential, component of quality of life. As discussed in other chapters in this volume and elsewhere (Pearlman & Uhlmann, 1991), quality of life also includes optimal mental functioning, emotional stability, satisfying and supportive social relations and environment, and a meaning to life that is characteristic and specific for each individual older person. All of these other factors interrelate and influence, and are influenced by, rehabilitative efforts and accomplishments. Thus, it may be well to refer to the component of quality of life being discussed in this chapter as "health-related quality of life" (Guyatt, Feeny, & Patrick, 1993).

Background: Functional Potentialities in Aging

Research advances in the past 10 years have provided a quite different understanding of the potentials for maintenance and restoration of function in old age and even very old age, in contrast to earlier views that aging was associated with inevitable declines in most functions. New understandings come from more carefully designed studies in which older human subjects have been carefully screened to permit measurements of function in those who are demonstrably free of disease conditions. Some of the most important observations have been made in longitudinal studies in which each subject is her or his own control. In such cases any changes or lack of changes are measured in the context of each individual rather than being potentially masked in cross-sectional averages.

The results indicate that critical organ functions such as maximum cardiac output, muscle strength and mass, brain metabolism and mental performance, and renal function may be maintained (or regained) in persons 80 or more years of age (Creary & Rapoport, 1985; Fiatarone, et al., 1990; Fleg et al., Lindeman, Tobin & Shock, 1985; Rodeheffer, et al., 1984; Schaie, 1989; Seals, Hagberg, Hurley, 1984), provided the individual has not acquired a chronic disabling disease. Sensible lifestyles are very important, including non-smoking (or stopping smoking), modest if any alcohol, adequate nutrition, and continuing physical and mental activity.

Indeed, there are only a relatively few changes with aging thus far identified that may be considered "intrinsic" changes (Williams, 1992), that is, changes that occur in virtually every person as the result

TABLE 6.1
Most Frequently Reported Chronic Conditions for People 65+.

Condition	Percentage reporting
Arthritis	48.3
Hypertension	38.1
Hearing impairment	28.7
Heart disease	27.9
Cataracts	15.7
Deformity of orthopedic impairment	15.5
Chronic sinusitis	15.3
Diabetes	8.3
Visual Impairment	8.2
Varicose veins	7.8

of common genetic inheritance. These include the genetically programmed onset of menopause in women, a decline in the mass and change in cell types in the immune system, an increase in cross-linking of proteins in supportive and connective tissues through the process of glycosylation with the result of general stiffening of these tissues, a decline in the supportive elements of the skin. In addition, any individual may have genetically determined predispositions to certain diseases or changes, which manifest themselves in the course of aging, such as adult–onset diabetes, Alzheimer's dementia, or increased risk of osteoporosis after menopause because of an individually determined smaller bone mass.

But the great preponderance of changes seen in the course of aging are better termed "extrinsic," in that they are the result of lifestyle choices and development of diseases and disabling conditions that vary considerably from person to person and may well be avoidable or modifiable. It is these extrinsic aging factors that present the opportunities and challenges for preventive and rehabilitative interventions to help assure a health-related quality of life in old age.

What are the most common significantly disabling chronic conditions appearing in older person? Table 6.1 summarizes the results of national survey data as reported by older individuals (National Center for Health Statistics, 1990). Arthritis is the most commonly reported problem, affecting almost 50% of older persons. This is followed in

TABLE 6.2
Principal Causes of Disability (Disabled Persons Ages 85 and Older)

Condition	Percentage
Dementia	19.43
Arthritis	16.75
Peripheral vascular disease	14.88
Cerebrovascular disease	12.86
Hip and other fractures	8.81
Ischemic heart disease	1.88
Hypertension	1.38
Diabetes	1.01
Cancer	0.91
Emphysema and bronchitis	0.26

frequency by hypertension; other common disabling conditions include impaired hearing and vision and orthopedic problems.

In the terminology recommended and generally accepted by the World Health Organization for impairments, disabilities, and handicaps, these chronic disabling conditions may become significant handicaps in many older persons and in particular in very old persons. National survey data, again, indicate that almost 40% of persons over the age of 85 are handicapped to the degree that they need some help from another person every day. This percentage is higher in women (45%) than in men (33%). The most commonly reported principal causes for such significant handicaps in very old persons are presented in Table 6.2 (Health Care Financing Administration, 1982).

Approaches to Rehabilitation in Older Persons

As already stated, the goal of rehabilitative efforts is to help a disabled and handicapped older person regain and maintain as much function and independence as possible. A fundamental principle in all of rehabilitative services, of particular importance for the geriatric population, is the need for a comprehensive and integrated approach, addressing medical, functional, and social aspects. This calls for contributions from a number of professional disciplines including medicine, nursing, social work, physical therapy, occupational therapy, psychology, and often other specialty areas working together in a truly interdisciplinary team approach to develop and implement a comprehensive individualized rehabilitative program. The disabled person and key family members or friends must be considered integral members of the team as well as the potential benefactors of the efforts. It is the disabled person, however, whose ultimate goals and desires for quality of life must be decisive.

Some Common Rehabilitative Challenges in Older Persons

Arthritis

As already noted, arthritic symptoms are the most common chronic complaint reported by older persons. Although there are a number of disease conditions that can lead to arthritis in older age, by far the most common is labeled osteoarthritis in the United States or osteoarthrosis in the United Kingdom. This condition affects typically joints that are most highly used and/or come under the most stress with long-term use, in particular the hips and knees, but also ankles and in some persons fingers and shoulders. Typically there is loss of and lack of replacement of the cartilage lining the joint surfaces, with eventual damage and changes in the bony surfaces of the joints. There may be some, or at times little or no, active inflammation but there is always pain, which is a major factor in limiting motion and use of the joints. There is a genetic predisposition to developing this condition in some persons, whereas others with similar lifestyles may have few or no problems. The symptoms, if not adequately treated, lead to a vicious cycle of less activity, which in turn results in loss of muscle strength through deconditioning and further decrease in level of regular activities.

After an adequate evaluation to establish the diagnosis, the key components of rehabilitative therapy consist of medications sufficient to control the pain and any inflammation that may be present, plus a well-defined, individualized program of physical therapy aimed at increasing muscle strength and maintaining joint flexibility. Nonsteroidal antiinflammatory drugs are usually effective in controlling any inflammation and contributing to relief of pain. It has recently been found that the analgesic drug acetaminophen, which has fewer side effects than the nonsteroidal drugs, may be just as effective in relieving the painful symptoms (Bradley, Brandt, Katz, Kalasinski, & Ryan, 1991). At times a time-limited course of corticosteroids (or injection into a joint) may be indicated. With corticosteroids or nonsteroidal drugs, caution needs to be taken to minimize the risk of gastrointestinal side effects, such as peptic ulceration.

Building strength in the muscles related to the function of an affected joint, such as a knee, is most important for stabilizing the joint and contributing to minimizing or avoiding pain with use, as well as improving functional ability. Typically, a daily program of muscle-building exercises is prescribed. The goal should be to see the affected older person regain and maintain the usual and desired level of functioning. The degree to which this is achieved would be the measure of health-related quality of life.

If pain and limitation of motion persist in an incapacitating degree despite the above efforts, joint replacement should be considered as a justifiable rehabilitative intervention.

Stroke

A thorough discussion of rehabilitation following a stroke is beyond the scope of this chapter; readers are referred elsewhere (Gibson & Caplan, 1984; Kelly, 1990). But certain principles, as well as aspects relating to quality of life may be summarized here.

In the first place, every person who suffers from the disabling effects of a stroke should be carefully evaluated by a multidisciplinary rehabilitative team. A comprehensive rehabilitation plan should be developed to address potential problems: complicating concomitant medical conditions such as hypertensive vascular disease; multiple organ systems affected by the stroke; significant depression present both as a direct central effect of the stroke itself plus the overall impact on the outlook of the affected person; and the social and economic implications for patient and family.

Immediately after a stroke, steps should be taken to minimize further loss of function as a result of confinement to bed and deconditioning of unaffected muscles and organ systems (Hayes & Carroll, 1986). The rehabilitation plan needs to be modified as progress in recovery is made.

Perhaps more than in almost any other condition calling for rehabilitation, the issue of motivation of the affected person is critical, and needs to be understood and addressed. As Kemp (1990) summarizes, motivation is determined by multiple factors: what a person wants to accomplish or regain (and the more focused this goal is, the better); what the person believes will happen (which depends on clear information about what is possible); what the rewards will likely be from a successful rehabilitative program; the costs of implementing the program in terms of investment of physical and emotional energy, plus the social and economic necessities. Older people may be willing to settle for less than might be possible in terms of restorative accomplishments, and may be more likely to accept the disability as inevitable and irreversible "at their age." Professionals may also undervalue the potential for restorative accomplishments.

Hip Fracture

Fractures of the hip become increasingly common with age, especially in Caucasian women who have thinner bones in general than do men, or women of other races. Unless gains are made in preventing hip fractures, by the age of 90, one in three Caucasian women are likely to be affected. Prevention is clearly the first goal, including measures to minimize loss of bone in later years as well as attention to risk factors for falls leading to injuries. The goal of a physically active lifestyle is also very important in the prevention of such problems as hip fractures. This would include adequate exercises of all types including weight-bearing exercises, in which comes into play in most specific rehabilitative programs which deconditioning is one of the abnormalities to be corrected. In terms of health-related quality of life, there really is no dividing line between most preventive and rehabilitative practices.

In older persons who have suffered hip fractures, the surgical repair of the fracture itself is a primary step in rehabilitation; the surgical details will not be discussed here. Of almost equal importance from the very first day after hip repair is the initiation of muscle-building exercises, which can be conducted reasonably vigorously in the unaffected extremities but can be initiated in a cautiously planned way in the leg that has been repaired. The older person should be out of bed and walking as soon as possible, with prosthetic assists such as walker or cane if indicated, but moving on to minimal use of such devices as soon as possible. The older person should be dressed in usual street clothes, eating at a table, visiting with family and friends, and in every way resuming all aspects of a normal life even while still in a hospital unit. A programmed increase in physical activity and exercise including performing all usual activity should be made a part of the specific rehabilitative plans. Recognition of appropriate treatment of any depression is important (Mossey, Mutran, Knott, & Craik, 1989).

"Deconditioning" is a potentially major hazard in many situations of chronic disability in older people in whom decreased physical activity is likely to occur or even be prescribed (Siebens, 1990), especially in the early days after an acute episode such as a hip fracture. The rapidity of loss of muscle strength and general physical function cannot be overemphasized: two days of vigorous physical activity is required to recover what is lost per day of bed rest. Studies including randomized clinical trials have also shown that involving older patients with hip fracture in a well-organized geriatric rehabilitative program immediately after the fracture, in a separate and special geriatric rehabilitation unit, produces more rapid recovery, more rapid discharge from hospital, less frequent admission to nursing homes, and a higher level of ultimate function than is typical for similar patients treated on a regular surgical unit after repair of fracture.

Again, the goal in rehabilitation for older persons suffering from hip fractures is return to their usual and preferred level of functioning, as a measure of health-related quality of life. In this situation, perhaps more than almost any other, the urgency of undertaking the rehabilitative efforts is perhaps most obvious.

Other Disabling Conditions

Other common disabling conditions in older people that should be discussed here include loss of hearing, loss of vision, and urinary incontinence. In each of these conditions, the basic principles of rehabilitation are the same although the specifics are obviously different. First, both the affected person, the family, and involved professionals should be helped to appreciate that such disabling conditions are not irreversible and that much improvement in function can usually be achieved. Second, the specific strategies for the problem at hand, including the most recent advances in rehabilitative steps for that problem, should be applied. And third, this effort needs to be undertaken in the context of the comprehensive medical, functional, and social characteristics and needs of each affected older person. Details of the rehabilitative strategies for these and other specific conditions can be found in a number of references (Kemp et al., 1990; Williams, 1984; Williams, 1990).

Adaptations of the Environment

Attention to environmental characteristics that may hinder or favor successful restoration of independent functioning is an essential element of every geriatric rehabilitative plan (Hiatt, 1990). The need for such attention is obvious when considering environmental risks for falls in the home or other settings frequented by older persons who are at risk for falling.

Another important aspect is the potential use of prosthetic devices and environmental modifications to assist a disabled person in being more functionally independent. This may involve addition of ramp access to homes or a mechanized chair on the stairway; it may also involve person-specific prosthetic devices to stabilize joints or assist in walking. In all such considerations, both the therapists and the affected older person must be very sensitive to the delicate line between providing help that increases independence and normal functioning and providing help that discourages more functional recovery and in fact leads to increased dependence.

Challenges for Further Research

As already indicated, much progress has been made in very recent years in understanding: (1) the characteristics of disabling conditions, (2) in appreciating the potentials for marked recovery of function with properly targeted regimens, and (3) in understanding and demonstrating how to accomplish the goals of maximum possible restoration of functioning and health-related quality of life through early interventions and sustained programs guided by multidisciplinary teams. But it is also clear that there is much more to learn. Given the high frequency of disabling conditions especially in very old people and the associated burdens and costs of care, it is most important that further research and demonstration efforts be vigorously pursued.

The needs for further research in geriatric rehabilitation were addressed as a major component of the work undertaken by the National Institutes of Health Task Force on Medical Rehabilitation Research, and the conclusions of that effort are presented in the report of that task force (Geriatrics, 1990). Challenges of high priority include:

- Further epidemiologic studies to obtain a better understanding of the interrelations between comorbidities in older persons as they

have an impact on loss of function and the potential for restorative accomplishments.
- Further research in identifying basic biomedical changes that increase the risks and hazards for injuries from such factors as falls, changes in bone density, and other risk factors that may be modified before loss of function occurs.
- Attention to identifying what may often appear to be "incongruent relationships" between the apparent functional capacity of older persons and their actual performance. In relation to this priority, more attention needs to be given to understanding the factors that enter into motivation and how these may best be addressed to achieve positive and sustained commitments.
- Much more research on issues of the role of differences in gender, race, nationality, educational level, and other cultural factors on both the likelihood of chronic disabilities and in the response to rehabilitative efforts needs to be undertaken. Such research will also necessarily address different and potential roles for informal as well as formal support in the rehabilitation program.
- Further research development and demonstration needs to be undertaken to determine the most effective ways to organize and deliver geriatric rehabilitative services—what settings, what teamwork approaches, what interrelations with other care providers and with families and social and health agencies, and what follow-up will best serve this population.

Acknowledgements

University of Rochester and Monroe Community HospitalRochester, New York.
The author wishes to acknowledge the expert assistance of Jeanne Soderberg.

References

Bradley, J.D., Brandt, K. D., Katz, B. P., Kalasinski, L. A., & Ryan, S. I. (1991). Comparison of an anti-inflammatory dose of ibuprofen, an analgesic dose of ibuprofen, and acetaminophen in the treatment of patients with osteoarthritis of the knee, *New England Journal of Medicine, 325*: 87–91.

Brummel-Smith, K. (1990). Introduction. In B. Kemp, et al., (Eds.), *Geriatric Rehabilitation*, (p. 3). Austin, TX: Pro-ed.

Creary, H., & Rapoport, S. I. (1985). The aging human brain. *Annals of Neurology*, *17*:2-10.

Fiatarone, M.A. Marks, E. C., Ryan, N. D., Meredith, C. N., Lipsitz, L. A. (1990). High-intensity strength training for nonagenarians, *Journal of the American Medical Association*, *263*:3029-3034.

Fleg, J.L. Gerstenblith, G., Zonderman, A. B., Boocker, L. C., Weisfeldt, M. L., Costa, P. T. (1990). Prevalence and prognostic significance of exercise-induced silent myocardial ischemia detected by thallium scintigraphy and electrocardiography in asymptomatic volunteers, *Circulation*, *81*:428-436.

Geriatrics. (June 28-29, 1990). Report of the Task Force on Medical Rehabilitation Research, (pp. 91-99). National Institutes of Health, Bethesda, MD, Administration Document.

Gibson, C.J., & Caplan, B.M. (1984). Rehabilitation of the patient with stroke. In T.F. Williams, (Ed.), *Rehabilitation in the Aging*, (pp. 145-160). New York: Raven Press.

Guyatt, G. H., Feeny, D. F., & Patrick, D. L. (1993). Measuring health-related quality of life. *Annals of Internal Medicine*, *118*:622-629.

Hayes, S.H. & Carroll, S.R. (1986). Early intervention care in the acute stroke patient. *Archives of Physical Medicine and Rehabilitation*, *67*:319.

Health Care Financing Administration (1982). Long Term Care Survey, presented by K.G. Manton at Annual Meeting of American Public Health Association. Washington, DC, 1985.

Hiatt, L.G. (1990). Environmental factors in rehabilitation of disabled elderly people. In S.J. Brody & L.G. Pawlson, (Eds)., *Aging and Rehabilitation II: The State of the Practice*, (pp. 154-164) New York: Springer Publishing.

Kelly, J.K. (1990). Stroke rehabilitation for elderly patients. In B. Kemp, et al., (Eds.). *Geriatric Rehabilitation*, (pp. 61-90) Austin, TX: Pro-ed.

Kemp, B. (1990). Motivational dynamics in geriatric rehabilitation: Toward a therapeutic model. In B. Kemp, K. Brummel-Smith, and J. W. Ramsdell, (Eds.), *Geriatric Rehabilitation*, (pp. 295-306). Austin, TX: Pro-ed.

Lindeman, R.D., Tobin, J., & Shock, N. (1985). Longitudinal studies on the rate of decline in renal function with age. *Journal of the American Geriatrics Society*, *33*:278-285.

Mossey, J.M. Murtan, E., Knott, K., and Crack, R. (1989). Determinants of 12 months after hip fracture: The importance of psychosocial factors, *American Journal of Public Health*, *79*:279-286.

National Center for Health Statistics. (1990). Current estimates from the National Health Interview Survey, 1989. *Vital and Health Statistics*, *10*, (176). Washington, DC; US Government Printing Office.

Pearlman, R.A. & Uhlmann, R.F. (1991). Quality of life in elderly, chronically ill outpatients. *Journal of Gerontology: Medical Sciences, 46* :M31–38.

Rodeheffer, R.J., Gerstenblith, G., Becker, L. C., Fleg, J. L., Weisfeldt, M. L. and Lakatta, E. G. (1984). Exercise cardiac output is maintained with advancing age in healthy human subjects: Cardiac dilatation and increased stroke volume compensate for a diminished heart rate. *Circulation, 69*:203–213.

Schaie, K.W. (1989). Perceptual speed in adulthood: Cross-sectional and longitudinal studies. *Psychology and Aging, 4*:443–453.

Seals, D.R., Hagberg, J. M., Hurley, B. F., Ehrani, A. A., and Hollozy, J. O. (1984). Effects of endurance training on glucose tolerance and plasma lipids levels in older men and women. *Journal of the American Medical Association, 252*:645–649.

Siebens, H. (1990). Deconditioning. In B. Kemp et al., (Eds.), *Geriatric Rehabilitation*, (pp. 177–192) Austin, TX: Pro-ed.

Williams, T.F. (1984). Introduction. In T.F. Williams, (Ed.), *Rehabilitation in the Aging*, (p. xiii) New York: Raven Press.

Williams, T.F. (1987). The future of aging. *Archives of Physical Medicine and Rehabilitation, 68*:335–338.

Williams, T.F. (1990). Introduction to rehabilitation and aging. In S. J. Brody & L. G. Pawlson. *(Eds.) Aging and Rehabilitation II: The State of the Practice*, (pp. 3–8) New York: Springer Publishing Co.

Williams, T.F. (1992). Aging versus disease: Which changes seen with age are the result of "biological aging"? *Generations: Journal of the American Society on Aging, 16* :21–26.

Chapter 7
Psychosocial Status in Cancer Patients

Barrie R. Cassileth

Cancer in the Elderly

Age is the major risk factor for cancer, with more than half of all cancers and 60% of all cancer deaths occurring in 12% of the population: people over age 65 (Kant et al., 1992., Kennedy, 1992). The risk of developing cancer doubles every five years after age 25 (Crawford and Cohen, 1987). Given the anticipated rise in the numbers of older people in the United States, the incidence of cancer can be expected to increase accordingly.

Thus, a discussion of cancer in a text about aging and quality of life is indeed appropriate. Psychosocial issues, of paramount importance to both aging and cancer, are especially so in geriatric oncology.

Deaths from coronary heart disease continue to drop as a result of improved diet, generally healthier lifestyle, and new drugs and treatment strategies. Thus, increasing numbers of people avoid or survive heart disease, leaving them vulnerable to degenerative diseases such as Alzheimer's disease and cancer (Kennedy, 1992). By this route as well, the incidence of cancer in the elderly will rise substantially in the next few decades, because most older people will be confronted by malignant disease.

Detection and Treatment of Cancer in the Elderly

Survival rates for almost all cancers are lower among older versus younger patients (Goodwin & Samet, 1992., Kant et al., 1992). Decreased survival could be attributable to underutilization of screening and early detection, suboptimal treatment, or physiologic conditions that accompany aging, such as decreased immune competence, decline in organ function, tumor behavior, or comorbidity.

The literature argues in both directions on each point, but there is a general consensus that broader use of screening should be encouraged (a special edition of the *Journal of Gerontology* [1992] reviews obstacles to wider screening) and, most important, that cancer treatment for the elderly should be much more aggressive.

Cost, the major obstacle, was removed only in the last few years when Medicare and private insurers began to provide coverage for mammography. Additional obstacles include the patient's wish to avoid the pain or discomfort of breast compression associated with mammography, fears of breast cancer treatment, which are especially evident among older women, inadequate physician prompting, difficulty reaching mammography centers at substantial distances from home, and so on.

The standard treatments for cancer include surgery, chemotherapy, and radiation therapy. Older age is associated with no treatment or less aggressive therapy, primarily, it is assumed, because clinicians fear that elderly patients cannot withstand the rigors of full-regimen therapy. Similarly, patients over 65 years of age are rarely included in cooperative group clinical trials, despite National Cancer Institute policy encouraging their participation (Kennedy, 1992). Age differences in the receipt of chemotherapy and radiation therapy persist even when comorbidity is controlled (Greenfield et al., 1987; Wetle, 1987).

Although the hazards of hospitalization for the elderly are well documented (e.g., Creditor, 1993), research data support policy and confirm that advanced age does not contraindicate appropriately aggressive treatment. A study of surgical response in patients aged 90 and older, for example, showed excellent outcome (Hosking et al., 1989). In another analysis of 19 studies collectively involving 780 patients with advanced cancer, all over age 69, comparative survival and response to chemotherapy were evaluated. Older and younger patients did not differ in response rates or survival (Begg & Carbone, 1986).

Perceived Meaning: The Basis of Psychosocial Response

In cancer medicine, psychosocial problems and age are connected. As age bias can influence therapy and thus survival itself in the elderly patient with cancer, so cancer and its treatments can generate psychosocial difficulties for the elderly. The meaning that is perceived and attributed to events and characteristics typically is more real and more important for the individual than is objective reality. Meaning determines understanding and implications, as well as emotional response and behavior, including whether one views treatment as reasonable and worthwhile.

Aging and cancer are two concepts that admit to multiple perceptions and meanings. In each case, the meaning held by an individual can deviate profoundly from generally agreed on public or scientific views. The meaning of "elderly" and of "cancer" can differ substantially across individuals and from one point in time to another. Attributed meaning can be a function primarily of one's idiosyncratic experience or beliefs. It can also be a matter of consensus in one's social group. Age, in particular, is a relative concept.

The Meaning of Age

At the turn of the current century, when average life expectancy was 49, people in their early and mid-forties were "elderly." Going back in time, differences between the meaning of various age groups then versus now become increasingly striking. Two thousand years ago, a 22-year-old was an "older" person, because the average life span at that time was 22 years (Kennedy, 1992). Today, age 22 connotes someone barely out of adolescence; a "young adult." A 45-year-old was a marvel of longevity during the middle ages, when the average person lived for 33 years, but that age today carries no shred of the sense of "elderly."

Along with the objectively increasing life span of Americans and the concomitant changes in accepted notions of youth, middle and old age, a new term, "down-aging," has entered the popular vocabulary. This term nicely captures the fact that, as people live longer, succeeding adult decades become associated with increasing youthfulness. "Down-aging," then, captures the changing meaning of age categories: someone aged 70 "is really" (that is, looks, acts, and feels) around 60; a 51-year old functions, feels, and appears like someone aged 40. The new phrase has linguistically captured and made more concrete the fact that chronologic age, along with the definition or meaning of "youth," "elderly," and so on, changes and will continue to change as time goes on both for society and for the individual.

The Meaning of Cancer

Similarly, the meaning attached to the word "cancer" is relative to one's experience and to the status of the disease. The status of the disease, in turn, relates not only to its treatability, potential for cure and symbolic connotations as a debilitating illness, but also to its relative meaning in the context of other dreaded illnesses and threats to life.

For centuries, "cancer" was synonymous not only with inevitable death, but also with prolonged misery, shame, and contagion. Similar to leprosy in terms of public reaction and social meaning, cancer was believed incurable, and facilities were constructed to house patients to keep them away from others to limit spread of the disease (Cassileth, 1983).

The stigma surrounding a diagnosis of cancer persisted well into the current century, taking the form of secrecy, euphemisms, and deception. Not until the late 1920s could cancer be discussed in books and magazines for the public. Not until the 1970s was a diagnosis of cancer routinely revealed (Cassileth, 1983). Prior to that time, few patients survived malignant disease. The greater openness and willingness to tell patients when cancer was diagnosed reflected the development of combination chemotherapy and multi-modality treatment, advances that greatly enhanced medicine's ability to manage cancer successfully. Prolonged remissions and cures became increasingly common.

These therapeutic advances, along with the start of open communication in cancer medicine that began not until the late 1970s, are consistent with a synchronous change in Federal policy. The shift from secrecy and timidity to aggressive attack was formalized when the United States officially declared war on cancer in 1970.

Older patients grew up before these positive changes were well entrenched. They learned about cancer during the time when people whispered the word; when we shrank away from this disease in fear and shame and searched our souls to uncover the sin that had merited so severe a punishment.

The meaning of cancer is shaped also by events external to the disease itself; by where cancer fits in the larger scheme of human ills. In a chronicle of personal experience with Alzheimer's disease, the diagnosing physician says, "I wish I could tell you it was cancer" (Davis, 1989). The implication of that statement is that some problems today are perceived to be worse than cancer. Aquired immune deficiency syndrome (AIDS) also fits in that category. In addition to the fact that it is not now curable, AIDS has replaced cancer as the reigning metaphor for the evil that disease can represent. Thus, from both medical and symbolic perspectives, cancer no longer carries the universally devastating meaning that it held previously. The increased possibility of successful cancer treatment, the terrifying and incurable nature of Alzheimer's disease and AIDS, and the fatal impact of these diseases on quality of life, and the shift of stigma from cancer to AIDS all contribute to today's reformulated meaning of cancer.

Communicating with the Elderly Patient with Cancer

Despite these major changes, remnants of cancer's symbolic and medical legacies remain in the memories of many older patients, mitigated to varying degrees by the changes that have since occurred, but often meriting attention. Adequate communication between physician and elderly cancer patient requires sensitivity to the possibly unique and harmful ideas that some older individuals continue to hold about malignant diseases.

People who secretly harbor the notion that they are being punished for past misdeeds, for example, need to be disabused of this notion. The only way to know is to ask: "What does this illness mean to you?"

Family members who want to protect patients from the reality of their diagnosis, or patients who do not want their spouses to know, similarly are reacting to cancer's past stigma. That once-common problem can be avoided by requesting that the spouse or other close family member attend the initial discussion of diagnosis and treatment. Regardless of the patient's age, the diagnosis and treatment plan always should be presented simultaneously. That is, the diagnosis should be discussed in the context of a treatment plan. This enables the patient and family member to think about treatment goals, rather than to be left dwelling only on the abstract and frightening news of a cancer diagnosis.

Beyond the necessary diagnosis and treatment plan, how much information do older patients want? Even in 1979, studies had documented cancer patients' preferences for maximum information and for the opportunity to participate in decisions about their care (Cassileth, Zupkis, Sutton-Smith, & March, 1980). Although data indicate an inverse relationship between age and amount of information preferred, the majority of older as well as younger patients indicated preferences for full communication and participation.

Interest in receiving as much information as possible about one's cancer and its treatment has intensified over time. This is a result of cancer's decreased stigma, of consumer education and activism in health care generally and cancer specifically, and the pervasive openness about cancer evident in frequent magazine articles. It stems also from frank discussion by public figures of their cancer diagnoses. The signs saying "cancer center" or "oncology program" over the doors through which patients pass on their way to appointments with their physicians also discourage euphemisms and efforts to avoid information.

The Fallacy of Homogeneity

Having cancer does not make people alike, especially from a psychosocial perspective. Similarly, older people are not necessarily like one another by virtue of shared chronologic age. Individuals and family members bring to age and to cancer a history of beliefs about illness and about the health care system, fate, and "appropriate" response to life's difficulties. From a clinical perspective, these realities translate to a time-honored tenet of medicine: That each patient requires individualized interaction, based on our best understanding of that person's unique preferences, problems, and needs. Across the span of individual differences, some problems and characteristics emerge as more common among older than younger patients with malignant diseases.

Social Resources and Functional Status

Life stages in our culture are associated with particular demands. The elderly are less likely than others to have pressing jobs and family responsibilities. Many elderly people, however, are the main caregivers of frail or ill spouses or even older parents or other relatives. For better or worse, the elderly generally are exempted by our society from demands that are implicit for younger people: The requirement that they function as productive, contributing members of the community. When illness appears, the elderly patient's time and energies are less torn than they are for younger patients between the demands of illness and treatment and those of caring for children, car pooling, maintaining jobs outside the home, and managing an often large household of spouse, children, and possibly an elderly parent.

The relative absence of these responsibilities is evident in the results of a study of 799 older people with newly diagnosed cancers, all of whom lived in New Mexico. Twenty-six percent of patients lived alone, and 39% had no children living in the area (Goodwin, Hunt, and Samet, 1991). These authors point to the problematic aspects of reduced job and family responsibilities, suggesting that absence of social support, which can have many negative social ramifications, also helps explain the undertreatment of elderly cancer patients.

Further, older patients are more likely to have multiple health problems or chronic illnesses with which they must contend, even as they grapple with cancer and its treatments. Imperfect health and reduced functional status may decrease independence among the elderly (Foreman & Kleinpell, 1990). Reduced independence may be more dramatic and more problematic for older people, especially if they lack the social resources and assistance needed to care for themselves and provide transportation to and from doctors' visits.

A large literature in oncology details the physical and physiologic deficits that follow cancer treatment. This literature addresses the reduced functioning specific to particular cancer diagnoses, and includes the study of various approaches to rehabilitation. The companion literature in surgical oncology describes new operative techniques aimed at minimizing the functional limitations that result from cancer surgery.

Range of motion limitations, for example, were a routine focus of rehabilitation during the decades when breast cancer surgery routinely involved radical mastectomy, including the removal of muscle mass. Today, less destructive surgical techniques along with well-studied exercises improve the speed and scope of recovered mobility. Older age, given physiologic realities, is associated with slower recovery (Vinokur, Threatt, Vinokur-Kaplan, & Satariano, 1990). Satariano Raaheb, Branch, and Swanson (1990) found that older women, following breast cancer treatment, had more difficulty completing tasks that involved upper-body strength than did same-age women who did not have breast cancer.

Psychosocial Status and Quality of Life

Studies consistently document a positive relationship between advancing age and better mental health or psychosocial status among patients with cancer. These effects are not necessarily sustained, and in fact they may be reversed, among older people in general. There is a striking psychological difference between the elderly as a group and elderly patients with cancer.

In an investigation of the psychosocial status of 758 patients with one of six different chronic illnesses, cancer among them, age offered a diagnosis-independent advantage. Better mental health was found with advancing age in each group of patients studied (Cassileth et al., 1984, 1985, 1986; Cassileth, Lusk, Brown, & Cross, 1992).

Psychosocial status is a major component of quality of life, but it is only one of several factors that comprise this construct in patients with cancer. Remaining factors include physical and occupational function; social interaction, which reflects the patient's capacity for interactions with family and others; and somatic sensation, which includes physical discomforts such as nausea and pain (Schipper, Clinch, McMurray, & Leavitt, 1984; Schipper, Clinch, & Powell, 1990). Quality of life among patients with cancer has been studied extensively, with primary emphasis placed on developing optimal measurements for application in cancer clinical trials (Cassileth, 1992).

There is general consensus concerning basic guidelines for quality of life among patients with cancer (Schipper et al; 1984; Slevin, Plant, Lynch, Frinkwater, & Gregory, 1988; Ware, 1987; Wartman, Morelock, Malitz, & Palm, 1983). Agreement reflects the essential subjective nature of quality of life, plus the understanding that quality of life must be evaluated over time, that it is multifactorial, and it must be illness-sensitive.

The subjective nature of quality of life is arguably its most crucial aspect. Only the individual can evaluate the quality of his own existence. That self-evident tenet is documented by the fact that proxy ratings produced by patients' family members, physicians, and other medical staff lack agreement with patient report (National Cancer Institute, 1990; Pearlman & Uhlmann, 1988. Schipper et al., 1984.

For decades, cancer medicine has utilized a measure of performance status, wherein the physician or other health professional rates the patient on a scale from 100% bedridden to 100% ambulatory and symptom free (Karnofsky & Burchenall, 1949). Performance status is all but universally applied in clinical oncology, because it permits quick, repeated, objective assessment of an important and readily quantifiable aspect of the patient's condition. Performance status also correlates well with survival, thus providing a predictive measure with substantial clinical utility. As noted above, performance status, or physical functioning, is one of the main factors shown to comprise quality of life.

Routine application of the performance status measure retarded acceptance of patient-assessed quality of life. Clinicians often perceived this important component as tantamount to quality of life per se. Further, the subjective nature of quality of life is not necessarily consistent with medicine's emphasis on objectively measurable indices of disease and well-being. It is only in recent years that patient-measured quality of life began to gain acceptance in cancer medicine as a viable, meaningful measure, inherently useful in addition to the evaluation of performance status.

Few studies have specifically examined quality of life among patients with cancer by age. Ganz, Lee, Sim, Polinsky, and Schag, (1992) report an investigation of 229 women with newly diagnosed breast cancer. The positive relationship observed between age and quality of life was most pronounced among married women and those who received segmental mastectomies. These results appear to highlight the contribution of social and physical factors to patient-perceived quality of life. They are also consistent with the larger literature documenting the previously noted direct correlation between age and psychosocial status or general well-being among older patients with cancer.

The interaction of age and chronic illness, the striking trend toward better psychosocial status and quality of life with advancing age among patients with cancer, despite the ravages of this disease and its treatment, represent intriguing issues that merit exploration.

Speculation concerning the reason for these positive results (Cassileth et al., 1984) includes the possibility that chronic illness, ironically, may offer social advantages that are less available to the healthy elderly, such as being surrounded by increased activity, interpersonal involvement, and concerned attention. The experience of years may confer on older patients more finely honed skills with which to manage life's stresses. Elderly patients as a group may have developed a perspective or a set of expectations that is more commensurate with adaptation to illness than is the case for younger patients. The biological advantage that confers longevity and cancer survival may simultaneously provide enhanced ability to cope adaptively with life stress. The apparent advantage that accompanies age among cancer patients raises questions that span basic science as well as social science areas of inquiry.

REFERENCES

Begg, C.B., & Carbone, P.P. (1986). Clinical trials and drug toxicity in the elderly. *Cancer*, 52, 1986–1992.

Cassileth, B.R. (1983). The evolution of oncology. *Perspectives in Biology and Medicine*, 26, 362–374.

Cassileth, B.R. (1992). Principles of quality of life assessment in cancer chemotherapy. *PharmacoEconomics*, 2, 279–284.

Cassileth, B.R., Lusk, E.J., Strouse, T.B., Miller, D.S., Brown L.L., & Cross, P.A. (1985). A psychological analysis of cancer patients and their next-of-kin. *Cancer*, 55, 72–76.

Cassileth, B.R., Lusk, E.J., Strouse, T.B., Miller, D.S., Brown L.L., Cross, P.A., & Tenaglia, A.N. (1984). Psychosocial status in chronic illness: A comparative analysis of six diagnostic groups. *New England Journal of Medicine*, 311, 506–511.

Cassileth, B.R., Lusk, E.J., Brown L.L., & Cross, P.A. (1986). Psychosocial status of cancer patients and next-of-kin: Normative data from the profile of mood states. *Journal of Psychosocial Oncology*, 3, 99–105.

Cassileth, B.R., Zupkis, R.V., Sutton-Smith, K., & March, V. (1980). Information and participation preferences among cancer patients. *Annals of Internal Medicine*, 92, 832–836.

Crawford, J., & Cohen, H.J. (1987). Relationship of cancer and aging. *Clinical Geriatric Medicine*, 3, 419–431.

Creditor, M. C. (1993). Hazards of hospitalization of the elderly. *Annals of Internal Medicine*. 118, 219-223.

Davis, R. (1989). *My journey into Alzheimer's disease.* Wheaton, IL: Tyndale House.

Foreman, M.D., & Kleinpell, R. (1990). Assessing the quality of life of elderly persons. *Seminars in Oncology Nursing*, 6, 292–297.

Ganz, P.A., Lee, J.J., Sim, M.S., Polinsky, M.L., & Schag, C.A. (1992). Exploring the influence of multiple variables on the relationship of age to quality of life in women with breast cancer. *Journal of Clinical Epidemiology, 45*, 473–485.

Goodwin, J.S., Hunt, W.C., & Samet, J.M. (1991). A population-based study of functional status and social support networks of elderly patients newly diagnosed with cancer. *Archives of Internal Medicine*, 151, 366–370.

Goodwin, J.S., & Samet, J.M. (1992). Factors affecting the diagnosis and treatment of older patients with cancer. In L. Balducci, G.H. Lyman, & W.B. Ershler (Eds.), *Geriatric oncology* (pp. 42–50). Philadelphia: J.B. Lippincott Company.

Costanza, M.E. (Guest Editor). (1992). Breast cancer screening in older women. *Journal of Gerontology, 47* (Suppl.)

Greenfield S., Blanco D.M., Elashoff, R.M., & Ganz, P.A. (1987). Patterns of care related to age of breast cancer patients. *Journal of the American Medical Association, 257,* 2766–2770.

Hosking, M.P., Warner, M.A., Lobdell, C.M., Offord, K.P., & Melton, L.J. (1989). Outcomes of surgery in patients 90 years of age and older. *Journal of the American Medical Association, 261,* 1909–1915.

Kant, A.K., Glover, C., Horm, J., Schatzkin A., & Harris, T.B. (1992). Does cancer survival differ for older patients? *Cancer, 70,* 2734–2740.

Karnofsky, D.A., & Burchenall, J.H. (1949). Clinical evaluation of chemotherapeutic agents. In C.M. MacLeod (Ed.), *Evaluation of chemotherapeutic agents in cancer* (pp. 191–205). New York: Columbia University Press.

Kennedy, B.J. (1992). Aging and cancer. In L. Balducci, G.H. Lyman, & W.B. Ershler (Eds.), *Geriatric oncology* (pp. 3–7). Philadelphia: J.B. Lippincott Company.

National Cancer Institute. (1990). *Quality of life assessment in cancer clinical trials*. Bethesda: United States Department of Health and Human Services.

Pearlman, R.A., & Uhlmann, R.F. (1988). Quality of life in chronic diseases: perceptions of elderly patients. *Journal of Gerontology, 43,* M25–30.

Satariano, W.A., Ragheb, N.E., Branch, L.G., & Swanson, G.M. (1990). Difficulties in physical functioning reported by middle aged and elderly women with breast cancer: A case-control comparison. *Journal of Gerontology, 45,* M3–11.

Schipper, H., Clinch, J., McMurray, A., & Levitt, M. (1984). Measuring the quality of life of cancer patients: The functional living index-cancer. *Journal of Clinical Oncology, 2,* 472–483.

Schipper, H., Clinch, J., & Powell, V. (1990). Definitions and conceptual issues. In B. Spilker (Ed.), *Quality of life assessment in clinical trials* (pp. 11–24). New York: Raven Press.

Slevin, M.L., Plant, H., Lynch, D., Frinkwater, J., & Gregory, W.M. (1988).

Who should measure quality of life, the doctor or the patient? *British Journal of Cancer, 57,* 109–112.

Vinokur, A.D., Threatt, B.A., Vinokur-Kaplan, D., & Satariano, W.A. (1990). The process of recovery from breast cancer for younger and older patients. *Cancer, 65,* 1242–1254.

Ware, J.E. (1987). Standards for validating health measures: Definitions and content. *Journal of Chronic Diseases, 40,* 473–480.

Wartman, S.A., Morlock, L.L., Malitz, F.E., & Palm, E. (1983). Impact of divergent evaluations by physicians and patients of patients' complaints. *Public Health Reports, 98,* 141–145.

Wetle, T. (1987). Age as a risk factor for inadequate treatment. *Journal of the American Medical Association, 258,* 516.

Chapter 8

Biopsychosocial Risks for Cardiovascular Disease in Spouse Caregivers of Persons with Alzheimer's Disease

Peter P. Vitaliano, Cynthia M. Dougherty, and Ilene C. Siegler

The recognition and diagnosis of Alzheimer's disease has increased dramatically in the past decade, with three to four million older Americans estimated now to suffer from this progressive, debilitating disease (Advisory Panel on Alzheimer's Disease, 1991; Anthony & Aboraya, 1992). AD is an important caregiving condition because of the special demands it places on family members. In the past decade more attention has been given to the daily stressors of older spouse caregivers of persons with AD. These include meeting daily physical and emotional demands as well as financial burdens encumbered by caring for a person with AD. To compound matters, caregivers lose the companionship and support of their spouse with AD. These experiences, coupled with prolonged distress and biobehavioral vulnerabilities, may make some spouse caregivers at risk for cardiovascular disease (CVD). Although correlations between cardiovascular variables and biopsychosocial factors have been examined in the general population, they have not been studied in caregivers. As such, this chapter describes a new line of research, namely the study of biopsychosocial factors as risks for and outcomes of CVD in older spouse caregivers.

Cardiovascular disease is the focus of this chapter because it is the leading cause of death worldwide in individuals over age 65 (American Heart Association, 1991) and it is related to psychosocial variables (Chesney & Rosenman, 1985). Spouse caregivers are important because: (1) their stress is chronic, generally without respite, and of rather long duration (≤ 15 years); (2) the population of older caregivers is of growing importance as the life expectancy of the general population increases; and, (3) caregivers are an identifiable population whose risks for distress may be reduced through intervention.

An explanatory model of stress sequelae (Vitaliano, Russo, Young, Teri, & Maiuro, 1991) proposes that:

$$\frac{\text{Biobehavioral Distress}}{} = \frac{\text{Exposure to Stressors} + \text{Vulnerability}}{\text{Psychological Resources and Social Resources}}.$$

When this model was applied to the study of burden in AD caregivers, it was shown that caregivers with high vulnerability (e.g., anger style, physical illness) and low resources (e.g., social supports, coping) had significantly higher burden scores 18 months after entering the study than did those with either low vulnerability or high vulnerability and high resources.

Here a path model is used to summarize literatures that bear on questions of interest (See Figure 8.1). The model refines the one presented above and includes feedback loops between the components, hence the arrows are bidirectional. Although the components are relevant to populations other than older caregivers, variables such as age (vulnerability) and caregiving (a prototypical stressor) may have synergystic effects so that the risks of CVD and impaired quality of life may become exacerbated in older adult caregivers. That is, aging may be correlated with mental and physical health problems, caregiving

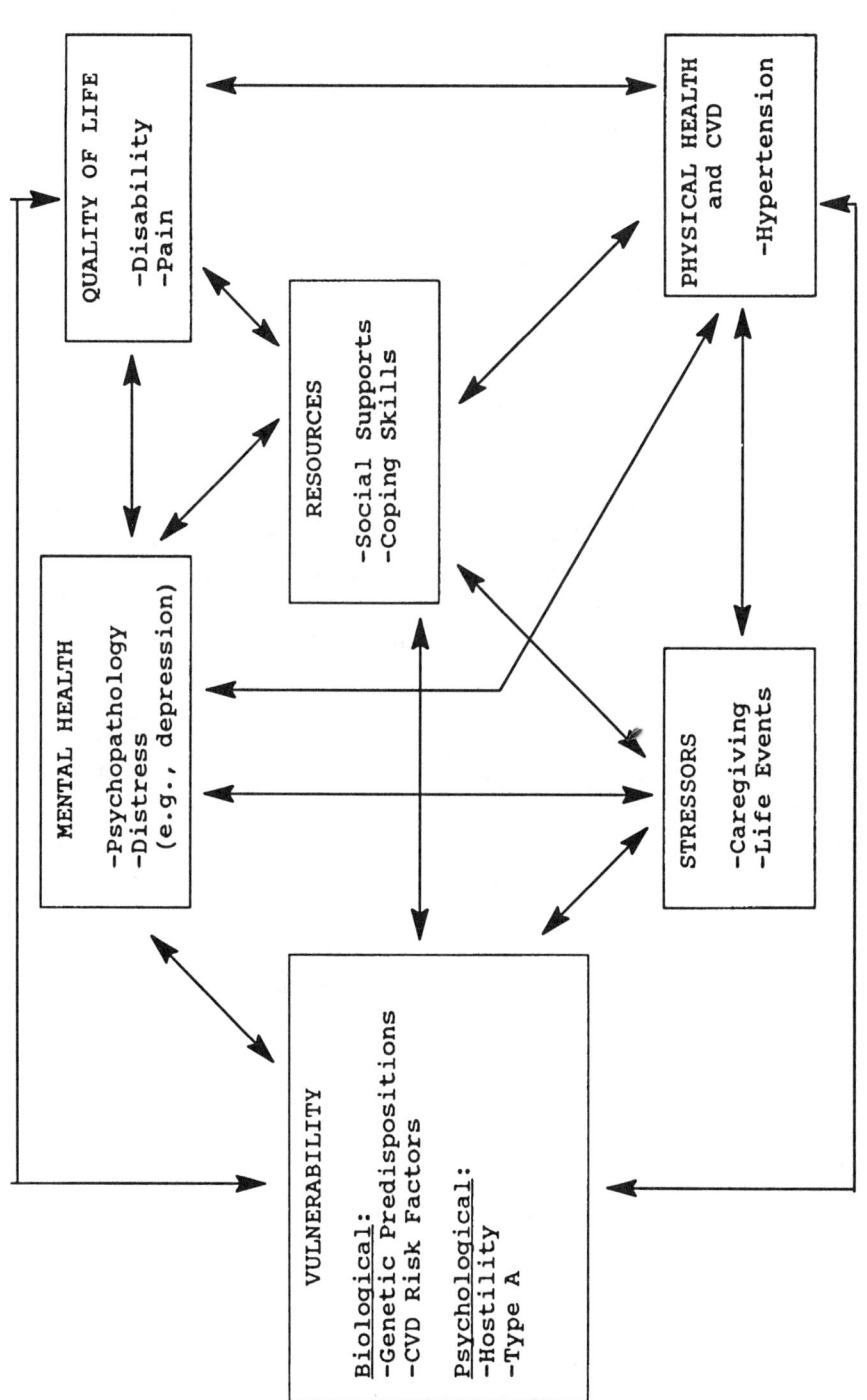

FIGURE 8.1 Path model of outcome of CVD and impaired quality of life.

may accentuate the problems of aging, and personality variables may further exacerbate the problems of caregiving. As such, the simultaneous presence of age-related biologic vulnerabilities, caregiving pressures, and more specific vulnerabilities (genetics, personality) may inflate one's risk for CVD.

Aging and Disease Vulnerability

Aging is not uniform across physiological systems (Fozard, Metter, & Brant, 1990). Whereas aging and disease appear to be distinct, they probably are not totally independent (Fozard et al., 1990). For example, disease is more common in older adults. The typical older person has 3.5 diseases and takes 13 prescription medications (Albert, 1989). Many diseases in later life begin earlier and are related to the practice of health-damaging behaviors over a lifetime (Siegler, 1989). Older persons may be more vulnerable to the physical and psychological effects of illness because of a decline in biopsychosocial capacities that occur with advancing age. Not all bodily functions decline with age, however, but older people are more likely to have multiple disorders or disorders that are both physical and psychological (Siegler & Costa, 1985). The more aged the person, the longer it takes to adapt to changes and stressors at the cellular and systemic levels. In fact, correlations between life stress and accelerated aging require further explanation (Eisdorfer & Wilkie, 1977). One interesting hypothesis is that one's sense of control may either mediate or modify relations between aging and health because correlations between health and control may grow stronger in old age (Rodin, 1986). This latter relationship could occur because the accumulation of different life experiences appears to increase the variability of perceived/desired control with age. Also, control may influence health maintenance behaviors or the seeking of medical care.

Aging and Cardiovascular Disease

In the U.S., 72% of persons over age 65 have some type of CVD (American Heart Association, 1991) and 12,000 of these people die annually (U.S. Department of Health and Human Services, 1982). By age 60, maximal coronary artery blood flow provides the CV system with 35% less blood than in previous years (Coyne & Hojlo, 1985). An older adult requires more time for heart rate to return to baseline once it is elevated (Ebersole & Hess, 1985). Reduced efficiency and contractile strength of cardiac muscle are reflected in a cardiac output that decreases by 1% per year from a baseline of 5 liters/minute. During nonstressful conditions, lowered cardiac output is adequate for an older person because metabolic demands are minimal, basal metabolic rate has declined, and the body in general is smaller. When an older adult is physically or mentally stressed, however, cardiac reserve becomes important because sudden demands for more oxygen are poorly tolerated. With advanced age, hormones that influence the force and speed of contractions decrease in amount, producing longer intervals between contractions, decreased cardiac force, and greater energy demands on the myocardium. Obesity, smoking, emotional states, lack of exercise, constant intake of calories and animal fats all can cause increased heart strain (Ebersole & Hess, 1985). Together, these changes cause an older person's heart to respond to increased oxygen demands with less efficiency and greater energy expenditure.

The Relevance of the CVD Path Model for Caregivers

In this section various components of the path model, their intercorrelations, and their specific relevance to caregiving are examined.

Mental Health

The progressively deteriorating nature of AD places demands on caregivers that may affect mental health (Schulz & Williamson, 1991). Estimates of depression among caregivers of frail elders have been as high as 43%-46% (Gallagher, Rose, Rivera, Lovett, & Thompson, 1989), three times the 14%-15% found among middle aged and elderly persons in the community (Eaton & Kessler, 1981). Schulz, Visintainer, and Williamson (1990) have cautioned, however, that "these studies provide little evidence about the population prevalence of either symptomatology or clinically defined psychiatric conditions attributable to caregiving" (p. 188). In fact, in a census tract study, Tennstedt, Cafferata, and Sullivan (1992) found that 33% of caregivers of frail elders were at risk for depression. This figure falls between the above-reported rates.

Anthony-Bergstone, Zarit, and Gatz (1988) found that caregivers had elevated hostility levels and Gallagher, Wrabetz, Lovett, Del Maestro, and Rose (1989) found that anger was the most common negative affect among AD caregivers. Other studies have found that caregivers high in criticism of their AD spouse were significantly more depressed, had lower life satisfaction, and reported more suppressed anger than caregivers low in spouse criticism (Vitaliano, Becker, Russo, Magana-Amato, & Maiuro, 1989). Criticism has also been useful in predicting negative patient behaviors (e.g., acting out, paranoia, etc.) 18 months after study entry even after relevant baseline covariates were controlled (Vitaliano, Young, Russo, Romano, & Magana-Amato, 1993). Caregiver suppressed anger assessed at baseline had a significant positive association with caregiver subjective burden both at baseline and 18 months later (Vitaliano, Russo, Young, Becker, & Maiuro, 1991).

Physical Health

Relatively few studies have examined the physical health of AD caregivers. Of the 34 caregiver studies reviewed by Schulz et al. (1990), only 11 examined physical health and only one used a biological marker (Kiecolt-Glaser et al., 1987). Robinson (1983) and Schulz, Tompkins, and Rau (1988) found health status to be between fair and good in AD caregivers. George and Gwyther (1986) found caregivers were similar to noncaregivers in physician visits and subjective health perceptions. In contrast, Haley, Levine, Brown, Berry, and Hughes (1987) found that caregivers rated their health as poorer, reported more physician visits and use of prescription medication, and endorsed more chronic illnesses than controls. The results of these studies may have differed because of varying definitions of health, measures of health status, and types of caregivers and patients.

The physical health of AD caregivers has been examined as a correlate of strain and depression. Robinson (1983) found no correlation between subjective health and strain (e.g., upset, burden, and psychological adjustment). In contrast, Schulz et al. (1988) found that chronic conditions, disabilities, and prescription drugs predicted depression in caregivers of stroke patients. Deimling and Poulshock (1985) found that AD caregivers who experienced a caregiving-related crisis reported significantly more health problems and depression. Caregivers who institutionalized patients reported more health problems than those who did not despite comparable levels of depression. The authors concluded that the decision to institutionalize had a more direct correlation with caregiver physical than mental health.

Vulnerability

As in the general population, vulnerable caregivers may become physically and/or mentally ill in response to stressful events by virtue of their genetic predispositions, environmental factors, familial environment, and individual development (Zubin & Spring, 1977). Such influences interact to produce risk factors for coronary heart disease. CVD risk factors are biological (age, gender, family history), biobehavioral (cholesterol, hypertension, obesity), and behavioral (smoking, sedentary lifestyle). CVD risk is determined by: smoking; family history of CVD; hypertension; obesity; and, hyperlipidemia. Genetic propensity for hyperlipidemias and hypolipidemias, hypertension, diabetes, obesity, and probably the lack of exercise all contribute to the likelihood of CVD. Risk profiles that predict CVD in persons < 65 years also predict CVD in those ≥ 65 years old (Kannel & Gordan, 1980).

Psychological variables such as Type A behavior, anger, and hostility may also make caregivers vulnerable to CVD problems. In the general population, such variables are associated with coronary-prone behavior patterns (Almada et al., 1991; Matthews & Rackaczky, 1988). In particular, Type A behavior and hostility covary with CVD (Barefoot et al., 1991; Siegler, Peterson, Barefoot, & Williams, 1992). Individuals respond to harassment with increased self-rated anger, but only high-hostility individuals have increased cardiovascular reactivity (Suarez & Williams, 1989). Anger and hostility are directly related to increased heart rate (Matthews & Rackaczky, 1988) and blood pressure (Gentry, Chesney, Gary, Hall, & Harburg, 1982). Hostility may contribute to health problems during an adult's life span through its influence on coronary risk behaviors (Siegler et al., 1992). Reactivity, over prolonged periods, may increase one's risk for coronary heart disease (Shekelle, Vernon, & Ostfeld, 1983) and hypertension (Gentry et al., 1982).

There is new evidence to suggest that Type A behavior, hostility, and anger may be associated with biological risks for CVD in older spouse caregivers. One study found higher systolic and diastolic blood pressure in response to an emotional task (discussion about one's spouse and their relationship) than to a spoken memory task. Moreover, after controlling for hypertension and gender, hostility, anger expression, and Type A behavior explained more blood pressure variability in response to the emotional than the memory task (Vitaliano, Russo, Bailey, Young, & McCann, 1993). Hypertensive caregivers had significantly higher blood pressure reactivities than normotensive caregivers, or hypertensive and normotensive controls. These data may be important because cardiovascular reactivity has been implicated in the development and exacerbation of CVD (Sparrow, Tifft, Rosner, & Weiss, 1984).

Another marker that may be important to CVD is recovery (Matthews, 1986). Recovery involves the degree to which an individual returns to prestress physiological levels following reactivity. Using the same samples as in the above study it was observed that individuals with poor recovery, in response to high levels of reactivity to the task, had significantly higher scores on depression and lower scores on life satisfaction/morale (Vitaliano, Paulsen, Russo, & Bailey, 1993). This may be important because in prospective studies depression appears to be a better predictor of coronary heart disease than is Type A behavior (Booth-Kewley & Friedman, 1987).

In another analysis of these samples, high density lipoprotein variability was explained by Type A behavior, controlled anger, and expressed anger (these were negatively associated with high density lipoprotein levels) after controlling for gender, body mass index, age, use of hypovolemic drugs, alcohol, and estrogen (Vitaliano, Young, Russo, & McCann, 1992). Because high density lipoprotein levels are negatively associated with CVD (Castelli, Doyle, & Gordon, 1977), these psychosocial variables may be CVD risk factors for older spouse caregivers.

How might biobehavioral vulnerabilities manifest themselves in caregivers? It is likely that feedback loops exist between all components of the path model given in Figure 8.1. For example, a caregiver's genetic and psychological (personality) vulnerabilities may increase mental (depression) and physical (hypertension) illness in response to caregiving demands, which may precipitate anger and hostility, which may reduce resources, which may, through a vicious cycle, exacerbate poor physical health, impaired quality of life, and perceived stress, etc.

Resources and Quality of Life

Vulnerability and resource variables are expected to interact to increase a caregiver's risk of mental and physical health problems. For example, hostility may influence social supports — hostile individuals may have lower levels of social support because they (1) judge their relationships harshly; (2) produce tension and conflict in their social environment; and, (3) emotionally drain their potential supports (Kessler, Price, & Wortman, 1985). Simultaneously, in older adults decrements in social supports may increase one's risk of psychological distress (Williamson & Schulz, 1992) and coronary heart disease (Antonucci & Johnson, 1992). As in the general population, caregivers in lower socioeconomic (SES) strata may experience higher levels of morbidity (e.g., CVD) and disability earlier than caregivers in a higher SES strata. Such differences may be explained in part by fewer social supports, more chronic/acute stress, and poorer health behaviors in lower SES groups (House et al., 1992). Spouse caregivers may be especially vulnerable to health problems, not only because of their age (Cantor, 1983; Noelker & Wallace, 1985), but because they lose their confidante to AD. The confidante relationship is thought to be the most essential dimension of social support (Lowenthal & Haven, 1968). Moreover, decrements in social supports are thought to be indicative of impaired quality of life (Pittman & Lloyd, 1988).

Relative to age- and gender-matched controls, caregivers have been shown to be at risk for impaired quality of life (e.g., lower life satisfaction) (Vitaliano et al., 1993). Unfortunately, impaired quality of life may be a risk factor for the early manifestation of CVD (via its correlation with CVD risk factors) as well as an outcome of CVD (via distress). Several studies have reported correlations between impaired life quality and CVD (Fletcher, Hunt, & Bulpitt, 1987). In a retrospective study, Siegrist (1987) found that quality of life variables (number of recent negative life events, poor social supports, and chronic interpersonal difficulties) significantly discriminated 190 myocardial infarction patients from 190 healthy matched controls. In a prospective study, Siegrist (1987) observed that the combination of impaired quality of life variables (stressful work context and subjectively appraised work load) explained significant variation in systolic blood pressure and the ratio of low-density lipoproteins to high-density lipoproteins in men who were initially free from coronary events.

What Can be Done about CVD Risk in Caregivers?

Many persons over age 65 die from CVD because it develops over extended periods and is related to prolonged health-damaging behaviors (Elias, Elias, & Elias, 1990; Siegler & Costa, 1985). Hence, modification of risk factors in later life may significantly reduce mortality (Kaplan, 1992). With the goal of prevention, it is recommended that caregivers with known biopsychosocial risk factors for CVD be routinely followed for CVD symptoms and be given interventions (Glueck, Laskarzewski, Rao, & Morrison, 1985). Previously, family screening for CVD risk factors has improved diagnostic and intervention strategies. Caregivers that do not have known risk factors may be difficult to identify. Many caregivers may not seek treatment for illnesses because, like older adults in general, they may tolerate symptoms and ailments because they: (1) expect poor health with old age, (2) worry that a serious condition may actually be found, and (3) fear the medical system (Besdine, 1980). If it can be shown that changes in behavior with advancing age are more health related than age related, more caregivers might seek treatment and this might improve their quality of life (Siegler & Costa, 1985).

Fortunately, communities, national organizations, and the federal government have been supporting the needs of older spouse caregivers through: (1) competent health care, (2) Alzheimer's support groups, and (3) respite care (Ory et al., 1985). Other interventions helpful for older spouses of AD patients include removing stressors, modifying the physical environment, teaching coping skills, providing social supports, and improving health practices (Gatz, 1992). Health care professionals familiar with the diagnoses and management of AD are central to families' support systems. Continuing education and National Institute of Health publications have been directed toward health care professionals, but these experts are not always available in many parts of the country. AD support groups can serve as a resource, reducing social isolation and providing practical information and coping strategies. Although respite care from community organizations provides support, such care is often not available or of poor quality (OTA, 1990). Because many families are likely to care for AD patients in the home, additional community resources are necessary.

Families have long provided the majority of long-term care for individuals suffering from AD and related disorders, often at tremendous financial and social costs. This chapter has presented a theoretical model for understanding how caregiver burdens can translate into physical health problems that affect the functioning and quality of life of caregivers. If family caregivers are no longer able to provide their selfless care, these burdens will fall to society as a whole. It is incumbent on us to identify ways to support family caregivers without incurring undue burdens or costs.

Acknowledgments

This research was supported by The National Institute of Mental Health, RO1 MH-43267; The National Institute of Aging, AG-O6770-62, AG-09276, and AG-10760; The National Heart, Lung and Blood Institute, HL-455702 and HL-36587; the National Institutes of Health, Clinical Nutrition Research Unit, DK38516; and the National Institutes of Health, Clinical Research Center, MO1-RR00037

References

Advisory Panel on Alzheimer's Disease. (1991). *Second report of the advisory panel on Alzheimer's disease.* DHHS Pub. No. (ADM) 91-1791. Washington, DC: Superintendent of Documents, U.S. Government Printing Office.

Albert, M.S. (1989). Assessment of cognitive dysfunction. In M.S. Albert & M.B. Moss (Eds.), *Geriatric neuropsychology.* New York: Guilford Press

Almada, S.J., Zonderman, A.B., Shekelle, R.B., Dyer, A.R., Davligus, M.L., Costa, P.T., Jr., & Stamler, J. (1991). Neuroticism and cynicism and risk of death in middle-aged men: The Western Electric Study. *Psychosomatic Medicine, 53,* 165-175.

American Heart Association. (1991). *Heart facts, 1991.* Dallas Texas: American Heart Association.

Aneshensel, C., Frerichs, R., & Huba, G. (1984). Depression and physical illness: A multiwave, nonrecursive causal model. *Journal of Health and Social Behavior, 25,* 350-371.

Anthony, J.C., & Aboraya, A. (1992). The epidemiology of selected mental disorders in later life. In J.E. Birren, R.B. Sloane, & G.D. Cohen (Eds.), *Handbook of mental health and aging* (2nd ed.). San Diego, CA: Academic Press, Inc.

Anthony-Bergstone, C.R., Zarit, S.H., & Gatz, M. (1988). Symptoms of psychological distress among caregivers of dementia patients. *Psychology and Aging, 3,* 245-248.

Antonucci, T.C., & Johnson, E.H. (1992). Conceptualization and methods in social support theory and research as related to cardiovascular diseases. In S.A. Schumaker, & S.M. Czajkowski (Eds.), *Support and cardiovascular disease.* New York: Plenum.

Barefoot, J.C., Peterson, B.L., Dahlstrom, W.G., Siegler, I.C., Anderson, N.B., & Williams, Jr., R.B. (1991). Hostility patterns and health implications: Correlates of Cook-Medley Hostility Scale scores in a national survey. *Health Psychology, 10,* 18–24.

Besdine, R.W. (1980). Geriatric medicine: An overview. In C. Eisdorfer (Ed.), *Annual review of gerontology and geriatrics* (pp. 135–153). New York: Springer Publishing Co.

Booth-Kewley, S., & Friedman, S. (1987). Psychological predictors of heart disease: A quantitative review. *Psychological Bulletin, 101,* 343–362.

Cantor, M.H. (1983). Strain among caregivers: A study of experience in the United States. *The Gerontologist, 23,* 597–604.

Castelli, W.P., Doyle, J., & Gordon, T, (1977). Alcohol and blood lipids: The Cooperative Lipoprotein Phenotyping Study. *Lancet, 2,* 153–155.

Chesney, M.A., & Rosenman, R.H. (Eds.). (1985). *Anger and hostility in cardiovascular and behavioral disorders.* New York: Hemisphere.

Coyne, M., & Hojlo, K. (1985). Physiological aspects of aging. *Occupational Health Nursing, 33,* 117–122.

Deimling, G.T., & Poulshock, S.W. (1985). The transition from family in-home care to institutional care. *Research on Aging, 7,* 563–576.

Eaton, W.W., & Kessler, L.G. (1981). Rates of symptoms of depression in a national sample. *American Journal of Epidemiology, 114,* 528–538.

Ebersole, P., & Hess, P. (1985). *Toward healthy aging: Human needs and nursing response* (pp. 168–239). St. Louis, MO: Mosby.

Eisdorfer, C., & Wilkie, F. (1977). Stress, disease, aging and behavior. In J.E. Birren & K.W. Schaie (Eds.), *Handbook of the psychology of aging* (pp. 251–275). New York: Van Nostrand Reinhold.

Elias, M.F., Elias, J.W., & Elias, P.K. (1990). Biological and health influences on behavior. In J.E. Birren & K.W. Schaie (Eds.), *Handbook of the psychology of aging,* (3rd ed.). New York: Academic Press.

Fletcher, A.E., Hunt, B.M., & Bulpitt, C.J. (1987). Evaluation of quality of life in clinical trials of cardiovascular disease. *Journal of Chronic Diseases, 40,* 557–566.

Fozard, J.L., Metter, E.J., & Brant, L.J. (1990). Next steps in describing aging and disease in longitudinal studies. *Journal of Gerontology 45,* 116–127.

Gallagher, D., Rose, J., Rivera, P., Lovett, S., & Thompson, L.W. (1989). Prevalence of depression in family caregivers. *The Gerontologist, 29,* 449–456.

Gallagher, D., Wrabetz, A., Lovett, S., Del Maestro, S., & Rose, J. (1989). Depression and other negative affects in family caregivers. In E. Light & B. Lebowitz (Eds.), *Alzheimer's disease treatment and family stress: Future directions of research* (pp. 218–244). Washington, DC: U.S. Government Printing Office.

Gatz, M. (1992). Stress, control, and psychological interventions. In M.L. Wykle, E. Kahana, & J. Kowal (Eds.), *Stress and health among the elderly* (pp. 209-222). New York: Springer Publishing Co.

Gentry, W.D., Chesney, A.P., Gary, H.E., Hall, R.P., & Harburg, E. (1982). Habitual anger-coping styles I: Effect of mean blood pressure and risk for essential hypertension. *Psychosomatic Medicine, 44,* 195-202.

George, L.K., & Gwyther, L.P. (1986). Caregiver well being: A multidimensional examination of family caregivers of demented adults. *The Gerontologist, 26,* 253-259.

Glueck, C.J., Laskarzewski, P.M., Rao, D.C., & Morrison, J.A. (1985). Familial aggregation of coronary risk factors. In W.E. Connor & J.D. Bristow (Eds.), *Coronary heart disease: Prevention, complications and treatment* (pp. 173-192). Philadelphia: Lippincott.

Haley, W.E., Levine, E.G., Brown, S.L., Berry, J.W., & Hughes, G.H. (1987). Psychological, social, and health consequences of caring for a relative with senile dementia. *Journal of the American Geriatric Society, 35,* 405-411.

House, J.S., Kessler, R.C., Herzog, A.R., Mero, R.P., Kinney, A.M., & Breslow, M.J. (1992). Social stratification, age, and health. In K.W. Schaie, D. Blazer, & J.C. House (Eds.), *Aging, health behaviors, and health outcomes.* Hillsdale, NJ: Erlbaum.

Kannel, W.B., & Gordon, T. (1980). Cardiovascular risk factors in the aged: The Framingham Study. In S.G. Haynes & M. Feinleib (Eds.), *Epidemiology of aging* (pp. 65-86). Washington, DC: USDHHS, PHS, NIH, NIA, NHLBI, NIH No. 80-969.

Kaplan, G.A. (1992). Health and aging in the Alameda County Study. In K.W. Schaie, D. Blazer, & J.C. House (Eds.), *Aging health behaviors and health outcomes.* Hillsdale, NJ: Erlbaum.

Kessler, R., Price, R., & Wortman, C. (1985). In M.R. Rosenzweig & L.W. Porter (Eds.), *Social factors in psychopathology: Stress, social support, and coping processes* (pp. 531-572). New York: Annual Reviews.

Kiecolt-Glaser, J.K., Glaser, R., Shuttleworth, E.C., Dyer, C.S., Ogrocki, P., & Speicher, C.E. (1987). Chronic stress and immunity in family caregivers of Alzheimer's disease victims. *Psychosomatic Medicine, 49,* 523-535.

Lowenthal, M.F., & Haven, C. (1968). Interaction and adaptation: Intimacy as a critical variable. *American Sociological Review, 33,* 20-30,

Matthews, K.A. (1986). Summary, conclusions, and implications. In K.A. Matthews, S.M. Weiss, T. Detre, T.M. Dembroski, B. Falkner, S.B. Manuck, & R.B. Williams, Jr. (Eds.), *Handbook of stress, reactivity, and cardiovascular disease.* New York: Wiley & Sons.

Matthews, K.A., & Rackaczky, C.J. (1988). Familial aspects of Type A behavior pattern and physiological reactivity to stress. In T.M. Dembroski, T.M. Schmidt, & G. Blumchen, (Eds.), *Biobehavioral bases of coronary heart disease*. Heidelberg: Springer-Verlag.

Noelker, L.S., & Wallace, R.W. (1985). The organization of family care for impaired elderly. *Journal of Family Issues, 6*, 23–44.

Office of Technology Assessment. (July, 1990). *Confused minds, burdened families: Finding help for people with Alzheimer's and other dementias* (OTA–BA–403). Washington, DC: U.S. Government Priting Office.

Ory, M.G., Williams, T.F., Emr, M., Lebowitz, B., Rabins, P.V., Salloway, J., Sluss-Radbaugh, T., Wolff, E., & Zarit, S.H. (1985). Families, informal supports, and Alzheimer's disease. *Research on Aging, 7*, 623–644.

Pittman, J.F., & Lloyd, S.A. (1988). Quality of family life, social support, and stress. *Journal of Marriage and the Family, 50*, 53–67.

Robinson, B.C. (1983). Validation of a caregiver strain index. *Journal of Gerontology, 38*, 344–348.

Rodin, J. (1986). Aging and health: Effects of the sense of control. *Science, 223*, 1271–1276.

Schulz, R., Tompkins, C.A., & Rau, M.T. (1988). A longitudinal study of the psychosocial impact of stroke on primary support persons. *Psychology and Aging, 3*, 131–141.

Schulz, R., & Williamson, G.M. (1991). A 2-year longitudinal study of depression among Alzheimer's caregivers. *Psychology and Aging, 6*, 569–578.

Schulz, R., Visintainer, P., & Williamson, G.M. (1990). Psychiatric and physical morbidity effects of caregiving. *Journal of Gerontology: Psychological Sciences, 45*, 181–191.

Shekelle, R.B., Vernon, S.W., & Ostfeld, A.M. (1991). Personality and coronary heart disease. *Psychosomatic Medicine, 53*, 176–184.

Siegler, I.C. (1989). Developmental health psychology. In M. Storandt & G.R. VanderBos (Eds.), *The adult years: Continuity and change* (pp. 119–142). Washington, DC: American Psychological Association.

Siegler, I.C., & Costa, P.T. (1985). Health behavior relationships. In J.E. Birren & K.W. Schaie (Eds.), *Handbook of the psychology of aging* (pp. 144–166). New York: Van Nostrand Reinhold.

Siegler, I.C., Peterson, B.L., Barefoot, J.C., & Williams, R.B. (1992). Hostility during late adolescence predicts coronary risk factors at mid-life. *American Journal of Epidemiology, 136*, 146–154.

Siegrist, J. (1987). Impaired quality of life as a risk factor in cardiovascular disease. *Journal of Chronic Diseases, 40*, 571–578.

Sparrow, D., Tifft, C.P., Rosner, B., & Weiss, S.T. (1984). Postural changes in diastolic blood pressure and the risk of myocardial infarction: The Normative Aging Study. *Circulation, 70*, 533–537.

Suarez, E.C., & Williams Jr., R.B. (1989). Situational determinants of cardiovascular and emotional reactivity in high and low hostile men. *Psychosomatic Medicine, 51*, 404–418.

Tennstedt, S., Cafferata, G.F., & Sullivan, L. (1992). Depression among caregivers of impaired elders. *Journal of Aging and Health, 4*, 58–76.

U.S. Department of Health and Human Services. (1982). Advance report of final mortality statistics. *Monthly Vital Statistics Report, 33*, 17.

Vitaliano, P.P., Becker, J., Russo, J., Magana-Amato, A., & Maiuro, R.D. (1989). Expressed emotion in spouse caregivers of patients with Alzheimer's disease. *The Journal of Applied Social Sciences, 13*, 215–250.

Vitaliano, P.P., Paulsen, V.M., Russo, J., & Bailey, S.L. (1993). Cardiovascular recovery and its biopsychosocial concomitants in older adults. Manuscript submitted for publication.

Vitaliano, P.P., Russo, J., Bailey, S.L., Young, H.M., & McCann, B.S. (1993). Psychosocial factors associated with cardiovascular reactivity in older adults. *Psychosomatic Medicine, 55*, 164–177.

Vitaliano, P.P., Russo, J., Young, H.M., Becker, J., & Maiuro, R.D. (1991). The Screen for Caregiver Burden. *The Gerontologist, 31*, 76–83.

Vitaliano, P.P., Russo, J., Young, H.M., Teri, L., & Maiuro, R.D. (1991). Predictors of burden in spouse caregivers of individuals with Alzheimer's disease. *Psychology and Aging, 6*, 392–401.

Vitaliano, P.P., Young, H.M., Russo, J., & McCann, B.S. (1992, August). *Psychosocial factors and health in older adults.* Paper presented at the meeting of the American Psychological Association, Washington, DC, Washington Hilton Hotel.

Vitaliano, P.P., Young, H.M., Russo, J., Romano, J., & Magana-Amato, A. (1993). Does expressed emotion in spouses predict subsequent problems among care-recipients with Alzheimer's disease. *Journal of Gerontology: Psychological Sciences, 48*, 202–209.

Williamson, G.M., & Schulz, R. (1992). Physical illness and symptoms of depression among elderly outpatients. *Psychology and Aging, 7*, 343–351.

Zubin, J., & Spring, B. (1977). Vulnerability— a new view of schizophrenia. *Journal of Abnormal Psychology, 86*, 103–126.

PART IV

Older People and Their Environments

Chapter 9
Social Support: Content, Causes and Consequences

Robert L. Kahn

Research on social support has had an unusual history. It entered the research literature in the 1970s and its attraction to researchers has increased since at a remarkable rate. The *Social Citation Index* for 1972 showed only two current articles on the subject, but the same index showed more than 50 articles for 1982 and hundreds in each of more recent years.

The popularity of the concept reflects its intuitive appeal rather than any consensus on definition or measurement; researchers agree about its importance for health and well-being but they have yet to agree on what support consists of, what makes it supportive, and how it should be measured. Thus, the effects of social support have been demonstrated without clear indication of the causal mechanisms involved. Furthermore, the few experimental efforts to increase social support have had mixed results, for reasons not yet well understood. It is as if the synthetic product sometimes lacks the potency of the natural one.

In this chapter these issues will be addressed, especially as they apply to older men and women. More specifically, (1) some of the more important evidence for the effect of social support on mortality and morbidity will be described; (2) a theoretical model of support throughout the life course will be proposed; (3) research that bears on the major components and relationships in that model will be reviewed; and (4) the attempts, successful and unsuccessful, to increase social support among older people most in need of it will be evaluated.

Social Support, Mortality, and Morbidity

Some of the most persuasive evidence for the life-sustaining effects of social support comes from a 9-year mortality study in Alameda County, California (Berkman, 1985; Berkman & Breslow, 1983; Berkman & Syme, 1979). The measures developed for that research did not assess supportive behavior directly, but were based instead on four kinds of social connections: marriage, contact with family and close friends, church group membership, and other group affiliations. Mortality rates over the 9 year period of the study showed a consistent pattern: greater overall risk of death among people who did not have these social connections. (Age-adjusted relative risks were 2.3 for men and 2.8 for women, respectively.) Moreover, the pattern held for many separate causes of death—ischemic heart disease, cancer, cerebrovascular and circulatory disease, and a residual category of other causes. The causal paths or mechanisms that might explain such effects could not be inferred from this study, however. Indeed, further analysis of these data showed that the increased mortality risk associated with lack of social connectedness persists even after the analysts controlled for such hypothesized causes as cigarette smoking, alcohol consumption, physical activity, obesity, life satisfaction, and use of preventive health services. Social support must have some of its effects through other paths.

A prospective community study of morbidity and mortality in Tecumseh, Michigan (House, Robbins & Metzner, 1982) replicated the main finding of increased mortality among men and women who scored low on measures of social relationships and activities. Moreover, the prospective design made it possible to control for the health of participants at the beginning of the 10-year study. The finding of increased mortality among men persisted after the imposition of this and other controls, although the increases among women became insignificant. Nevertheless, the overall findings suggest that the relationship of social support to well-being involves causality rather than mere association.

A third major study of social support and mortality was conducted in Durham County, North Carolina (Blazer, 1982), and all participants were 65 years of age or older. Consistent with the Alameda County and Tecumseh studies, the Durham research showed increased mortality over a 30-month period for older men and women with low social connectedness. (The relative mortality risk was 2.04 for people with impaired roles and attachments and 1.88 for those with impaired frequency of social contacts).

Other studies, which concentrated on morbidity rather than mortality, show that lack of social connectedness is related to heart disease (Seeman & Syme, 1987; Antonucci, 1990). Among Japanese-Americans in California, prevalence of coronary heart disease was lower for those who scored high on an index of social affiliation composed of marital status, attendance at religious services, and membership in organizations. (Analyses in Hawaii yielded similar findings.) In a 5-year prospective study of ischemic heart disease among men in Israel, the incidence of angina was predicted by the incidence of family problems and conflicts, which could be interpreted either as lack of support or as an indication of the supportive aspects of family relations being overwhelmed by negative factors (Medalie & Goldbourt, 1976). This study also showed that expressions of love and support by the wife buffered (reduced) the effect of anxiety in increasing incidence of angina. Finally, the Framingham Study of Heart Disease showed that women clerical workers who had nonsupportive supervisors were at increased risk of developing coronary heart disease during an 8-year follow-up period (Haynes, Feinleib, & Kannel, 1980).

The similarities in findings across these studies is impressive, although some inconsistencies do exist (Berkman, 1985). However, despite differences in measures and concepts of social support and connectedness, despite differences in the outcome variables of choice, and despite differences in design and statistical procedures, all these studies show that membership in a social network of family, friends, or co-workers is health protective and life extending.

Additional evidence for the importance of social support and connectedness comes from research at specific life stages—studies of infant attachment, child development, adolescence, and mid-life transitions, for example. They are complemented by studies of support at times of particular stress or challenge—job loss (Cobb & Kasl,

1977) and illness (Cobb, 1976; Janis, 1983), for example—and by research in particular settings, especially the work setting.

Thus, membership in a support-giving network of family and friends seems important for health and well-being throughout the life course. The still unanswered questions are what aspects of social relations are support-providing, by what specific behaviors support is conveyed, by what causal paths support exerts its effects on health and the prolongation of life, and how the answers to these questions change as an individual moves through the life course.

The Convoy of Social Support

A framework within which such questions can be addressed has been proposed by Kahn and Antonucci (Figure 9.1). The central concept is this model is the *convoy*, which for each individual represents those other people who provide any form of support during the life course. The set of such people at any given time can thus be regarded as a network, defined in terms of supportive relationships with the same individual. Past research on the structure of supportive relationships has relied heavily on the concept of networks (Barnes, 1972; Fischer, Jackson, Stueve, Gerson, & Jones 1977, Harary, 1969; Wellman, 1981). Most studies of social support attempt to characterize the support that individuals receive from members of their networks (family, friends, colleagues, and others). This can be done both in terms of the dyadic relationships that link an individual to the various members of his or her network and in terms of properties that describe the network as a whole. Properties of dyadic links within networks include frequency of interaction, type of support given, the amount of support, whether or not it is reciprocated, and the like. Properties of the network as a whole include such factors as size, stability, homogeneity, internal connectedness, and symmetry; of these variables, however, only size has been much studied as a predictor of individual well-being.

Research on networks has tended to be cross-sectional and static, as has research on social support. The life-course perspective, however refers to changes over time and reminds us that the size and structure of networks must be subject to such changes. People move in and out of neighborhoods, in and out of jobs and, not infrequently, in and out of marriages. Interests change with age and changing circumstances; people die. It is important to recognize the consequent

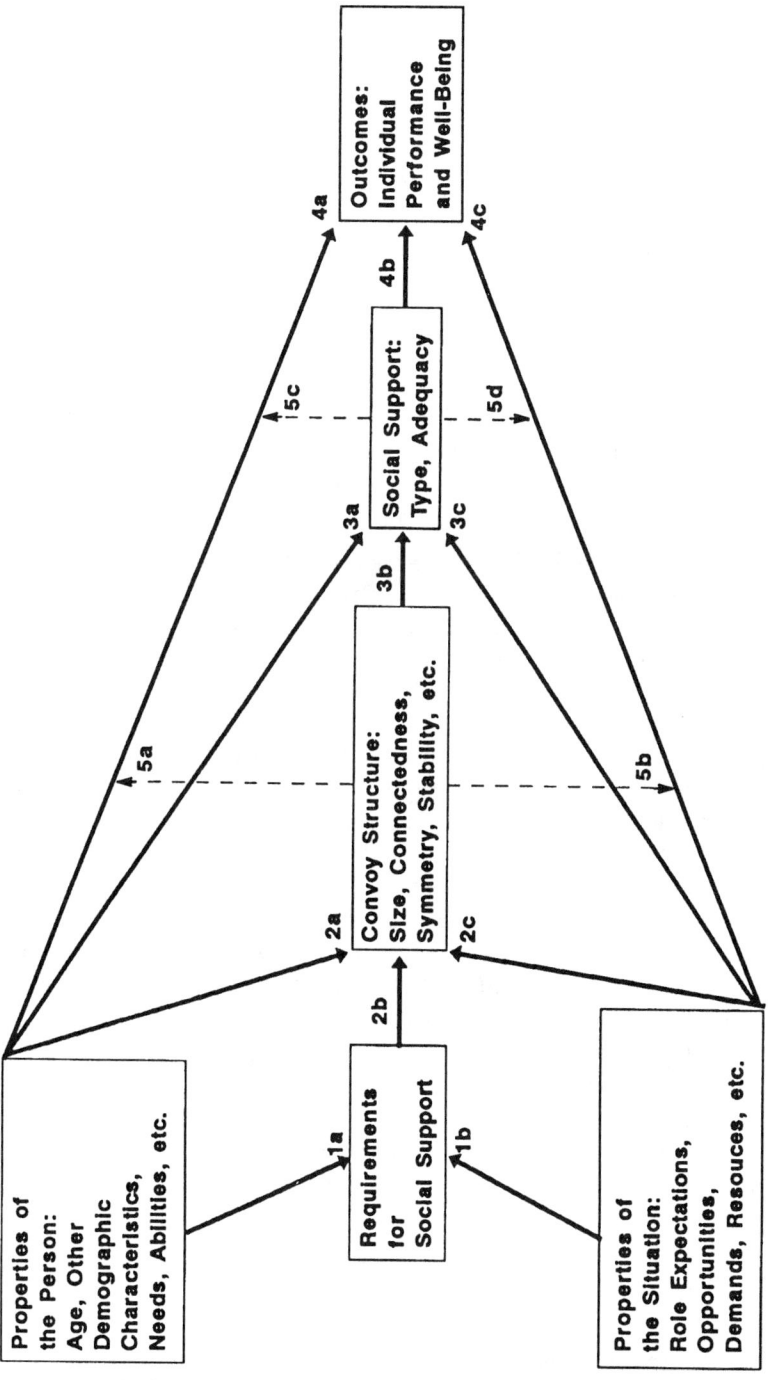

FIGURE 9.1 The Convoy Model of Social Support: Hypothetical determinants and effects.

fluidity of each individual's support network and to designate the dynamic networks of social support with a unique term: the *Convoy** of social support.

Choosing this metaphorical label implies that each person can be thought of as moving through the life course surrounded by a set of other people to whom he or she is related by the giving and/or receiving of social support (Kahn & Antonucci, 1984). Each property of the convoy and its separate dyadic links can then be regarded both in static and dynamic terms. With respect to size, for example, it is important to know not only whether the convoy is large or small, but also whether it is growing or reducing. Both characteristics are hypothesized to have effects on individual well-being.

As Figure 9.1 shows, the convoy is the central concept in an explanatory framework proposed for the study of social support (Kahn, 1979; Kahn & Antonucci, 1984). It is a structural concept, shaped by the interaction of situational factors and properties of the person and in turn affecting the adequacy of support and thus the person's well-being and performance of life roles. These relationships and the others represented in Figure 9.1 can be described in terms of five general propositions, each of which identifies a category of more specific hypotheses:

1. A person's requirements for support at any given time are determined jointly by enduring properties of that person (age, other demographic characteristics, personality, etc.) and by properties of the situation (expectations and demands of work, family, and other roles): Arrows 1a and 1b in Figure 9.1.
2. The structure of a person's convoy (size, connectedness, stability, etc.) is determined jointly by enduring properties of the person, by the person's requirements for social support, and by properties of the situation: Arrows 2a, 2b, and 2c in Figure 9.1.
3. The adequacy of social support received by a person is determined by the properties of the convoy, and by properties of the person and situation: Arrows 3a, 3b, and 3c in Figure 9.1.
4. Life outcomes, including measures of well-being and performance in major roles, are determined jointly by enduring proper-

---

*A similar use of the term *convoy* first came to our attention in the work of David Plath, who in turn credits Loki Madan for his use of the term in an ethnographic study of Kashmir.

ties of the person, adequacy of social support, and properties of the situation: Arrows 4a, 4b, and 4c in Figure 9.1.
5. The influence of personal and situational factors on criteria of performance and well-being is moderated by the convoy structure and by the adequacy of social support: Arrows 5a, 5b, 5c, and 5d in Figure 9.1.

Thus, if the convoy is regarded as the core of the model, the remainder of it consists of the hypothesized causes and effects of convoy structure, including its moderating or interactive effects as well as its direct outcomes. The model itself, however, should be viewed as a set of proposals or hypotheses, rather than as a schematic summary of research findings already in hand. Research on social support has examined some, but by no means all, of these hypothesized relationships. The remainder of this chapter provides a discussion of that research.

The Research Evidence

Research on social support has generated many findings relevant to the model. Some of them can be regarded as providing a partial test of the proposed hypotheses, but some of the earlier findings contributed to the formulation of that model. Conspicuously absent in almost all of this research are the dynamic measures that would require longitudinal research designs or, as a far less satisfactory substitute, systematic development of retrospective data. At present, many of the inferences about change in social support across the life course must be made from comparisons across age groups, with inevitable confounding of cohort and historical effects. With those cautions, we turn to some research findings relevant to the model. Unless otherwise cited, they come from a nationwide two-wave study of social networks and support among people aged 50 and older (Kahn & Antonucci, 1984) and its more recent derivatives (e.g., Antonucci, Kahn, & Akiyama, 1989).

Properties of the Person

Among people of middle age and beyond who continue to live in private households, age does not appear to have strong effects on the size of social networks. A nationwide study of men and women aged

55 or more found typical network size in the range of 7 to 10 persons, with networks of people aged 75 and over smaller by only one person than the networks of those in the age range of 55–64 (Antonucci, 1985, 1990). Similar findings are reported by Babchuk (1978–1979), and Cantor (1979).

Gender makes more of a difference than age in network size; at every age, women report larger networks than men (Antonucci, 1985, 1990). This finding is from a national survey in which the measurement of network size involved a three-step iterative process that required respondents to identify individuals "who are important to you because of what they do for you or what you do for them." The tendency for women's networks to be larger than those of men was also found by Harris et al. (1981) and by Veroff, Douvan, and Kulka (1981).

Gender appears to affect satisfaction with one's network, as well as network size. Women are more satisfied than men with the support provided by friends and other network members. They are more likely than men to mention children, family, and friends as sources of support. The pattern holds also for sibling relations; sisters are closer than brothers. It is reversed, however, for spousal support; men are more likely to cite their wives as sources of support than women their husbands, and men are more satisfied than women with support from their spouses.

For both men and women, marital status affects network size, perhaps because both partners tend to bring members into the network or perhaps because, at least in middle age and beyond, married couples have more opportunities for social interaction than single men or women. Socioeconomic status also confers some advantage in the size of support networks, as it does in so many other respects. As one goes higher on the socioeconomic scale, networks become not only larger but more diverse in their membership, less likely to be restricted to family and immediate neighbors.

Other personal characteristics do not have clear effects on network characteristics. Some scattered evidence suggests that people of Italian and Hispanic backgrounds have larger networks, and this is certainly consistent with folklore and casual observation, but the data are neither powerful not consistent (Antonucci, 1990; Markides, Liang, and Jackson, 1990). Personality characteristics, at least within the normal range of functioning adults, are also not strong predictors of network characteristics.

Properties of the Situation

It is plausible that network properties should be dependent on situational factors in substantial part, but research evidence is limited. Two variables, however, emerge significantly in the national survey cited earlier—residential arrangements—single versus multiple dwelling units, for example—and geographical proximity (Kahn & Antonucci, 1984). Proximity is of major importance; in spite of modern methods of travel and communication, 67% of persons identified as network members lived "within an hour's drive" of the respondent. The physical characteristics of residential arrangements predict network size and frequency of contact, but appear to be less important in themselves than as indicators of whether or not an intact couple is in residence.

Types of Social Support

No study has compared different types of social support across a broad range of specific hypothesized effects. In theory, however, one would expect that positive effects would be maximized when the kind of support offered was congruent with the requirements of the situation and the needs of the person. What constitutes such congruence remains to be specified, but some evidence for the importance of situation-appropriate forms of social support is reported by Antonucci, Kahn, and Akiyama (1989) in a study of social support in response to the discovery of cancer-suspicious symptoms.

In re-interviews of the national sample previously cited, conducted 4 years after the original study, older men and women were asked whether they had experienced any of a list of 19 physical symptoms at any time since the previous interview. Thirteen of these symptoms had been rated by a medical expert as cancer-suspicious and therefore deserving of medical attention. One hundred and ten of the respondents reported at least one such symptom. The research question was whether these individuals sought medical diagnosis, how soon after the symptom onset the appointment was made, and what interactions with network members preceded the call to a doctor. Interviews were also conducted with network members named by these respondents, in order to test the validity of their answers.

The single strongest predictor of the decision to see a doctor was instrumental support from a network member—that is, direct pragmatic assistance such as offering and providing transportation, making telephone calls to set appointments, and the like. Other forms of social support, socio-emotional and informational, did not in themselves have significant effects. It is plausible that well-meant amateur reassurance about a symptom, however supportive, would not increase the likelihood of prompt action.

Unpacking the Concept of Social Support

That social support in general tends to generate a broad range of positive effects is no longer in dispute. Limitations and inconsistencies in the research findings, however, imply that the effects of social support are conditioned or moderated by other factors. We need to know, in other words, *how, when* and *why* social support is supportive.

To answer those questions requires research specification of support in three respects—substantive, spatial, and temporal. Substantive specification means identifying and measuring the properties of supportive interpersonal transactions, discovering what is said and done. Spatial specification means locating those supportive transactions in a structure of relationships and a sequence of other exchanges. Temporal extension of the support concept means charting support patterns across the life course, thus making the concepts of support and network dynamic rather than static. The concept of the convoy and the model represented as Figure 9.1 are attempts to extend the concept and emerging theory of social support along these lines, although not all of these ideas are represented in the figure.

For example, it seems useful to include at least four kinds of interpersonal transactions under the more general rubric of social support—emotional, informational, instrumental, and appraisal (House, 1981; House & Kahn, 1985). Emotional support includes expressions of esteem, liking, or concern. Informational support includes the giving of advice, suggestions, directives, or relevant data. Instrumental support consists of more tangible forms of aid—money, time, or other resources. Support that takes the form of appraisal could be considered a subcategory of information; its primary content is feedback or assessment of a person's behavior and its effects. Not all such assessments are supportive, as many an unsuccessful program of supervisory appraisal has demonstrated, but appraisal and affirmation can be supportive.

Specifying supportive transactions in a contextual or spatial sense requires that they be located in a causal sequence that includes the events or conditions that evoke them and the immediate effects of the support-giving transactions themselves. Figure 9.1 identifies two main categories of support-evoking variables, properties of the person (demographic and psychological) and properties of the situation (demands, opportunities, resources, etc.). Together these personal and situational characteristics determine both the individual's requirements for support and the social structure within which support is provided. These in turn determine the adequacy of support given in relation to need, and thus affect the more distal outcomes of individual performance, health, and well-being.

Extending the concept of social support in a temporal sense means treating it as a dynamic variable as well as a persisting condition. There are losses and gains in supportive relations as individuals change roles, jobs, residences. And increasingly in old age, the structure of one's support network is altered by the death of a friend or family member. As proposed earlier in this chapter, each descriptive variable should be treated both in static and dynamic terms.

Stress and Strain: The Buffering Hypothesis

One line of research addresses indirectly the element of individual need in supportive relations. It developed out of an effort to improve results already in hand. The epidemiological studies already cited show the link between social support and morbidity and mortality, and other studies link social support to psychological indicators of well-being. All these relationships, however, although of considerable consistency, are of modest magnitude. Correlations of .35 or a bit higher are the norm. The question of whether social support had significant effects thus gave way to the question why they were not stronger.

Speculative answers to this question began with the plausible assumption that social support might have major effects on well-being only when the need for support was high, either for individual or situational reasons. This possibility is commonly referred to as "the buffering hypothesis," the prediction that social support reduces the amount of strain experienced under conditions of high stress, but that the effect is less pronounced or wholly absent under conditions of low stress.

Empirical investigation of the buffering hypothesis thus became a search for statistical interactions. Numerous studies of this kind have now been conducted, but the results are varied and the hypothesis is still in dispute. Kasl (1984), in reviewing this work, is characteristically cautious but notes a number of sizable, quantitative studies that reported significant buffering effects. These include evidence that supervisory support buffers the effects of job stressors on diastolic blood pressure (Caplan et al., 1980; French, Caplan, & Harrison, 1982; Winnbust, Marcelissen, & Kleber, 1982), on the probability of developing ulcers (House & Wells, 1978), on serum glucose and cortisol levels (Caplan, Cobb, French, Harrison, & Pinneau, 1980; French, Caplan, & Harrison, 1982), on symptoms of depression and low satisfaction with life (Karasek, Triantis & Chandhry, 1982). Fewer studies in work settings measured support from other sources than the supervisor, but several reported significant buffering effects. For example, House and Wells (1978) found that the impact of job stress on self-reported neurotic symptoms was buffered by support from one's spouse, and Caplan et al. (1980) reported that the effects of job stressors on blood pressure and blood chemistry were buffered by positive interpersonal relations with co-workers and subordinates as well as with supervisors. Kasl's research on the stresses of unemployment showed that social support buffered effects on perceived deprivation and insecurity but not on other negative outcomes. The buffering hypothesis persists, but the reasons for its confirmation in some studies and not in others remain to be explained despite some attempts at reconciliation (LaRocco, House, & French 1980; Kahn & Byosiere 1992).

Social Support and Aging

The buffering hypothesis, with its emphasis on the importance of support at times of major stress and intensified need, leads naturally to an interest in stressful life transitions and events. Thinking in these terms points up the uniquely stressful nature of life events that disrupt support structures, and thus both intensify the need for support and reduce the means of meeting that need.

In adult and later life, at least three classes of life events have this dual nature:

bereavement, which involves the loss of spouse support and of couple-defined friendships;
involuntary retirement or job loss which, in addition to its economic impact, involves the loss of support from co-workers;
compulsory residential relocation, which is often imposed on older people after bereavement or illness and which brings the additional disruption of support from friends and neighbors.

Bereavement

Higher age-specific mortality rates among widowed men and women as compared to those still married had long been noted in cross-sectional data (Kraus & Lilienthal, 1959; March, 1912). Longitudinal studies in more recent decades confirmed these early findings and added to their specificity. Thus, Parkes, Benjamin, and Fitzgerald (1969) reported excess mortality among widowers during the first 6 months of bereavement, but a gradual reduction of that effect, so that after 5 years mortality among the widowed subjects in their research was not greater than in the control group. Helsing, Szklo, and Comstock (1981), in a large and well-controlled mortality study of men over a 12-year period, confirmed the finding of higher overall mortality rates among those widowed but not the finding of a significant decline beginning 6 months after bereavement.

Other studies have replicated both the finding of higher mortality among those widowed and the tendency of mortality among both widows and widowers to revert to "normal" with the passage of time. They have also demonstrated some gender differences in bereavement effects, although the negative impact of bereavement holds for both men and women (Rees & Lutkins, 1967; Ward, 1985).

The interaction of age with bereavement has been less researched, but there is some evidence that the effects on health and mortality are less when widowhood comes relatively late (Heyman & Gianturco, 1973). The tentative explanation emphasizes the concepts of greater psychological preparation and consequently less stress when negative events are seen as age-appropriate. Almost none of the research on widowhood and health uses biomedical as well as self-reported measures, and almost none of it utilizes full prospective research designs. A study now under way in the Detroit area (Wortman & House, 1991) will provide such data for a large, representative community sample.

Retirement

Findings on the health effects of retirement are mixed. Among men, especially blue-collar workers, there is some evidence for increased mortality after retirement (Haynes, McMichael, & Tyroler, 1977), for increased illness (Martin and Doran, 1966), and for lowered satisfaction with life (Stokes & Maddox, 1967). These findings have been interpreted as loss of social support, presumably by co-workers. However, other studies have found no effects of retirement on health and a few have even reported health improvements (Shanas, 1979; Eckerdt, 1987; Eckerdt, Baden, Bosse, & Dibbs, 1983).

This mixture of findings might lead to the conclusion that no generalization is possible, but the search for explanatory "third variables" suggests that the effects of retirement depend substantially on whether it is voluntary or involuntary (unpublished data, Institute for Social Research). The same national data set further indicates that the negative impact of retirement is dependent on the extent to which retirement disrupts one's social support networks, and that this disruption may be greater among blue-collar than white-collar workers, presumably because nonwork sources of social support may be more numerous in the white-collar population.

Yet to be investigated is the extent to which the apparent effects of retirement depend on its coincidence with other stressful life events—for example, economic problems, residential moves, or disability. Studies of plant closings and job loss, which have a long research tradition, involve experiences that in some respects resemble involuntary retirement, and their negative effects, both physical and psychological, have been frequently described. Some of those effects, but not all, have been shown to be buffered by social support, especially from the spouse (Cobb & Kasl,1977; Price, 1992; Turner, Kessler, & House, 1991).

Involuntary Residential Relocation

Changes in residence, compelled by economic pressures, failing health, or family insistence, are common in old age. Their effects have been well summarized by Minkler (1985), who distinguished between moves within the community or private households and moves into (or between) nursing homes. She found that such moves within the "community of private households" resulted in lower self-ratings of health and increased numbers of physician visits; no increase in mortality was apparent, however. Moves from private households to nursing homes, on the other hand, were associated with subsequent increases in mortality. Minkler interprets the findings as reflecting different degrees of disruption of support networks. Other investigators have put more emphasis on individual differences in need and tolerance for social stimulation, and have invoked such concepts as optimization (Lawton, 1983) or congruence (Kahana, 1982) to explain the empirical range of relocation effects.

In summary, all three classes of stressful life events—bereavement, involuntary retirement, and involuntary residential change—have been shown to have adverse effects on mortality, morbidity, and/or quality of life. Those effects, however, are not unvarying, and they appear to be linked to individual networks of social support as well as to other individual characteristics. The negative effects of involuntary relocation in old age are probably caused in part by disruption of support networks and they may be minimized to the extent that sources of social support remain and offer assistance, or new sources of support are mobilized.

All three event categories—bereavement, involuntary retirement, and compulsory change in residence—become more likely with increasing age. A mitigating factor, however, is also age-related; some stressful life-events appear to be less damaging when they are seen as somehow age-appropriate and in that sense not unexpected.

Prospects for Intervention

For both scientific and pragmatic reasons, it is important not only to observe social support but to create or increase it. Can people be taught to behave supportively? Can people learn how to evoke supportive behavior from others? Can "designated" sources of support (those created by intervention) substitute for "natural" sources? Not many well-designed experiments have attempted to answer such questions, and those that have been done offer a qualified rather than an unambiguous affirmative conclusion, such as yes but, or maybe, or sometimes.

For example, a field study of adherence to medical regimens for hypertension (Caplan, Cobb, French, Caldwell, & Shinn, 1976) showed that the presence and involvement of a spouse or "true partner" increased adherence. However, a subsequent field experiment to provide such support by choosing a person to take the role of "true partner" did not have the same adherence-enhancing effect (Flowers, 1978). One is reminded of Mark Twain's description of an elderly prudish acquaintance who was trying to learn to curse effectively: "She had the words but not the music."

On the other hand, a few support-enhancing interventions have been unequivocally successful. One such experimental study (Raphael, 1977) involved 200 recently bereaved widows, who were randomly assigned to experimental or control groups. The experimental treatment consisted of support and encouragement initiated by the group leader (experimenter) and continued over the period of 3 months during which the groups met. After 13 months, widows who had been in the experimental groups showed lower overall morbidity than those in the control groups.

A recent large field experiment with unemployed workers also showed positive effects of a supportive intervention, although it could be argued that the experimental treatment went beyond the usual notions of support (Caplan, Vinokur, Price, & van Ryn, 1989). Subjects were recruited from queues at four unemployment compensation offices in Michigan. A population of 628 people was chosen, in approximately equal numbers from three broad occupational categories—professional and managerial, service and clerical, and blue collar. These subjects were formed into experimental groups of 25 persons, with two trainers, a man and a woman, assigned to each group.

Assignment of individuals to an experimental or control group was randomized, and the groups met eight times, for three hours each time, over a two-week period. The experimental treatment had four main components—modeling of social support and positive regard by the trainers, instruction in problem-solving and decision-making processes, learning and practicing the skills of job seeking, and provision of information designed to inoculate job seekers against setbacks in the search.

Interviews at two subsequent times showed that over a period of 30 months the members of experimental groups had significantly higher rates of re-employment, a higher quality of working life in the jobs obtained, a higher proportion working in what they considered their main occupation, and higher monthly earnings. They rated themselves higher in motivation for job seeking and efficacy in it. Not surprising in light of their better employment experience, they also scored higher in self-esteem and subjective quality of life, and lower in such negative affects as anxiety, anger, and depression.

Conclusion

It can be argued that the experimental intervention with the unemployed was not only supportive but empowering; the use of role-playing, for example, to teach effective behavior in an employment interview goes beyond the usual definition of social support. The combination of support with increased control and autonomy is not inappropriate, however. They are related, and not simply.

Interpersonal behaviors considered supportive typically include expressing respect and affection, giving information and advice, and providing tangible assistance. These behaviors can be performed in ways that either increase or decrease the autonomy and control of the individual being "supported." Support, in other words, can consist of teaching, encouraging, and enabling another person, but it can also take the form of constraining, warning against, and doing for another. We would predict greater positive effects for support that is also autonomy-enhancing, and the unemployment experiment involved support of that kind.

A nursing-home experiment conducted more than 10 years ago is almost unique in comparing these two kinds of social support, one that also increased autonomy and another that reduced it (Avorn & Langer, 1982). Seventy-two residents of a nursing home, with an average of 78, were given the task of completing a simple jigsaw puzzle. They were told that there would be four 20-minute practice sessions, after which there would be a trial in which their performance would be timed and evaluated. For the practice sessions, the subjects were divided into three groups—one to receive verbal encouragement as they worked, one to receive direct assistance, and the third to be left to themselves as a control group. Comparative performance before and after the experimental "practice sessions" showed improvement for those who were only encouraged, deterioration for those who were directly assisted during practice, and no change for the control group.

More work is needed on the interactions of supportive and autonomy-developing behavior, but the evidence on both permits an informed conclusion if not yet a scientific generalization: to maximize the quality of life among older people, policy and professional practice must enhance autonomy and control as well as provide support. This is not a task for gerontologists alone; child-rearing, teaching, and the leadership of organizations (when it rises above bureaucracy) require that support be given in ways that increase the abilities of those who receive it.

Providing such support is almost always time-consuming and frequently difficult; it asks for a societal commitment of resources and effort. Nor is this all; even if such commitment were already in place, much has yet to be learned about how best to provide support that also increases autonomy and thus enhances self-efficacy. That learning requires a sustained process of intervention, experimentation, and research evaluation. And as this review suggests, that process has only begun.

References

Antonucci, T. C. (1985). Personal characteristics, social support, and social behavior. In R. H. Binstock & E. Shanas (Eds.), *Handbook of aging and the social sciences* (2nd ed., pp. 94–128). Princeton, NJ: Van Nostrand-Reinhold.

Antonucci, T. C. (1990). Social supports and social relationships. In R. H. Binstock, & L. K. George (Eds.), *Handbook of aging and the social sciences* (3rd ed., pp. 205–225). Orlando, FL: Academic Press.

Antonucci, T. C., Kahn, R. L., & Akiyama, H. (1989). Psychosocial factors and the response to cancer symptoms. In R. Yancik & J. W. Yates (Eds.), *Cancer in the elderly: Approaches to early detection and treatment* (pp. 40-52). New York: Springer Publishing Co.

Avorn, J., & Langer, E. J. (1982). Induced disability in nursing home patients: A controlled trial. *Journal of the American Geriatrics Society, 30*, 397–400.

Babchuk, N. (1978-1979). Aging and primary relations. *International Journal of Aging and Human Development, 9*, 137–151.

Barnes, J. A. (1972). *Social networks*. New York: Addison-Wesley.

Berkman, L. F. (1985). The relationship of social networks and social support to morbidity and mortality. In S. Cohen & S. L. Syme (Eds.), *Social support and health* (pp. 241–262). Orlando, FL: Academic Press.

Berkman, L., & Breslow, L. (1983). *Health and ways of living: Findings from the Alameda County Study*. New York: Oxford University Press.

Berkman, L., & Syme, S. L. (1979). Social networks, host resistance, and mortality: A nine-year follow-up study of Alameda County residents. *American Journal Epidemiology, 109*, 186–204.

Blazer, D. (1982). Social support and mortality in an elderly community population. *American Journal of Epidemiology, 115*, 684–694.

Cantor, M. H. (1979). Neighbors and friends: An overlooked resource in the informal support system. *Research on Aging, 1*, 434–463.

Caplan, R. D., Cobb, S., French, J. R. P., Jr., Caldwell, J. R., & Shinn, M. (1976). *Adhering to medical regimens: Pilot experiments in patient education and social support*. Ann Arbor, MI: The Institute for Social Research.

Caplan, R. D., Cobb, S., French, J. R. P., Jr., Harrison, R. V., & Pinneau, S. R., Jr. (1980). *Job demands and worker health: Main effects and occupational differences*. Ann Arbor, MI: Institute for Social Research.

Caplan, R. D., Vinokur, A. D., Price, R. H., & van Ryn, M. (1989). Job seeking, reemployment, and mental health: A randomized field experiment in coping with job loss. *Journal of Applied Psychology, 74*(5), 759–769.

Cobb, S. (1976). Social support as a moderator of life stress. *Psychosomatic Medicine, 38*, 300–314.

Cobb, S., & Kasl, S. V. (1977). *Termination: The consequences of job loss*. Cincinnati, OH: DHEW (NIOSH) Publication No. 77-224.

Eckerdt, D. J. (1987). Retirement. In G. L. Maddox (Ed.), *The encyclopedia of aging* (pp. 577–580). New York: Springer Publishing Co.

Eckerdt, D. J., Baden, L., Bosse, R., & Dibbs, E. (1983). The effects of retirement on physical health. *American Journal of Public Health, 73*, 779–783.

Fischer, A., Jackson, R., Stueve, C., Gerson, K., & Jones, L. (1977). *Networks and places: Social relations in the urban setting*. New York: The Free Press.

Flowers, R. (1978). *Effects of social support on adherence to therapeutic regimens*. Unpublished doctoral dissertation. University of Michigan, Ann Arbor, MI.

French, J. R. P., Jr., Caplan, R. D., & Harrison, R. V. (1982). *The mechanisms of job stress and strain*. Chichester: John Wiley & Sons.

Harary, F. (1969). *Graph theory*. New York: Addison-Wesley.

Harris, L., & Associates (1981). *Aging in the eighties: America in transition*. Washington, DC: The National Council on the Aging.

Haynes, S., Feinleib, M., & Kannel, W. (1980). The relationship of psychosocial factors to coronary heart disease in the Framingham Study. III Eight year incidence of coronary heart disease. *American Journal of Epidemiology, 111*, 37–58.

Haynes, S. G., McMichael, A. J., & Tyroler, H. D. (1977). The relationship of normal involuntary retirement to early mortality among U. S. rubber workers. *Social Science and Medicine, 11*, 105–114.

Helsing, K., Szklo, M., & Comstock, G. (1981). Factors associated with mortality after widowhood. *American Journal of Public Health, 71*, 802–809.

Heyman, D., & Gianturco, D. 91973). Long-term adaptation by the elderly to bereavement. *Journal of Gerontology, 28*(3), 359-362.

House, J. S. (1981). *Work, stress, and social support*. Reading, MA: Addison-Wesley.

House, J. S., & Kahn, R. L. (1985). Measures and concepts of social support. In S. Cohen & S. L. Syme (Eds.), *Social support and health* (pp. 83-108). Orlando, FL: Academic Press.

House, J. S., Landis, K. R., & Umberson, D. (1988). Social relationships and health. *Annual Review of Sociology, 14*, 293-318.

House, J. S., Robbins, C., & Metzner, H. (1982). The association of social relationships and activities with mortality: Prospective evidence from the Tecumseh Community Health Study. *American Journal of Epidemiology, 116*, 123-140.

House, J. S., & Wells, J. A. (1978). Occupational stress, social support, and health. In A. McLean, G. Black, & M. Colligan (Eds.), *Reducing occupational stress: Proceedings of a conference*. U. S. Department of Health, Education and Welfare, HEW (NIOSH) Publication No. 78-140.

Janis, I. L. (1983). The role of social support in adherence to stressful decisions. *American Psychologist, 38*, 143-160.

Kahana, E. (1982). A congruence model of person-environment interaction. In M. P. Lawton, P. G. Windley, & T. O. Byerts (Eds.), *Aging and the environment: Theoretical approaches* (pp. 97-121). New York: Springer Publishing Co.

Kahn, R. L. (1979). Aging and social support. In M. W. Riley (Ed.), *Aging from birth to death* (pp. 77-91). Boulder, CO: Westview Press.

Kahn, R. L., & Antonucci, T. C. (1984). *Social supports of the elderly: Family/friends/professionals*. Final report to the National Institute on Aging, Grant No. AG01632-01.

Kahn, R. L., & Byosiere, P. (1992). Stress in organizations. In M. D. Dunnette & L. M. Hough (Eds.), *Handbook of industrial and organizational psychology* (2nd ed., vol. 3, pp. 571-650). Palo Alto, CA: Consulting Psychologists Press.

Karasek, R. A., Triantis, K. P., & Chandhry, S. S. (1982). Coworker and supervisor support as moderators of associations between task characteristics and mental strain. *Journal of Occupational Behavior, 3*, 181-200.

Kasl, S. V. (1984). Stress and health. *Annual Review of Public Health, 5*, 319-341.

Kraus, S., & Lilienfeld, A. M. (1959). Some epidemiologic aspects of the high mortality rates in the young widowed group. *Journal of Chronic Disease, 10*, 207-217.

LaRocco, J. M., House, J. S., & French, J. R. P., Jr. (1980). Social support, occupational stress, and health. *Journal of Health and Social Behavior, 21*, 202–216.

Lawton, M. P. 91983). Environment and other determinants of well-being in older persons. *The Gerontologist, 23*, 349–357.

March, L. (1912). Some researches concerning the factors of mortality. *Journal of the Statistical Society, London Journal Series A, 75*(5), 505–538.

Markides, K. S., Liang, J., & Jackson, J. S. (1990). Race ethnicity, and aging: Conceptual and methodological issues. In R. H. Binstock, & L. K. George (Eds.), *Handbook of aging and the social sciences* (3rd ed., pp. 112–129). Orlando, FL: Academic Press.

Martin, J., & Doran, A. (1966). Evidence concerning the relationship between health and retirement. *Sociological Review, 14*, 329.

Medalie, J., & Goldbourt, V. (1976). Angina pectoris among 10,000 men: II. Psychosocial and other risk factors as evidenced by a multivariate analyses of a five year incidence study. *American Journal of Medicine, 60*, 910–921.

Minkler, M. (1985). Social support and health of the elderly. In S. Cohen & S. L. Syme (Eds.), *Social support and health* (pp. 199-216). Orlando, FL: Academic Press.

Parkes, C. M., Benjamin, B., & Fitzgerald, B. G. (1969). A broken heart: A statistical study of increased mortality among widows. *British Medical Journal, 1*, 740–743.

Price, R. H. (1992). Psychosocial impact of job loss on individuals and families. *Current Directions in Psychological Science, 1*(1), 9–11.

Raphael, B. (1977). Preventive intervention with the recent bereaved. *Archives of General Psychiatry, 34*, 1450–1454.

Rees, W. P., & Lutkins, S. G. (1967). Mortality of bereavement. *British Medical Journal, 4*, 13–16.

Seeman, T. E., & Syme, S. L. (1987). Social networks and coronary artery disease. *Psychosomatic Medicine, 41*, 340–353.

Shanas, E. (1979). The family as a social support system in old age. *The Gerontologist, 19*, 169–174.

Stokes, R. G., & Maddox, G. L. (1967). Some social factors on retirement adaptation. *Journal of Gerontology, 22*, 329–333.

Turner, B. J., Keller, R. C., & House, J. S. (1991). Factors facilitating adjustment to unemployment: Implications for intervention. *American Journal of Community Psychology, 19*, 521–542.

Veroff, J., Douvan, E., & Kulka R. (1981). *The inner American*. New York: Basic Books.

Ward, R. A. (1985). Informal networks and well-being in later life: A research agenda. *The Gerontologist, 25*, 55–61.

Wellman, B. (1981). Applying network analysis to the study of support. In B. Gottlieb (Ed.), *Social networks and social support*. Beverly Hills: Sage.

Winnbust, J. A. M., Marcelissen, F. H. G., & Kleber, R. J. (1982). Effects of social support in the stressor-strain relationship: A Dutch sample. *Social Science and Medicine, 16,* 475–482.

Wortman, C. B., & House, J. S. (1991). *Widowhood, bereavement, and coping*. Unpublished research proposal, University of Michigan, Institute for Social Research, Ann Arbor, MI.

Chapter 10

Aging Well and Institutional Living: A Paradox?

Margret M. Baltes

The question posed in the title of this chapter is of importance only if long-term care institutions will be an integral part of our future societal structures and institutions. Mainly due to demographic factors, severe chronic impairment and illness will remain a significant characteristic of the next cohorts of elderly. The old-old population will grow faster than the young-old. By 2050, demographic projections suggest that about one-third of the elderly population will be over the age of 80. Thus, because of the sheer increase of the elderly population, the number of the ill and sick elderly will most likely increase. Furthermore, the growing proportion of people living alone in industrialized Western societies, as well as the declining birth rates, may make informal care systems such as family caregivers less available (Myers, 1990). The ongoing need for institutions does not necessarily support the gloomy demographic predictions of the "apocalyptic demography," as Binstock (1992) has called it. It does not deny at all the more optimistic scenarios for the future proposed, for instance, by Fries (1990).

The question of whether institutions can be designed in ways that facilitate "successful aging" or whether institutions and successful aging are contradictory and mutually exclusive seems a valid one and one in need of answer. Society is confronted with a major task of improving the quality of life for the institutionalized elderly. As a consequence, the institutional environment needs to be designed to permit successful aging in order to maintain the highest possible quality of life for elderly even in this living context.

A Model of Successful Aging

Criteria of Success

The notions of successful aging, aging well and other similar terms have recently attracted considerable attention (Baltes, Kohli, & Sames, 1989; Baltes & Baltes, 1990a). This surge has been brought about by research on latent or unused potentials and reserves in old age be it in the cognitive, social, or biological area. This has created optimism about old age and an interest in understanding the conditions under which potentials can be activated and quality and quantity of life increased. Obviously, questions about indicators or criteria for successful aging have been tackled, but are far from being resolved. Researchers have become aware that single-criterion solutions are obsolete. Instead the quest is for an *array of criteria*—including quantitative and qualitative as well as subjective and objective criteria (see i.e., Baltes & Baltes, 1990a; Ryff, 1989). Figure 10.1 summarizes the most often mentioned criteria defining the goals or standards towards which successful aging is aimed.

It seems that a general agreement on the priority or weight of these criteria can never be reached. This is so because goals or outcomes of successful aging are dependent not only on scientific knowledge but also on social and cultural norms and values. This suggests that the goals of aging are culture-specific, even subgroup-specific within a culture and subject to change concomitant with changes in norms, values, and knowledge. We propose, therefore, to characterize successful aging as the process(es) of reaching the criteria or goals, which, in turn, then ensure the maintenance of quality of life.

Examples of Indicators of Successful Aging

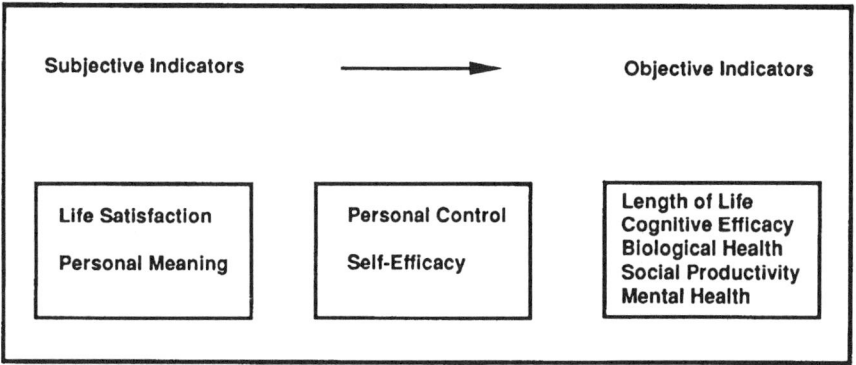

FIGURE 10.1 Examples of indicators of successful aging used in the literature ranging from rather subjective to more objective criteria.

Successful Aging from a Process-Oriented Perspective

Baltes and Carstensen (in preparation) have argued that both theory and empirical research about successful aging might benefit from a shift in perspective. The shift from a product- or outcome-oriented to a process-oriented perspective would produce a change in research questions away from a concentration on *what* is successful aging to focusing on *how* is it achieved. Looking more intently for strategies or mechanisms that facilitate successful aging and not exclusively for the goals or outcomes defining successful aging might allow us to overcome the deadlock in this research domain (see Baltes & Carstensen, in preparation). The model of selective optimization with compensation (Baltes & Baltes, 1990b) is an attempt to specify processes that facilitate successful aging in light of losses and deficits, regardless of the environmental context.

The Model of Selective Optimization with Compensation

In the model proposed by Baltes and Baltes (1990b), successful aging is facilitated via three components or processes, selection, compensation, and optimization. These three components taken by themselves are not new but have not previously been proposed in concert. Their activation and interplay guarantee successful management of the ups and downs of aging and are based on three major phenomena of human aging. First is an increasing negative balance between gains and losses. Development at any phase in the life cycle encompasses both gains and losses. The dynamic between gains and losses in old age, however, becomes more pressing and demanding because losses start to outnumber gains.

The second phenomenon is the existence of plasticity or latent reserves that can be activated, and of limits to these reserves. Although there are large unused potentials that can be activated given age-friendly environments, there is at the same time increasing biological vulnerability, which reduces the scope and breadth of existing reserves. Plasticity and its constraints become particularly salient as the balance between gains and losses tips toward losses with advancing old age. In the face of the many losses with aging, an elderly person may have to use his or her reserves to their limits and, thus, be increasingly in need of supportive, less-demanding environments to achieve successful adaptation.

Finally, development and aging involve a process of specialization and individuation. The considerable heterogeneity in the elderly illustrates this life-long process (Schaie, 1983, 1990). The effects of genetic and learning history as well as environmental history accumulate over time and contribute to another particularity of old age, namely an increase in diverse patterns of pathologies modulating the course of normal aging (Rowe & Kahn, 1987).

A model of successful aging needs to take into account both gains *and* losses in order to reflect the enormous adaptive performance required of the elderly. The Selective Optimization with Compensation (SOC) model describes three processes facilitating this adaptive task.

Definition of the Three Processes. An example from real life will serve to introduce the three processes of the SOC model. In a television interview, Arthur Rubinstein was once asked about the secret that ensured his ability to remain such an accomplished pianist in his old age. Rubinstein, jokingly or not, explained that he has restricted his repertoire (selection), practices the fewer pieces more often (optimization) and uses a trick to cover up the loss in the flexibility of his fingers; he slows down just before fast movements, thereby creating the impression of playing faster than he actually does (compensation).

In general, then, *selection* refers to an increasing restriction of one's life world to fewer domains of functioning as a consequence of or in anticipation of losses in personal and environmental resources. Selection may mean avoidance of one life domain, goal, task, or activity altogether or it can mean a restriction in domains, tasks, or goals within one domain. Thus, an elderly person managing a chronic illness might avoid and give up the domain of sexuality altogether, might cut down on goals and involvements in the social network at large, but might make no changes in the domain of family involvement. It is the adaptive task of the person to concentrate on and select those domains, tasks, goals, and expectations that are of high priority, a process that involves a convergence of environmental demands, individual motivations, skills, and biological capacity.

Selection can be either proactive or reactive. Proactively, the person can monitor his or her functioning, predict future changes and losses (e.g., death of the spouse), and make efforts to search for tasks and domains that will remain intact after losses. Selection is reactive when unpredicted or sudden changes force the person to make a choice or when the environment sets limits, like it does in long-term care institutions. In addition, selection can reflect active behavior changes initated by the person (i.e., choosing to stay committed in the social arena) or passive adjustment (accepting the assistance offered or avoiding driving a car).

Compensation, the second component factor facilitating adaption to losses, becomes operative when specific behavioral capacities or skills are lost or reduced below the level required for adequate functioning. Compensatory efforts can be automatic or planned. If a domain is defined by a large number of activities and means and, thus, is well elaborated, the person will not experience much trouble in counterbalancing or compensating for a specific behavioral deficiency. If the deficiency is large in scope (i.e., paralysis) or if the domain and goal is defined by one or very few activities, compensation will be more difficult. If, for instance, a farmer defines his work domain only by tending to his fields, it will be hard for him to compensate for an impairment, such as a loss of vision or severe arthritis, that hampers mobility. If, however, he defines his work domain by a number of additional activities aside from tending the fields, he may compensate for his impairment by becoming a gardener in his backyard or by teaching his children about farming.

Compensation is not necessarily dependent on already existing activities or means. Compensation might sometimes require the acquisition of new skills or new means not yet in a person's repertoire. An avid reader of literature who becoms blind might learn Braille in order to continue reading literature or might be diverted to listening to "books on tape."

The component of compensation, thus, differs from selection in that the target, the domain, the task, or the goal is maintained, but other means are selected to compensate for a behavioral deficiency in order to maintain or optimize prior functioning. The element of compensation involves aspects of both the mind and technology. Psychological compensatory efforts include, for example, the use of new mnemonic strategies (including external memory aids) when internal memory mechanics or strategies prove insufficient. A hearing aid is an example of compensation by means of technology. The world of the handicapped is full of technical means that compensate for impairments and make a more or less independent and successful life possible. In addition to technical means, human means are often needed to compensate as well. In this sense, the assistance of a hand or arm when walking, an aide to do the cooking, or a companion to do the writing may by compensatory means, which enable the elderly to pursue his or her life as fully as possible. Thus, selection and compensation guarantee, foremost, the maintenance of functioning. They also participate, however, in optimizing functioning.

Optimization, the third component factor, reflects the view of plasticity; that is, aging also represents a time of growth, enrichment, and engagement. Elderly persons may still augment reserves or resources and maximize their chosen life courses with regard to both quantity and quality of life through the optimizing strategies of practice, training, or other attempts at improvement. These optimizing strategies may relate to further development of already existing goals and expectations (see the example of Rubinstein) or may reflect new goals and expectations in line with developmental tasks of the third phase of life (such as acceptance of one's own finality). Without a doubt, the process of optimization—the opportunity to practice, train, etc.—is contingent to a large extent on stimulating and enhancing environmental conditions (Lawton, 1987; Riley, this volume; Rosenmayr, 1983).

It seems important to realize that, in old age, optimization will often have to occur in a situation of restraints or losses. Thus "optimal" will always be constrained by what is possible. There is not one ideal or one standard for what is optimal; it will always be gauged against the possibilities of a specific person with specific personal and environmental resources and reserves. Let us now ask the question of whether the processes of selection, compensation and optimization can be activated in institutions. Will elderly persons be able, and will the institution be designed, to select, compensate, and optimize?

Successful Aging in Institutions

Institutions and Selection

Ideally, entering an institution is the result of a decision to select a low-demanding environment that provides compensatory support for weaknesses and lost competencies. If selecting an institution is part of successful aging, such moves should have positive effects. What is known about the effects of institutionalization and relocation?

When reviewing the literature on this topic (for a more detailed account see Baltes, Wahl, & Reichert, 1991), it seems fair to conclude that institutionalization reflects selection only under certain conditions. As early as 1977, Schulz and Brenner attempted to resolve the equivocal findings in terms of the degree of controllability and predictability of the move by the elderly. When the elderly can control and predict their move, positive effects are more likely. Thus, institutionalization may, indeed, have positive effects and be part of successful aging when and if the selection process is under the control of the elderly or at least expected by them.

Institutions and Compensation

Compensation is required when skills are waning or lost altogether and other means and avenues are needed to reach the intended goals, or expectations. The question, therefore, is whether residents need compensatory means and whether the institutional environment provides such compensatory means to the residents.

Summarizing the empirical literature with regard to the existence of needs on the part of elderly entering or living in institutions (see also

Baltes, Wahl, & Reichert, 1991), two major needs for compensation are revealed. Everyday competencies that are critical for maintaining an independent life in the community seem to be, on average, significantly reduced both before and after institutionalization and are in need of compensation. Aside from person-related weaknesses, there are weaknesses, losses, and limitations in the social network and the informal care system of the elderly. For instance, caregivers often express relief after a family member is institutionalized, reflecting the institution's role in compensating for exhausted support in the family system.

Does the institution provide technical, medical, and human assistance and thus facilitate compensatory efforts? On a microecological level, research on the conditions for dependency of the elderly in institutions (for reviews see Baltes, 1988; Baltes & Reisenzein, 1986; Baltes & Wahl, 1987, 1991) demonstrates how the process of compensation can operate in the social interactions between elderly residents and staff.

Specifically, the behavioral stream associated with dependence and independence of elderly residents in the social world of nursing homes has been studied by observing interactions between residents and staff members during daily routines over a period of 2 to 3 weeks in quite diverse institutional settings. To date, about 230 elderly and their interaction partners have been observed (for a summary of details see Baltes, 1988, 1994). Analyzing these detailed observations of interaction patterns between elderly residents and staff, a "dependency-support script" as well as an "independence-ignore script" can be seen as dominating the institutional world: Dependent self-care behaviors are followed most likely by social actions and attention, independent behaviors are most likely ignored (see Figure 10.2). Thus, the staff provides assistance that represents a compensatory mechanism for the elderly to accomplish self-care activities. Whether these compensatory mechanisms are, indeed, needed is a different question. More often than not, they are provided based on the expectation, rather than real existence, of incompetence in the elderly (Reichert, 1993).

On the macro-level, evidence dating back two decades supports the facilitating and hindering influences of environments' physical characteristics on behaviors of the elderly (e.g., Pastalan & Carson, 1970; Lawton, 1977; 1980). Not surprisingly, environmental designers and architects of special housing for the elderly have always placed their major emphasis on creating environmental prosthetics (Parmelee & Lawton, 1990). In this sense, long-term care institutions can be

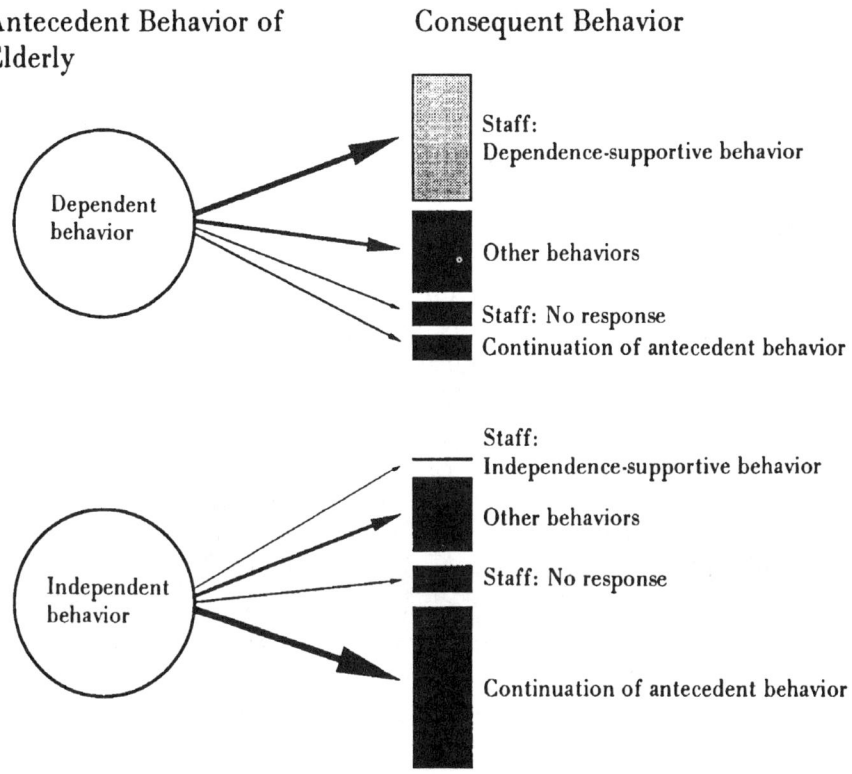

FIGURE 10.2 The dependence-support script in nursing homes: Dependent behavior of the elderly is firmly linked to supportive and reinforcing behavior of staff. Independent behavior, in contrast, is ignored (data from M. Baltes & Wahl, 1991).

described as relatively nondemanding and secure living spaces with rather easy access to a number of services and aids that may be used by the elderly to compensate for losses and weaknesses. Aside from compensation, however, there may be room for improvement or activation of latent reserves (Baltes, 1988) and thus for optimization in long-term care settings.

Institutions and Optimization

For an elderly person, being involved in selection and compensation aimed at successful aging means seeking opportunities to not only maintain but also to optimize living. In the face of decreased competencies in the institutionalized elderly, it seems plausible that domains, skills, or goals selected for optimization should serve both physical survival and psychological well-being, thereby enhancing quantity and quality of life, the essence of successful aging. Four domains for optimization can be discerned in the literature: health, life mastery (personal control), independence/autonomy, and social relationships.

A great number of intervention studies have attested to the potential for change *in health* status and the effect such changes can have for the optimization of residents' functioning. Physical exercise has been shown to improve biological functioning and well-being (for a review see Baltes & Reichert, 1992; Krauss Whitbourne, 1985); cognitive intervention increases well-being (Dittman-Kohli, 1986) and can help to ameliorate the impact of dementia on daily living (Wiedl, Schöttke, & Gediga 1987); behavioral interventions are shown to reverse chronic dependent behaviors and thus increase autonomy (see Mosher-Ashley 1986–1987; Smyer, Zarit, & Qualls, 1990).

Personal control has been labeled a basic need by Rodin (1986, see also Baltes & Baltes, 1986; Langer, 1983). Yet institutions for the aged are still very much associated with what Goffman (1961) called the "total institution," a setting that seems to be diametrically opposed to personal control. The initial studies of control-enhancing interventions by Langer and Rodin (1976; Rodin & Langer, 1977) have become classics despite, or perhaps because of, the often raised methodological criticisms (Munson, 1989; Schultz, 1976). But even if these interventions did not raise personal control beliefs (which we don't know because they were never assessed), they demonstrated dramatic effects on activity level, health, and life satisfaction.

Moreover, the research on dependency alluded to before suggests that the dependence-support script enables elderly residents to have instrumental, albeit passive control over social contact. When elderly residents engage in dependent behaviors (e.g., requests for bodily care), these elicit prompt and reliable responses on the part of the staff, involving not only care but also social attention. Therefore, although dependent behavior may result in a diminution of certain self-care behaviors, it provides elderly nursing home residents with a strategy for exerting control over their social environment, improving their social contacts, and avoiding isolation (Baltes, 1988; Baltes & Wahl, 1987). This is not to say that control might not be better attached to independent behaviors or, in other words, that as much autonomy as possible should be encouraged even within a prosthetic setting.

Independence/autonomy. For this reason, Baltes, Neumann and Zank have sought to change the institutional context from one that focuses on the dependence-support script to one that embraces an independence-support script. To activate such a script, a training program for caregivers was directed at creating greater sensitivity of the importance of a balance between dependency and autonomy (Parmelee & Lawton, 1990) for the elderly. Results confirm the malleability of social environmental conditions (caregiver behavior) responsible for a great amount of the dependency in the elderly. Specifically, long-standing staff behavior can be changed to optimize conditions supporting autonomy for elderly residents. Staff, when given the required skills (e.g., insight into aging conditions and behavior management strategies), are apt and willing to pay attention to and reinforce the strengths and competencies of the elderly rather than their weaknesses. The autonomy-enhancing perspective is readily adopted and in line with the helping role when helping is understood as "help toward self-help."

Social contacts and activities. Just as aging is commonly associated with pathology and helplessness, it is also frequently associated with loneliness (Baltes & Tesch-Römer, in press). Obviously, the sole criterion is not mere quantity of social interactions (Greene & Monahan, 1982; Harel, 1981; Parmelee, 1982; Tesch, Whitbourne, & Nehrke, 1981). Differentiation between quantity and quality of social interactions (see Quevillon & Lee, 1983), self- and other-initiated interactions (see Parmelee, 1982), and peripheral and close contacts (Carstensen, 1991) have been proposed as significant dimensions.

Intervention research aimed at increasing and optimizing the level of social activity and social interaction of residents by manipulating and rearranging the institutional environment has a long tradition (Carstensen, 1987). Overall, these efforts can be judged to have minimal effects of short duration. Carstensen (1987, 1991) provides an explanation for the lack of increase in social interactions in terms of selection processes enacted by the elderly (the socioemotional selectivity theory). She demonstrates that elderly people are not interested in increasing just any contact, but only contacts that promise emotional benefits.

Discussion and Conclusion

The aim of the present chapter was to address the question of whether successful aging is possible in long-term care institutions. In answering this question, the model of selective optimization with compensation was presented and empirical support for the possibility of realizing this model in institutions was summarized. The enaction of the three processes, selection, compensation, and optimization is based on a dynamic interplay between person and environmental conditions.

On a macro-level, institutions can be seen, in principle, to create an age-friendly world that facilitates adaptation in that they provide a less demanding physical and social ecology. Elderly in selecting this world reduce the demands of everyday life. They also gain access to a great variety of compensatory means via technological, medical, and social systems that support functioning in the face of diminished reserve capacities. The elderly, because of the decrease in demands from the environment, can invest time and energy in a few selected domains, if the institution provides enhancement possibilities.

On the micro-level, though, a highly *individualized* approach is needed in order not to "over-" or "underdemand" the elderly. Overcompensation is a frequent phenomenon because the general tendency of nursing home staff is to perceive the institutionalized elderly as predominantly weak and helpless. This expectation of incompetence can, in turn, lead to an overemphasis on compensation in long-term care institution. Karuza, Rabinowitz, and Zevon (1986) have described such a professional orientation as reflecting a medical model of helping. According to the medical model, the elderly are responsible neither for the cause nor for the solution of their problems. Karuza et al. argue that a helping model that attributes no responsibility for the occurrence of a problem but full responsibility for its solution to the individual is more desirable because it yields both support and autonomy or control to the elderly residents.

Moreover, staff frequently are the main people with whom institutionalized elders interact (Baltes, 1988). In such cases, any negative expectations and stereotypes on the part of the staff can easily be internalized by the elderly, thus opening the door for negative self-fulfilling prophecies, which, in turn, reinforce staff and societal beliefs (Butler, 1987; Kuypers & Bengtson, 1973). In any case, negative expectations and stereotypes, whether held by the environment or by the elderly, may prevent maintenance of capacities and optimal functioning. Overcompensation for extant or imagined deficits is one such condition.

In contrast, there is risk of "overdemand" when optimization is the target. In the case of health and daily activities, it seems highly appropriate to provide institutionalized elderly with the full range of possibilities for using all their competencies and reserve capacities. However, there are limits to the elderly's reserves, including functional health limitations. Because of large interindividual differences, the guiding principle should be the idea of the "just manageable difficulty level" (Brim, 1988) or Lawton's (1977) environment–person fit model. Both conceptions speak to the expectation that only environmental "press" or demands that are attainable can serve optimization. Beyond that point, environmental press causes stress and may have detrimental rather than beneficial effects for the elderly.

A differential approach with regard to optimization is also necessary in the area of personal agency of the institutionalized elderly. Here, too, limits can be observed. Control enhancement can have negative effects when it leads people to blame themselves for the occurrence of negative events, for example, an accident. Hence, one should bear in mind the possibility that control enhancement may lead to an overload of responsibility and emotional stress in the face of health-related events. Attention also has to be paid to the discrepancy between ability to control and possibility of control (Schulz, 1976). If the setting provides no opportunity to exert control, any effort at control enhancement will have negative effects.

Thus, successful aging can mean different things for different people. We should not define success against an absolute standard. Instead, it is the adaptation level of individual people measured against a specific environment and its demands that determines success. The "just manageable difficulty" standard (Brim, 1988) differs from person to person and needs to be balanced against each person's resources and competence level for successful optimization.

The concept of person–environment fit thus gains special importance. Parmelee and Lawton (1990) introduced the idea of a basic dialectic between security and autonomy. Environments, including institutional settings, need to provide as much security as necessary with as much autonomy as possible. Although the competence level of the elderly person seems to be the critical factor in deciding how much autonomy versus security, often no objective assessment of that level is made. On the contrary, meaningful assessment is replaced all too often by conventional negative stereotyping and expectations of incompetence. As long as this is the case, care runs the risk of being "excessive" and thus harming rather than helping elderly residents. Ensuring quality of life in institutions requires striking a balance between autonomy and security, not necessarily an easy organizational task, but one that is nonetheless vitally important for maximizing successful aging.

ACKNOWLEDGMENTS

Some parts of this chapter have been discussed previously in Baltes, Wahl, & Reichert (1991). I would like to thank Ann Horgas and Ron Abeles for a careful and critical reading of this paper.

References

Baltes, M. M. (1988). The etiology and maintenance of dependency in the elderly: Three phases of operant research. *Behavior Therapy, 19*, 301–319.
Baltes, M. M. (in press). Dependencies in old age: Gains and losses. *Current Directions in Psychological Science.*
Baltes, M. M., & Baltes, P. B. (1986). *The psychology of control and aging.* Hillsdale, NJ: Lawrence Erlbaum.
Baltes, P. B. & Baltes, M. M. (Eds.) (1990a). *Successful aging: Perspectives from the behavioral sciences.* New York: Cambridge University Press.
Baltes, P. B. & Baltes, M. M. (1990b). Selective optimization with compensation. In P. B. Baltes & M. M. Baltes (Eds.), *Successful aging: Perspectives from the behavioral sciences* (pp. 1–34). New York: Cambridge University Press.
Baltes, M. M. & Tesch-Römer, C. (in press). Einsamkeit im Alter. (Loneliness in the elderly). In D. Todt (Ed.), *Zur Natur sozialer Beziehungsgefüge* (The nature of social relational systems). Berlin: Parey.
Baltes, M. M., & Carstensen, L.L. (in preparation). The process of successful aging.
Baltes, M. M., Kohli, M., & Sames, R. (1989). *Erfolgreiches Altern: Bedingungen und Variationen.* Bern: Hans Huber.
Baltes, M.M., Neumann, E.M., & Zank, S. (in press). Maintenance and rehabilitation of independence in old age: An intervention program for staff. *Psychology and Aging.*
Baltes, M. M. & Reichert, M. (1992). Successful aging: A product of biological factors, environmental quality, and behavioral competence. In J. George & S. Ebrahim (Eds.), *Health care for older women* (pp. 236–256). Oxford: Oxford University Press.
Baltes, M. M., & Reisenzein, R. (1986). The social world in long-term care

institutions: Psychosocial control toward dependency. In M. M. Baltes & P. B. Baltes (Eds.), *The psychology of control and aging* (pp. 315–343). Hillsdale, NJ: Erlbaum.

Baltes, M. M., & Wahl, H.-W. (1987). Dependence in aging. In L. L. Carstensen & B. A. Edelstein (Eds.), *Handbook of clinical gerontology* (pp. 204–221). New York: Pergamon Press.

Baltes, M.M., & Wahl, H.-W. (1991). The behavior system of dependency in the elderly: Interactions with the social environment. In M. Ory, R.P. Abeles, & P.D. Lipman (Eds.), *Aging, health, and behavior* (pp. 83–106). Beverly Hills, CA: Sage.

Baltes, M.M., Wahl, H.-W., & Reichert, M. (1991). Successful aging in long term-care institutions? *Annual Review of Gerontology and Geriatrics, 11*, 311–337.

Binstock, R. (1992). *Implications of aging for the individual and society.* Paper presented at the Conference on Aging: The quality of life. Washington, DC, February.

Brim, O.G., Jr. (1988). Losing and winning: The nature of ambition in everyday life. *Psychology Today, 9*, 48–52.

Butler, R. N. (1987). Ageism. In G. L. Maddox (Ed.), *The encyclopedia of aging* (pp. 22–23). New York: Springer Publishing Co.

Carstensen, L. L. (1987). Age-related changes in social activity. In L. L. Carstensen & B. A. Edelstein (Eds.), *Handbook of clinical gerontology* (pp. 222–237). New York: Pergamon Press.

Carstensen, L.L. (1991). Socioemotional selectivity theory: Social activitiy in life-span context. In K. W. Schaie & M. P. Lawton (Eds.), *Annual Review of Gerontology and Geriatrics* (Vol. 11, pp. 195–217). New York: Springer Publishing Co.

Dittmann-Kohli, F. (1986). Die trainingsbedingte Veränderung von Leistungsselbstbild und kognitiven Fähigkeiten im Alter. (Changes in the perception of one's cognitive functioning and self). *Zeitschrift für Gerontologie, 19*, 309–322.

Fries, J. F. (1990). Medical perspectives upon successful aging. In P. B. Baltes & M. M. Baltes (Eds.), *Successful aging: Perspectives from the behavioral sciences* (pp. 35–49). New York: Cambridge University Press.

Goffman, E. (1961). *Asylums: Essays on the social situation of mental patients and other inmates.* Garden City, NY: Doubleday.

Greene, V. L., & Monahan, D. J. (1982). The impact of visitation on patients well-being in nursing homes. *The Gerontologist, 22*, 418–423.

Harel, Z. (1981). Quality of care, congruence and well-being among institutionalized aged. *The Gerontologist, 21*, 523–531.

Karuza, J., Rabinowitz, V. D., & Zevon, M. A. (1986). Implications of control and responsibility on helping the aged. In M. M. Baltes & P. B. Baltes (Eds.), *The psychology of control and aging* (pp. 373–396). Hillsdale, NJ: Erlbaum.

Krauss Whitbourne, S. (1985). *The aging body.* New York: Springer Publishing Co.

Kuypers, J. A,. & Bengtson, V. L. (1973). Social breakdown and competence. *Human Development, 16,* 181–201.

Langer, E. J. (1983). *The psychology of control.* New York: Sage.

Langer, E. J., & Rodin, J. (1976). The effects of choice and enhanced personal responsibility for the aged: A field experiment in an institutional setting. *Journal of Personality and Social Psychology, 34,* 191–198.

Lawton, M. P. (1977). The impact of the environment on aging and behavior. In J. E. Birren & K. W. Schaie (Eds.), *Handbook of the psychology of aging* (1st ed., pp. 276–301). New York: Van Nostrand Reinhold.

Lawton, M. P. (1980). *Environment and aging.* Monterey, CA: Brooks/Cole.

Lawton, M. P. (1987). Environment and the need satisfaction of the aging. In L. L. Carstensen & B. A. Edelstein (Eds.), *Handbook of clinical gerontology* (pp. 33–40). New York: Pergamon Press.

Mosher-Ashley, P. M. (1986–87). Procedural and methodological parameters in behavioral-gerontological research: A review. *International Journal of Aging and Human Development, 24,* 189–229.

Munson (1989). Control and dependency in residential care settings for the elderly: Perspectives on intervention. In P. S. Fry (Ed.), *Psychological perspectives of helplessness and control in the elderly* (pp. 187–215). Amsterdam: Elsevier.

Myers, G. C. (1990). Demography of aging. In R. H. Binstock, & L. K. George (Eds.), *Handbook of aging and the social sciences* (3rd ed., pp.19–44). New York: Academic Press.

Parmelee, P. A. (1982). Social contacts, social instrumentality, and adjustment of institutionalized aged. *Research on Aging, 4,* 269–280.

Parmelee, P. A., & Lawton, M. P. (1990). The design of special environments for the aged. In J. E. Birren & K. W. Schaie (Eds.), *Handbook of the psychology of aging* (pp. 465–488, 3rd edition). New York: Academic Press.

Pastalan, L. A., & Carson, D. H. (1970). *Spatial behavior of older people.* Ann Arbor: University of Michigan-Wayne State University, Institute of Gerontology.

Quevillon, R. P., & Lee, H. C. (1983). Social involvement as a predictor of subjective well-being among the rural institutionalized aged. *International Journal of Behavioral Geriatrics, 1,* 13–19.

Reichert, M. (1993). *Hilfeverhalten gegenüber alten Menschen: Eine exper-*

imentelle Überprüfung der Rolle von Erwartungen. (Helping behavior towards elderly people: An experimental analysis of expectations). Essen: Blaue Eule.

Rodin, J. (1986). Health, control, and aging. In M. M. Baltes & P. B. Baltes (Eds.), *The psychology of control and aging* (pp. 139–165). Hillsdale, NJ: Erlbaum.

Rodin, J., & Langer, E. (1977). Long-term effects of a control-relevant intervention with the institutionalized aged. *Journal of Personality and Social Psychology, 35,* 897–902.

Rosenmayr, L. (1983). *Die späte Freiheit* (The late freedom). Berlin: Severin & Siedler.

Rowe, J. W., & Kahn, R. L. (1987). Human aging: Usual and successful. *Science, 237,* 143–149.

Ryff, C. D. (1989). Beyond Ponce de Leon and life satisfaction: New directions in quest of successful ageing. *International Journal of Behavioral Development, 12,* 35–55.

Schaie, K. W. (1983). The Seattle Longitudinal Study: A twenty-one year exploration of psychometric intelligence in adulthood. In K. W. Schaie (Ed.), *Longitudinal studies of adult psychological development* (pp. 64–135). New York: Guilford.

Schaie, K. W. (1990). Intellectual development in adulthood. In J. E. Birren & K. W. Schaie (Eds.), *Handbook of the psychology of aging* (3rd Ed., pp. 291–309). New York: Academic Press.

Schulz, R. (1976). The effects of control and predictability on the physical and psychological well-being of the institutionalized aged. *Journal of Personality and Social Psychology, 33,* 563–573.

Schulz, R., & Brenner, G. (1977). Relocation of the aged: A review and theoretical analysis. *Journal of Gerontology, 32,* 323–333.

Smyer, M. A., Zarit, S. H., & Qualls, S. H. (1990). Psychological intervention with the aging individual. In J. E. Birren & K. W. Schaie (Eds.), *Handbook of the psychology of aging* (pp.375–404). New York: Academic Press.

Tesch, S., Whitbourne, S., & Nehrke, M. (1981). Friendship, social interaction and subjective well-being of older men in an institutional setting. *International Journal of Aging and Human Development, 13,* 317–377.

Wiedl, K. H., Schöttke, H., & Gediga, G. (1987). Reserven geistiger Leistungsfähigkeit bei geriatrischen Psychiatriepatienten und Altenheimbewohnern (Reserves of cognitive abilities in geriatric patients and nursing home residents). *Zeitschrift für klinische Psychologie, 16,* 29–42.

Chapter 11

Human Factors and Aging: The Operator-Task Dynamic

Robin A. Barr

Many of us remember when indoor plumbing was by no means universal, when washing clothes involved much more than selecting the right detergent and water temperature, and when adding up the month's bills required mental arithmetic, a sharp pencil, and carrying-over little figures on paper. Quality-of-life has been improved immeasurably by easily-accessible plumbing, automatic washing machines, and affordable, reliable calculators.

These and other daily activities have seen the strong influence of technology. Yet technology can marginalize some lives just as it improves others. Calculators are no use if the contrast in the display is beyond the contrast sensitivity of a user's eyes. Confusing instructions and displays on washing machines can frustrate and intimidate whole

---

This chapter was prepared in my capacity as a government employee. Therefore it is in the public domain.

groups of potential users. A bath tub might as well not be there if the bather cannot step over the side.

The discipline of human factors seeks to improve the match between human capabilities and the demands of the environments in which people live and work. The focus is on equipment, tasks, and other aspects of the physical environment. The discipline has a 50 year history in military and industrial applications. Recently the field has burgeoned into new areas encompassing communication, transportation, rehabilitation, and aging.

Within the field, methodologies exist to analyze tasks into component units and to match them to abilities in potential users, to select and train personnel for specialized tasks, and to use existing physical and functional anthropomorphic measurements (tables of normative data on static and dynamic measurements, e.g., height, reach, grip strength, etc.) to aid the design of new equipment. Many of these techniques, data, and procedures are reviewed and described in available handbooks and reference sources (NASA, 1978; Salvendy, 1987; Stoudt, Damon, McFarland, & Roberts, 1965, 1973). However, as Charness and Bosman (1990) and Czaja (1990) have pointed out, data pertaining to older adults in these handbooks and reference sources remain scarce and of questionable quality.

What can human factors offer aging? The single most encompassing answer is that it offers a dynamic conceptualization of the relation between older adults and the tasks and technologies they face. The operator–task dynamic is at the heart of that conceptualization. It is the instrument of change. Human factors researchers seek to enhance performance and eliminate age-associated difficulties in completing everyday tasks by altering that dynamic. Their methods involve training the operator or changing the task conditions. If applied well, human factors techniques can design a calculator that suits older eyes and hands, arrange washing machine instructions so that they assist older users instead of confuse them, and design a bath that permits access to older adults whose mobility is impaired. The topics described below (instrumental activities of daily living, medication adherence, driving, and paid work) give some sense of the diverse areas in which human factors researchers are already seeking ways to change the operator–task dynamic and improve functioning and quality of life among older adults.

Instrumental Activities of Daily Living

The 1986 Functional Limitations Supplement to the National Health Interview Survey indicated that 41.9% of women over the age of 75 report difficulty doing heavy housework and 26.6% report difficulty shopping (Van Nostrand, Furner, & Suzman, 1993). If these figures, and similar numbers for other instrumental activities, are seen as unchangeable they represent a huge cost. Some—often costly—aid is necessary to accomplish the tasks or they do not get done, or, worse, an older adult is injured trying to complete the task. On the other hand, using a human factors framework, these figures represent the result of current values of the operator–task dynamic. If that dynamic is understood, then interventions become possible that improve the fit between the user and the task.

Instrumental activities of daily living (IADLs) previously have been divided only into broad functional categories (e.g., heavy housework, meal preparation; Lawton & Brody, 1969). For a human factors approach to succeed in improving the above statistics, these broad categories must be divisible into a relatively uniform set of demands on the person. If this latter analysis succeeds then interventions to make the demands match the abilities of the operator can also succeed.

To investigate this question, Czaja and her colleagues (Czaja & Nair, 1992; Clark, Czaja, & Weber, 1990) sought to use "task analysis" to identify the demands made by everyday tasks, and those particular aspects of the environment that contribute to problems completing these tasks. They videotaped older men and women performing each of 25 activities, including getting into and out of bed, dressing, grocery shopping, preparing meals, and washing dishes. From the videotapes, the activities were decomposed into (1) components; (2) environmental demands associated with the components; and (3) person-actions generated by the environmental demands. For example, *meal preparation* (an activity), includes as a component *retrieve food from storage*. That component is associated with environmental demands, (e.g., *repositioning an object*) and the environmental demands generate person actions (e.g., *reach*, *lift*). Note that the person actions and environmental demands are not unique to meal preparation.

Certain person-actions were evident across many IADLs. In fact, lifting and lowering actions, together with push/pull actions accounted for about 60% of all actions across all IADLs. Repositioning was the most common environmental demand across IADLs. Therefore, one important requirement for a human factors analysis was satisfied. Despite variation in the equipment used and the situations encountered, common actions and demands were identified that were an important part of the operator–task dynamic.

The physical abilities of these older people varied widely and that variability was reflected in some of the results. For example, the presence of arthritis was associated with difficulties in manipulating objects. Nevertheless common problems were identified across the sample. The most common problem was fatigue. The excessive standing time and physical actions required by meal preparation, grocery shopping, and doing laundry appear responsible.

These findings suggest guidelines for reducing task demands and thereby improving performance. Reducing the need for lifting and lowering, pushing and pulling, and standing should improve performance. Reducing the time needed to complete these tasks will also reduce their burden on older adults. Physical strength training and stamina training are likely to reduce fatigue while completing these tasks. Thus Czaja and her collaborators have revealed ways both to alter operator characteristics (strength and stamina training) and task characteristics (more efficient design) that, in turn, should reduce difficulties with activities of daily living. The results also suggest that human factors methods can be applied successfully to a notoriously vague problem area—instrumental activities of daily life.

Medication Adherence

Adherence to medication schedules is a major problem among older old adults (Kendrick & Bayne, 1982; Park, Morrell, Frieske, & Kincaid, 1992; Parkin & Henney, 1976; Wandless, Mucklow, Smith, & Prudham, 1979). Though the causes of nonadherence are many (Blackwell, 1973; Bloch, Rosenthal, Friedman, & Caldarolla, 1977; Drury, Wade, & Woolf, 1976), recent evidence, using a new measurement technology, has implicated memory problems as a substantial contributor to nonadherence (Leirer, Morrow, Pariante & Sheikh, 1988; Park et al., 1992).

The discovery that memory plays a role in adherence problems implies that such problems may be reduced through cognitive factors interventions. Cognitive factors research (Card, Moran, & Newell, 1983) focuses on analyzing tasks in terms of the cognitive demands they place on operators, and on interventions that better match the task and the cognitive capabilities of the operator. It is a subspecialty of human factors, which deals more generally with physical, sensory, motor, and cognitive functioning and their relation to task characteristics.

Relevant industries have not been slow to recognize the memory burden associated with medication compliance and drug-store shelves offer a selection of aids to assist taking medication. Are these aids effective? A number of organizers sold in drug-stores require that medications be taken out of their initial packaging and placed in compartments in the organizer. The "aid," thus adds a new task—loading—with its own chance of associated error. Indeed Park, Morrell, Frieske, Blackburn, and Birchmore (1991) found that of three organizers tested, two led to significant numbers of loading errors. They recommended only one device as having the potential to increase medication adherence.

If there is an error in the "organizer" approach it is that the inventors of the devices failed to consider how the adherence task was changed by their devices. Human factors methods require that the whole task be considered when any one part of it is changed. Consistent with this human factors (or more specifically, cognitive factors) emphasis, Leirer, Morrow, Tanke, and Pariante (1991) first identified an environmental demand that causes problems in adherence (need to recall prospectively) and then redesigned the task to eliminate that demand. The investigators used a computer voice mail system to remind older adults to take medications. The adults received a phone call with a prerecorded voice indicating that it was time to take a particular medication. The voice mail system thus removed the need to rely on prospective recall—and it reliably reduced adherence errors.

Driving

Driving is an increasingly important activity for older adults. Large numbers of older adults view continuing to drive as critical to maintaining their quality of life (Persson, 1993). At the start of the 1980s 43% of women over 65 held driving licenses. By the end of the decade 57% held licenses (computed from statistics reported in U.S. Federal Highway Administration, 1981; U.S. Federal Highway Administration, 1990; U.S. Bureau of the Census, 1990). Most men of that age and older do drive (U.S. Federal Highway Administration, 1990).

These trends reflect both cohort changes in driving at younger ages and changes in the residency pattern of older adults. Increasingly older adults live in suburbs (Rosenbloom, 1988). These suburbs have been designed for a population that relies on personal cars. Many developments have no sidewalks. Public transportation is geared toward the journey to and from work rather than grocery shopping, going to a physician's office, or visiting a pharmacy. The placement of such offices and stores relative to most private housing frequently necessitates a trip by car or other vehicle. Specialized transportation services can address only a small part of the mobility needs of this population. The services would be overwhelmed if large numbers of suburban older adults were to stop driving and rely solely on them (Rosenbloom, 1988).

Unfortunately driving fatalities among older adults have increased along with their increased use of cars. On average, a 70 year old is three times as likely to die in a crash of given severity as is a 20 year old. Adults older than 70 are even more vulnerable (Evans, 1988). In the 1980s, deaths among drivers over 65 increased by 43% even as fatalities for the driving population as a whole fell by 8% (Barr, 1991).

The operator–task dynamic in driving involves both the relation between the driver and the car and also the relation between the driver and the external highway environment. Can either cars or the highway environment be better designed to suit older drivers? Can the skills of high-risk older drivers be improved so that they better match the environmental demands of driving? The examples below illustrate two approaches to these questions.

Drivers over 65 years old are over-represented in intersection crashes (Insurance Institute for Highway Safety Facts, 1986). A working hypothesis might be that improvements in intersection design may particularly benefit their crash history. Staplin and Fisk (1991) offer one approach to improving intersection layout that may benefit older drivers. They propose that some older drivers find the information demands at an intersection beyond their cognitive capacity. These demands include: finding which of several signal lights is relevant, paying attention to the relevant signal and ignoring the others, scanning the approach to the intersection to look for approaching traffic, and checking the intended direction of travel to make certain the way is clear and no pedestrians are entering the road. Staplin and Fisk attempted to reduce these demands by indicating on a sign which signal configuration to expect. The sign was placed on the approaches to the intersection.

They provide data to suggest that such advance warning of the kinds of decision needed to determine whether it is safe to make a left turn at an intersection aids both young and older drivers. They also recommend against a particular sign configuration, currently in use at some intersections, that appears especially troublesome for older drivers. The sign states "left turn yield on green" and shows a green filled circle. The problem appears to be that the sign pairs information to yield the right-of-way with a signal that characteristically indicates that it is appropriate to proceed (the green filled circle).

However, a change in highway design is enormously expensive if it is to be implemented at all intersections. Any such change is likely to be implemented gradually and, for the forseeable future, older and younger drivers will continue to confront some intersections that present the same degree of hazard as those of today.

Parasuraman and Nestor (1991) review a number of studies that take an alternative approach to human factors issues involved in driving. The studies together make a preliminary case for the view that selective attention is related to several measures of driving competence. Owsley, Ball and their colleagues (Owsley, Ball, Sloane, Roenker, & Bruni, 1991; Ball, Owsley, Sloane, Roenker, & Bruni, in press) have continued in that tradition, using a concept termed "useful field of view" (UFOV) (Sanders, 1970). UFOV measures aspects of perception and attention as well as reaction time.

In two separate studies (Owsley et al., 1991; Ball et al., in press) a strong relationship has emerged between performance on this test and at-fault driving crashes among samples of drivers aged 55 and over. That relationship establishes the case that UFOV measures component skills involved in driving. The test offers promise as an assessment instrument.

However, the major promise of this approach lies in its potential to reduce the mismatch between these perceptual and attentional skills in at-risk older drivers and the driving environment they encounter. Ball and her colleagues have shown one way to change this dynamic. They found that UFOV could be expanded through training and that the training-related expansion in field was retained over a 6-month testing interval (Ball, Beard, Roenker, Miller, & Ball, 1988). It remains to be determined whether this change in the dynamic reduces driving crashes.

Work and Aging

Although research on older workers contributed early to the field of human factors and aging (McFarland, 1943; Murrell, 1962; Welford, 1958), the topic received scant attention in the ensuing 30 years. However, the younger workforce of that era is now aging and this latest demographic trend will likely promote new studies in how to make a middle-aged and older workforce more productive (Warr, 1993).

The earlier wave of research focused on the then dominant kinds of employment. Thus, Heron and Chown (1961) reported that in manufacturing industries, workers over 45 were more likely to move to easier work or leave the industry altogether. Murrell (1962) observed that middle-aged and older workers were most likely to leave jobs putting heavy demands on perception.

In the succeeding 30 years both the distribution of jobs and the nature of the work in particular jobs has changed. Hard, manual labor that was characteristic of agriculture and manufacturing is now very much less common within these industries. In turn, manufacturing and agriculture now account for a smaller percentage of the workforce than service-related work. Job-related skills are now more important than physical strength and stamina. These skills can be performance-oriented, cognitive, or interpersonal. As the workforce is aging, the issues of design for older workers in these new jobs become concerns related to productivity and output for the workforce as a whole.

The few examples described here focus on ways in which the operator–task environment can be assessed and improved with regard to older workers. Excellent reviews of the age and employment literature can be found in Warr (1993) and in Sterns, Laier, and Dorsett (1993).

Increasingly work tasks involve computer operations. Though the redesign of tasks into computer operations brings numerous advantages (in speed of operation, record keeping, and error-checking), such redesign can also place heavier cognitive demands on the computer operator. These tasks require that operators master new procedures and a new lexicon, and force them to rely on mental models and memory to retrieve documents or access information. Czaja and Sharit (in press, a,b) investigated performance and stress reactions to computer tasks of varying complexity as a function of age. The tasks were chosen to be representative of jobs that are widely performed in industrial settings (in increasing order of complexity, data entry, file modification, and inventory management). The subjects had varying amounts of computer experience and were novices in the particular computer tasks they were given. In general, the older subjects both performed more poorly than the younger subjects and showed evidence of heightened stress reactions. Performance was worse, stress reactions were more severe, and age differences were greater in the most complex task (inventory management). These differences are consistent with a broad body of evidence in cognitive aging research identifying a relationship between the size of age differences observed in a task and the complexity of cognitive operations, processes or resources needed to complete that task [e.g., Birren, 1956; Hoyer & Plude, 1982; Salthouse, 1982; see Salthouse (1991) for an overview].

From a human factors perspective, then, the issue becomes how to reduce the cognitive complexity of a work-related computer task in order to reduce age differences—and improve performance—across the age-spectrum of workers. Providing on-screen cues is potentially effective in reducing these demands. However, such cues also increase the visual complexity of the computer display, and thus, could exacerbate differences in performance. Careful task analyses of such computer-based jobs will identify where demands are particularly high and offer a rationale for selecting the kinds of support that will most facilitate performance. These analyses remain to be done.

Experience accumulates with age. Experience is most often an advantage in work settings, and elsewhere. Indeed Czaja and Sharit (in press a,b) found that self-rated experience with computers was associated with better performance on the computer tasks in their study. One important issue is whether specific job-related experience compensates for possible age-associated declines in job-related abilities. In natural settings, that pattern has been reported several times. Thus, Murrell, Powesland, and Forsaith (1962) found that although older novice British engineering drillers were slower than younger workers, older experienced workers were as fast as younger experienced workers. Among American office workers, Kutscher and Walker (1960) found that performance improved slightly with increasing age. However, this trend was confounded with amount of experience. Younger experienced workers were as effective as older experienced workers.

The nature of work changes over time. In some professions obsolescence is a very potent underside to the otherwise positive benefits of expertise. For example, Dubin (1990) defined the "half-life" of knowledge in a given profession as that time after which only 50% of acquired knowledge is applicable. In an acknowledgeably unscientific survey of different professionals, he reports half-lives ranging from 8 years in physics, economics, and sports physiology to 1 to 2 years in computers and software systems.

Thus, an issue confronting anyone employed in a technology-dependent job is the ability to adapt to new technologies and associated work tasks as they are introduced into the work setting. For human factors researchers, the issue is how to identify ways to facilitate the introduction of these new tasks and technologies in order to capitalize on the existing skills of the workforce. Techniques of task-analysis can contribute both to designing the task so that it optimally fits older operators, and designing training programs so that they optimally benefit older trainees (Sterns & Doverspike, 1989). Can older workers adapt to these new technologies as well as younger workers? Must extra steps be taken to ensure that workers of all ages can gain the most from such new technologies? Unfortunately little is known now that can directly answer these important questions.

Summary

Human factors research has enormous potential across a variety of domains to identify the task components and environmental demands that create most difficulty for older adults. The above examples illustrate what progress has been achieved and where more progress is needed. Within the human factors framework older adults' performance is the product of current values of the operator-task dynamic. By changing the values in that dynamic, the discipline can do much to dispel the myth that older adults are necessarily disadvantaged in the tasks of daily life. Through altered task-environments and through training, older adults can become equal participants in all human activity and thereby continue to appreciate all of life's true quality.

Acknowledgments

I very much appreciate the assistance of the editors of this book, Ronald Abeles, Helen Gift, and Marcia Ory. I am also indebted to the good efforts of Sara Czaja, Jan Dorsett, Von Leirer, Dan Morrow, Denise

Park, and Harvey Sterns. Without their keen reading this chapter would have suffered substantially.

References

Ball, K., Beard, B., Roenker, D., Miller, R., & Ball, D. (1988). Visual search: Expanding the useful field of view. *Journal of the Optical Society A, 5(12)*, 2210–2219.

Ball, K., Owsley, C., Sloane, M., Roenker, D., & Bruni, J. (in press). Visual attention problems as predictors of vehicle crashes in older drivers. *Investigative Opthalmology and Visual Science*.

Barr, R.A. (1991). Recent changes in driving among older adults. *Human Factors, 33*, 597–600.

Birren, J.E. (1956). The significance of age changes in speed of perception and psychmotor skills. In J.E. Anderson (Ed.), *Psychological Aspects of Aging* (pp. 97–104). Washington, DC: American Psychological Association.

Blackwell, B. (1973). Drug therapy: Patient compliance. *New England Journal of Medicine, 289*, 249–252.

Bloch, S., Rosenthal, A.R., Friedman, L., & Caldarolla, P. Patient compliance in glaucoma. *British Journal of Opthalmology, 61*, 531–534.

Card, S., Moran, T.P., & Newell, A. (1983). *The psychology of human-computer interaction*. Hillsdale, NJ: Lawrence Erlbaum Associates.

Charness, N. & Bosman, E.A. (1990). Human factors and design for older adults. In J.E. Birren & K.W. Schaie (Eds.) *Handbook of the Psychology of Aging*, 3rd Ed. San Diego, CA: Academic Press.

Clark, M.C., Czaja, S.L., & Weber, R.A. (1990). Older adults and daily living performance. *Human Factors, 32*, 537–550.

Czaja, S. J. (Ed.) (1990). *Human Factors Research Needs for an Aging Population*. National Research Council. Washington, D.C: National Academy Press.

Czaja, S.J. & Nair, S. (1992). Difficulties encountered by older adults in the performance of everyday activities. In S. Kuma (Ed.) *Advances in Industrial Ergonomics and Safety*. London: Taylor & Francis.

Czaja, S.J. & Sharit, J. (in press, a). Age differences in the performance of computer work. *Psychology and Aging*.

Czaja, S.J. & Sharit, J. (in press, b). Stress reactions to computer-interactive tasks as a function of task structure and individual differences. *International Journal of Human Computer Interaction*.

Drury, V.W.M., Wade, O.L., & Woolf, E. (1976). Following advice in general practice. *Journal of the Royal College of General Practitioners, 26,* 712–718.

Dubin, S.S. (1990). Maintaining competence through updating. In S.L. Willis & S.S. Dubin (Eds.), *Maintaining professional competence* (pp. 9–43). San Francisco: Jossey-Bass.

Evans, L. (1988). Risk of fatality from physical trauma versus sex and age. *Journal of Trauma, 28,* 368–378.

Heron, A. & Chown, S.M. (1961). *Aging and the semi-skilled: A survey in manufacturing industry on Merseyside.* London: Her Majesty's Stationery Office.

Hoyer, W.J., & Plude, D.J. (1982). Aging and the allocation of attentional resources in visual information processing. In R. Sekuler, D. Kline & K. Dismukes (Eds.), *Aging and Human Visual Function* (pp. 245–263). New York: Alan R. Liss.

Insurance Institute for Highway Safety. (1986). *Elderly.* Insurance Institute for Highway Safety Facts. Arlington, VA: Insurance Institute for Highway Safety.

Kendrick, R., & Bayne, J.R. (1982). Compliance with prescribed medication by elderly patients. *Canadian Medical Association Journal, 127,* 961–962.

Kutscher, R.E., & Walker, J.F. (1960). Comparative job performance of office workers by age. *Monthly Labor Review, 83,* 39–43.

Lawton, M.P., & Brody, E. (1969). Assessment of older people: Self-maintaining and instrumental activities of daily living. *The Gerontologist, 9,* 179–186.

Leirer, V.O., Morrow, D.G., Pariante, G.M., & Sheikh, J.I. (1988). Elders' nonadherence, its assessment, and computer assisted instruction for medication recall training. *Journal of the American Geriatrics Society, 36,* 877–884.

Leirer, V.O., Morrow, D.G., Tanke, E.D., & Pariante, G. (1991). Elder's nonadherence, its assessment, and medication reminding by voice mail. *The Gerontologist, 31,* 514–520.

McFarland, R.A. (1943). The older worker in industry. *Harvard Business Review, 21,* 505–520.

Murrell, K.F.H. (1962). Industrial aspects of aging. *Ergonomics, 5,* 148–153.

Murrell, K.F.H., Powesland, P.F., & Forsaith, B. (1962). A study of pillar-drilling in relation to age. *Occupational Psychology, 36,* 45–52.

National Aeronautics & Space Administration (NASA) (1978). *Anthropometric Source Book (vol. 1); Anthropometry for designers (vol. 2); A handbook of anthropometric data (vol. 3); Annotated Bibliography* (NASA Ref. Pub. 1024).

Owsley, C., Ball, K., Sloane, M., Roenker, D.L., & Bruni, J.R. (1991). Visual perceptual/cognitive correlates of vehicle accidents in older drivers *Psychology and Aging, 6,* 403–415.

Parasuraman, R., & Nestor, P.C. (1991). Attention and driving skills in aging and Alzheimer's disease. *Human Factors, 33,* 539–557.

Park, D.C., Morrell, R.W., Frieske, D.A., Blackburn, A.B., & Birchmore, D. (1991). Cognitive factors and the use of over-the-counter medication organizers by arthritis patients. *Human Factors, 33,* 57–67.

Park, D.C., Morrell, R.W., Frieske, D., & Kincaid, D. (1992). Medication adherence behaviors in adults: Effects of external cognitive supports. *Psychology and Aging, 7,* 252–256.

Parkin, D. M., & Henney, C.R. (1976). Deviation from prescribed drug treatment after discharge from hospital. *British Medical Journal, 2,* 686–688.

Persson, D. (1993). The elderly driver: Deciding when to stop. *The Gerontologist, 33,* 88–91.

Rosenbloom, S. (1988). The mobility needs of the elderly. In *Transportation in an Aging Society: Improving Mobility and Safety for Older persons. Special Report: 218.* Washington, DC: Transportation Research Board, National Research Council.

Salthouse, T.A. (1982). *Adult cognition. An experimental psychology of human aging.* New York: Springer Verlag.

Salthouse, T.A. (1991). *Theoretical perspectives on cognitive aging.* Hillsdale, NJ: Lawrence Erlbaum Associates.

Salvendy, G. (Ed.) (1987). *Handbook of human factors.* New York: Wiley.

Sanders, A.F. (1970). Some aspects of the selective process in the functional field of view. *Ergonomics, 13,* 101–117.

Staplin, L.K., & Fisk, A.D. (1991). Left-turn intersection problems: A cognitive engineering approach to improve the safety of young and old drivers. *Human Factors, 33,* 559–571.

Sterns, H.L., & Doverspike, D. (1989). Aging and the training and learning process. In I.L. Goldstein (Ed.), *Training and development in organizations* (pp. 299–332). San Francisco: Jossey Bass.

Sterns, H.L., Laier, M.P., & Dorsett, J.G. (1993). Enhancing the work and retirement experience of older adults. In B.R. Bonder & L. Wagner (Eds.) *Functional performance in the elderly.* F.A. Davis: Philadelphia.

Stoudt, H.W., Damon, A., McFarland, R.A., & Roberts, J. (1965). *Weight, height, and selected body dimensions of adults. Vital and health statistics,* Series 11, No. 8. Rockville, MD: Public Health Service.

Stoudt, H.W., Damon, A., McFarland, R.A., & Roberts, J. (1973). Skinfolds, body girths, biacromial diameter and selected anthropometric indices of adults. Vital and health statistics. *Vital and health statistics*, Series 11, No. 35. Rockville, MD: Public Health Service.

U.S. Bureau of the Census. (1990). *Current Population Reports*, No. 1057. Washington, DC: U.S. Government Printing Office.

U.S. Federal Highway Administration. (1981). *Highway statistics, 1980.* Washington, DC: U.S. Government Printing Office.

U.S. Federal Highway Administration. (1990). *Highway statistics, 1989.* Washington, DC: U.S. Government Printing Office.

Van Nostrand, J.F., Furner, S.E., & Suzman, R. (Eds.) (1993). Health data on older Americans: United States, 1992. *National Center for Health Statistics, Vital Health Statistics, 3(27)*.

Wandless, I., Muckow, J.C., Smith A., Prudham, D. (1979). Compliance with prescribed medicines: A study of elderly patients in the community. *Journal of the Royal College of General Practitioners*, 29, 391–396.

Warr, P. (1993). Age and employment. In M. Dunnette, L. Hough, & H. Triandis (Eds.) *Handbook of Industrial and Organizational Psychology*, volume 4. Palo Alto: Consulting Psychologists Press.

Welford, A.T. (1958). *Aging and human skill.* Oxford: Nuffield Foundation.

Chapter 12

Maintaining a Sense of Control in Later Life

Margie E. Lachman, Mauri A. Ziff, and Avron Spiro III

It is indeed fitting that a chapter on control should be included in a volume inspired by the celebration of Columbus' discovery of America, because control was at the very heart of his journey. Columbus and other explorers of his time were after control in a very grand sense—control of the world, its resources, and its people. The primary goal of the explorers was mastery of the environment and control was what motivated their expeditions. This theme is well-captured in Kirkpatrick Sale's (1990) volume about Columbus. Sale (1990) concluded that the reason for why the precise island where Columbus made landfall is unknown was that he felt if he kept the site to himself, only he would *control* the routes to the Indies and only he would get the gold.

Control remains an important motivating force in our time. One of the challenges of later life is to maintain a sense of control in the midst of the changing balance of gains and losses (Baltes & Baltes, 1990). The importance of control for maintaining a high quality of life is considered first. Next, control is defined and its developmental course in later life is examined. Finally, the impact of control beliefs on aging and possible interventions to enhance the sense of control are discussed.

Control and the Quality of Later Life

Control has been identified repeatedly as an important ingredient for successful aging (Baltes & Baltes, 1986; Brandtstädter & Renner, 1990; Brim, 1992; Rodin, 1986; Rowe & Kahn, 1987; Schulz, Heckhausen, & Locher, 1991). "Sense of control and quality of life for older people are intimately interrelated. Sense of control is a pivotal contributor to a wide variety of behaviors and to both mental and physical well-being, which are essential elements of quality of life" (Abeles, 1991, p. 297).

A recent poll by the Alliance for Aging Research found that although most Americans said they want to live to be 100, they are afraid of losing their independence as they age (*Boston Globe*, 1991, p. 3). Although Americans are optimistic that scientific research will lead to increased longevity, they fear losing their personal independence. Two-thirds of the respondents said they wanted to see their 100th birthdays, but 75% said they worry about losing control of their lives. Nearly 80% said they fear ending up in a nursing home more than dying a quick death from a sudden disease. The report concluded, "We need to advance scientific research into healthier and more independent lives for people as they age." Thus, extending the life span is not sufficient; maintaining a sense of control is indeed a necessary condition for enhancing one's quality of life.

Definition of Control

The term "control" has many meanings. In the popular press, magazine articles and books on how to control every aspect of life (romance, weight, physical appearance, health, career advancement, etc.) are proliferating. In the context of aging, however, control is typically associated with loss: losing independence, losing control of one's bladder, or losing control of one's mind.

The focus of this chapter is on the sense of control, that is, the perception that one can take charge of what happens in one's life. It includes beliefs or expectations about the extent to which one's actions can bring about desired outcomes. Two main sources affect control: one's own efficacy (internal) and the responsiveness of the environment, other people, or random forces (external). This definition focuses on the subjective sense of control rather than on the objective reality. One's beliefs, whether accurate or not, do influence behaviors. Although the veridicality of control beliefs is important (Weisz, 1983), the evidence suggests it is typically more adaptive to overestimate than to underestimate control (Bandura, 1977; Taylor, 1989).

Assessment. Locus of control has typically been assessed with self-report instruments ever since Rotter's (1966) inventory was published. Several key changes in the format have occurred over the past two decades. First, Rotter's scale measured control with a unidimensional internal–external scale. Now locus of control is considered a multidimensional construct with a number of key dimensions: primary, secondary, vicarious, internal, external, etc. (Schulz, Heckhausen, & Locher, 1991). The multidimensional conception used in this chapter is derived from Levenson's (1981) model, which includes three dimensions: internal or personal mastery ("It's due to me"), chance ("It's due to fate or luck"), and powerful others' ("It's due to others") control. Second, the preferred response format is no longer a dichotomous one. Whereas Rotter asked respondents to choose between a pair of items, one representing an internal view and one an external view, newer multidimensional conceptions ask respondents to rate their extent of agreement or disagreement with both internal and external statements on a Likert scale (typically with six points).

Third, a distinction is now made between domain-specific vs. general control beliefs. Rotter treated control beliefs as generalized expectancies, akin to a personality trait. More differentiated views now exist which acknowledge that control beliefs differ across diverse areas of life such as health, intellectual functioning, or memory (Lachman, 1986; Rodin, Timko, & Harris, 1985; Wallston & Wallston, 1981). This domain-specificity is an important consideration for a developmental perspective because trajectories of change across the life span differ by domain. Sample items from multidimensional, general and domain-specific control scales are presented in Table 12.1.

Correlates of Control

What areas of life are related to control beliefs? To paraphrase *Poor Richard's Almanac*: Having a sense of control makes a person healthy, wealthy, and wise. Actually, such a causal statement is too strong because most of the evidence is correlational. Those with a more internal sense of control also have: better health, fewer and less

TABLE 12.1
Sample Items from Locus of Control Scales

General Control (Levenson, 1981)
When I make plans, I am almost certain to make them work. (Internal)
When I get what I want it's usually because I'm lucky. (Chance)
Getting what I want requires pleasing those people above me. (Powerful Others)

Health Control (Wallston & Wallston, 1981)
If I take care of myself, I can avoid illness. (Internal)
No matter what I do, if I am going to get sick, I will get sick. (Chance)
Regarding my health, I can only do what my doctor tells me to do. (Powerful Others)

Intellectual Control (Lachman, 1986)
If I studied a map carefully I could figure out how to get around in a strange place. (Internal)
I have little control over my mental state. (Chance)
I couldn't learn to solve novel word problems without a teacher's help. (Powerful Others)

Interpersonal Control (Paulhus & Christie, 1981)
I have no trouble making and keeping friends.
I find it easy to play an important part in most group situations.

Political Control (Paulhus & Christie, 1981)
By taking an active part in political and social affairs we, the people, can control world events.
The average citizen can have an influence on government decisions.

---

severe illnesses or health problems, higher socioeconomic status, higher educational level, better memories, and higher intellectual functioning (Rodin et al., 1985). Control is also related to mental health; those who say they feel in control of their lives are less depressed, less neurotic, less anxious, more open-minded, and more assertive (Lachman & Lewkowicz, in preparation).

Epidemiological studies have shown that a sense of control, along with social support (see Chapter 9 in this volume), is among the most important psychosocial predictors of morbidity, mortality, and psychological well-being (Rodin, 1986; Rowe & Kahn, 1987). In recent studies of two separate samples [HMO members and the Normative Aging Study participants (Bossé, Ekerdt, & Silbert, 1984)], the interactive effects of sense of control and social support (having friends or family to rely on in a crisis) on health were explored (Ziff & Lachman,

1992; Ziff, Spiro, & Lachman, 1993). Significant interactions between measures of sense of control and social support were found in relation to a variety of health outcome measures including self-rated health, number of reported health problems, number of cardiovascular risk factors, illness severity, and health-related quality of life (Ware & Sherbourne, 1992).

The nature of the interactions found was such that higher levels of social support compensated for or buffered the effect of a lower sense of control on the various health outcomes. As depicted in Figure 12.1, those who had a higher sense of control and greater social support had fewer reported health problems. However, those who had a low internal control did not suffer from more health problems if they had high levels of social support. Thus, although a high internal sense of control is related to better health, an external sense of control can be compensated by other factors, such as strong social support.

It is hard to dispute that a sense of control is an important component of functioning in later life. But how does sense of control change with aging and what can be done about decrements in perceived control?

Aging and the Sense of Control

Over two dozen studies have examined age differences in control beliefs, either cross-sectionally or longitudinally (Lachman, 1986; Rodin et al., 1985). The results from studies using unidimensional scales are conflicting, whereas those using multidimensional scales provide a clearer consensus. Internal control beliefs remain relatively stable or decrease slightly, whereas external control beliefs increase markedly (Lachman, 1991). Perhaps this is not surprising given that the probability of uncontrollable events increases in later life (e.g., retirement, illness or death of spouse, siblings, friends, self). The focus of the current discussion, however, is on perceived control, which may vary across individuals even when describing the same objective situation. Typically, correlations between objective and subjective aspects of control are low, in the .20 to .30 range.

In a recent study (Lachman, 1991), a battery of generalized and domain-specific locus of control instruments was administered to a sample of 200 healthy, community-residing men and women aged 20 to 89. The respondents were randomly selected from four town registers in west suburban Boston and stratified by age and gender. Two of the

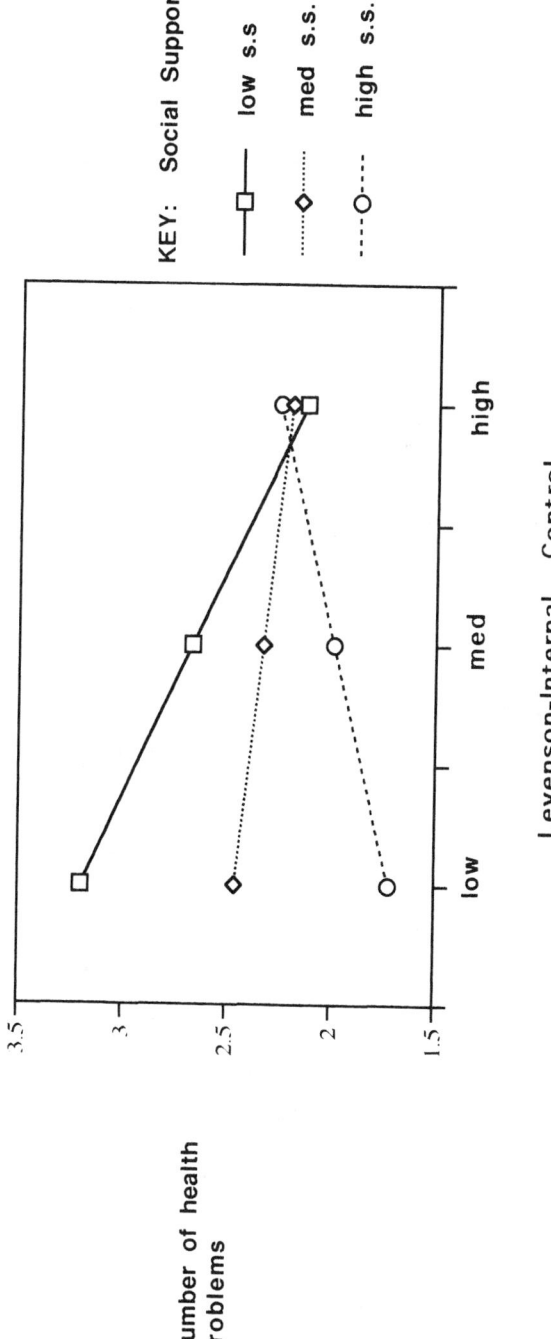

FIGURE 12.1 The interactive effects of internal control and social support on the number of reported health problems (From Ziff, Spiro, & Lachman, 1993).

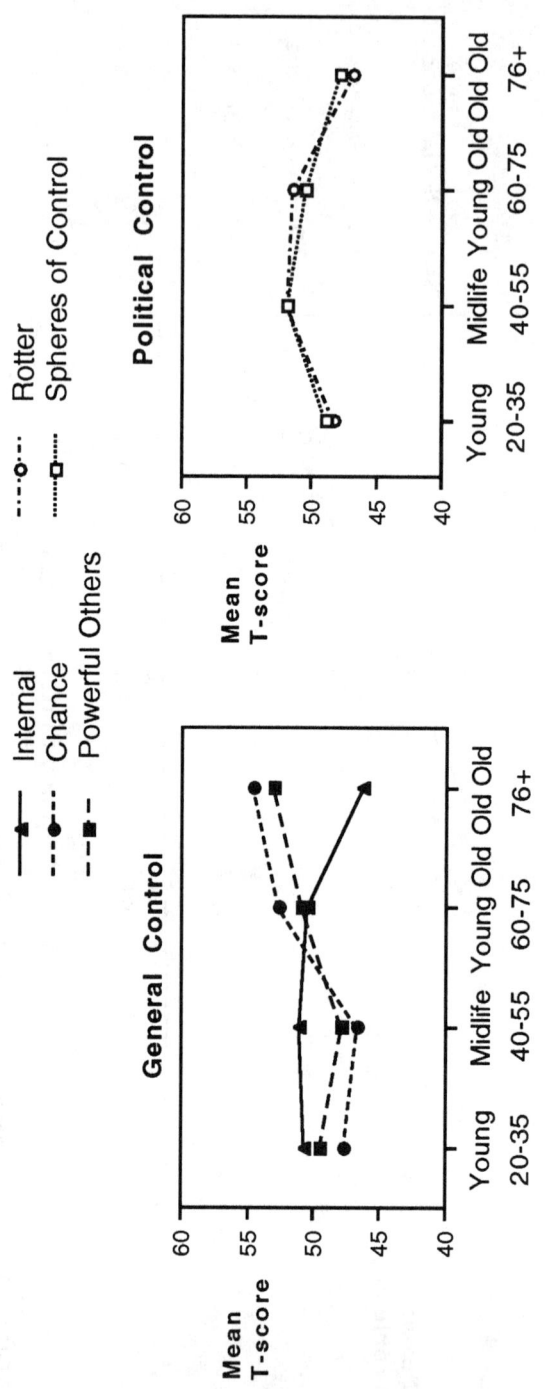

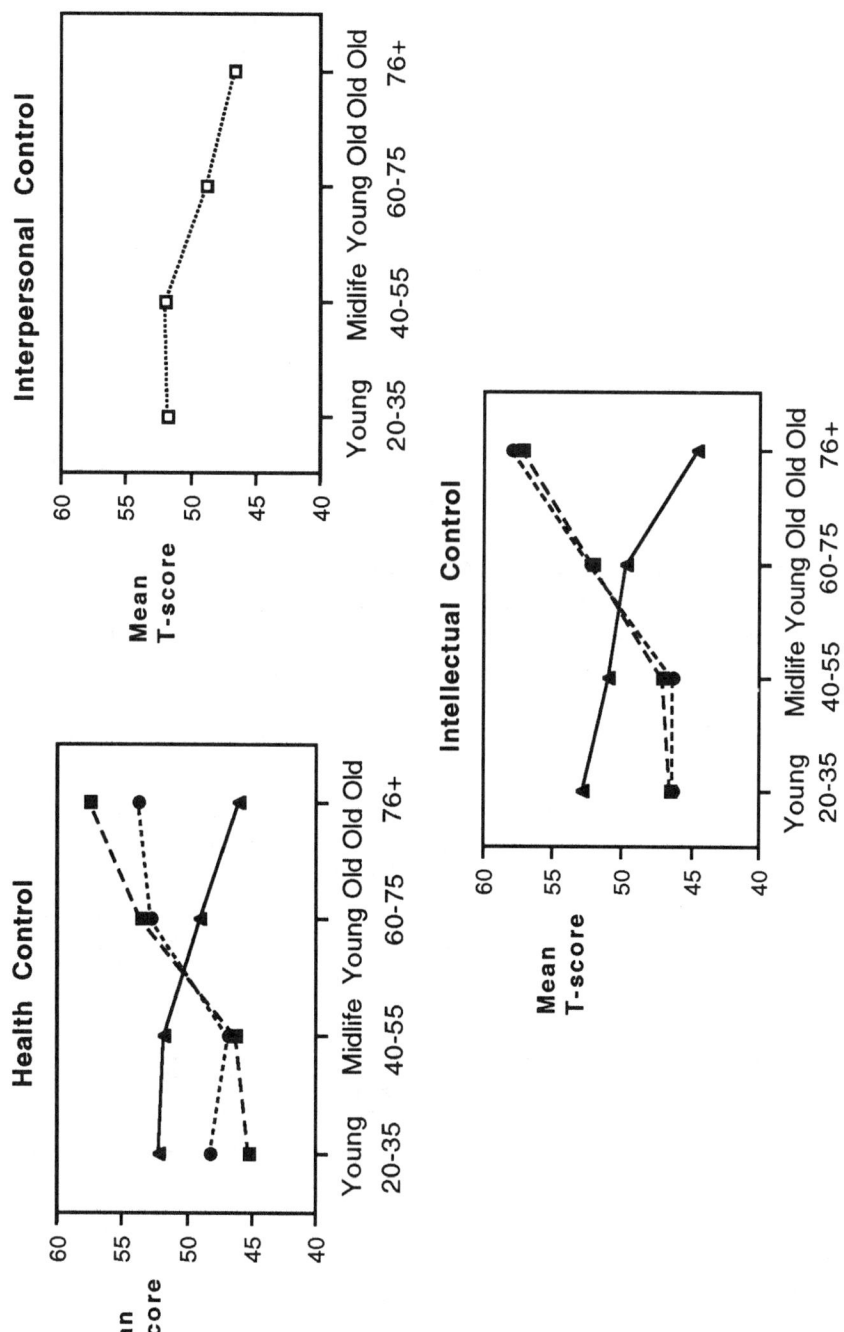

FIGURE 12.2 Age differences in general and domain-specific control beliefs. (Adapted from Lachman, 1991).

towns had a median educational level between 12 and 13 years, and two had a median educational level between 15 and 16 years. The sample was divided into four age groups: young adults (M age = 29.2, range 20–39), middle-aged adults (M age = 47.0, range 40–59), young-old (M age = 66.5, range 60–75), and old-old (M age = 80.6, range 76–89).

The findings revealed a relatively consistent pattern of age differences in control beliefs, although there were individual differences within age groups. Although internal beliefs decreased and external beliefs increased, the changes were not uniform. Patterns of change varied as a function of the specific dimension and domain (see Figure 12.2). Changes in internal dimensions were relatively small, whereas changes in external dimensions were greater. For the general sense of control changes were also small, although in the expected direction. Perceived control over health and cognitive functioning remained relatively stable across young adulthood and middle age, but showed changes in old age. Beliefs in internal control over health and cognitive functioning declined, whereas beliefs in the roles of external forces sharply increased in later life. In contrast, beliefs in political and interpersonal control showed minimal changes across the adult life span (Lachman, 1991).

These results are based on relatively healthy samples of community-residing and well-educated older adults. It is important to note that control beliefs vary by gender, socioeconomic status (SES), race, and educational level. Women and racial minorities, along with those of lower education and SES, report lower levels of internal control (Gurin & Gurin, 1976; Lachman, 1985). Patterns of age differences are similar across gender and SES groups, even though absolute levels of sense of control may vary (Lachman, 1985).

Dynamic Processes of Aging and Control

In light of the aging-related patterns of control and the correlations with different aspects of functioning, an often asked question is which comes first—the control beliefs or the changes in functioning? Theoretically, the emphasis has been on the role that beliefs (efficacy, control, attributions) play in influencing performance decrements (Abramson, Seligman, & Teasdale, 1977; Bandura, 1977). Empirically, however, the evidence suggests that the experience of aging-related changes and decrements sets the process in motion (Lachman & Leff,

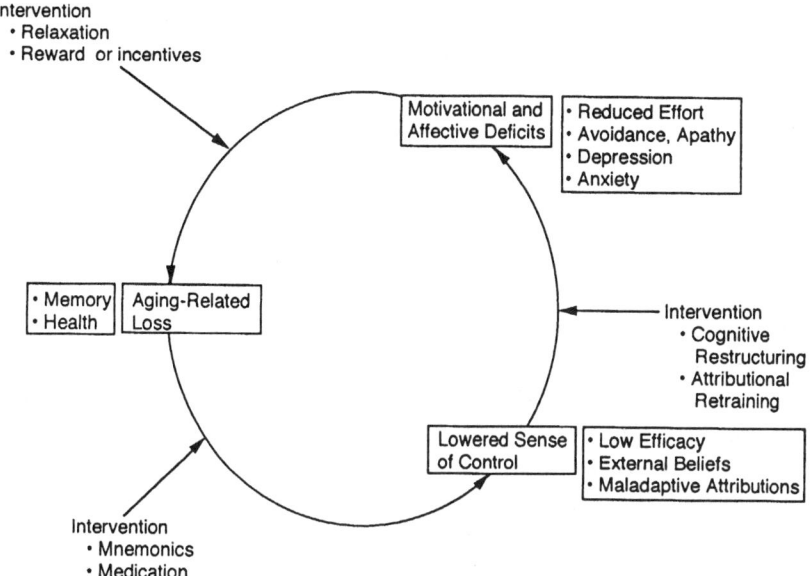

FIGURE 12.3 Sense of control and aging-related loss: Points for intervention.

1989). Viewed from a developmental perspective, the relations between control beliefs and changes in functioning are seen not as a unidirectional, one-step process, but rather as an ongoing process that unfolds over time. It is less important to determine which changes first than it is to look at their ongoing reciprocal relationship over time.

Although a sense of control may decline in response to some objective changes in cognitive functioning or health, it is crucial to consider the implications of a lowered sense of control for future functioning. For example, a sense of control affects whether someone engages in health-promoting behaviors, which in turn may affect health (Ziff, Lachman, & Lewkowicz, 1992). Also, sense of control affects choice and effort in challenging situations such as those involving memory problems (Perlmuter, Monty, & Chan, 1986).

The relationship between control beliefs and functioning can be depicted by a circular model that captures the cyclical nature of aging (see Figure 12.3). Similar to the social breakdown syndrome proposed by Kuypers and Bengtson (1973), this model examines the relationship between internalized negative expectations and aging-related declines. This cycle may begin at any point in the model. Note that interventions are also possible at several points. Typically, however, interventions focus on only one segment of the model without considering the whole process.

For purposes of illustration, assume that an age-related decline in memory triggers the cycle. The traditional response is to teach a mnemonic strategy or other technique that focuses directly on improving memory performance (Yesavage, 1985). However, this is often ineffective. What is often ignored is that changes in self-efficacy and sense of control accompany aging-related losses. Unless these negative beliefs are also tackled, the mnemonic strategy interventions are unlikely to be effective (Elliott & Lachman, 1989). If older adults believe that their memory is not good and that there is nothing they can do to improve it, they are unlikely to use effort to learn or implement new strategies! If, however, control beliefs are enhanced along with teaching new skills, this combination is likely to increase effort and persistence as well as to reduce depression and anxiety (Bandura, 1977; Rodin, 1983), thereby maximizing the effectiveness of skill learning.

Intervention Programs

Research by Lachman and her colleagues has focused on changing efficacy and control beliefs using cognitive restructuring techniques (Lachman, 1991; Lachman, Weaver, Bandura, Elliott, & Lewkowicz, 1992). They found that many older adults not only believe that their capacity is declining, but also that they have no control over this decline (i.e., it is inevitable and irreversible). They then developed a cognitive restructuring intervention to educate people about two competing conceptions of memory aging and to promote the more adaptive view. The effectiveness of this intervention was examined alone and in combination with a memory-training condition.

In the memory skills training condition, participants were instructed in basic skills (e.g., concentration, visualization) applicable to a wide range of memory tasks. In addition, participants were asked to apply these skills using their own self-strategies for remembering the materials to be learned. This approach was adopted both because of the poor track record of mnemonic techniques in past research and for theoretical reasons. Based on past research (Dittmann-Kohli, Lachman, Kliegl, & Baltes, 1991; Willis, 1990), however, it was expected that (1) experience with memory tasks alone would not be sufficient to increase beliefs about efficacy and control over memory and that (2) additional instruction about self-defeating versus self-enhancing attitudes would be necessary to increase self-efficacy and control beliefs.

The cognitive restructuring treatment was administered in two 1.5 hour group sessions conducted by two clinical psychologists. These sessions included viewing a videotape of older adults modeling adaptive responses for dealing with laboratory and real world memory tasks. There was no practice on memory tasks, per se, but the instructors presented difficult memory problems and the participants were asked to note and discuss their reactions to them. This intervention had three main components:

1. *Education about adaptive and maladaptive conceptions of memory.* Two views of memory were presented: One view emphasized inevitable loss and deterioration of memory with age; the other portrayed memory as a body of skills and knowledge that can be maintained and improved through effort. These views were demonstrated in a videotape, in which older adult actors coped with memory problems from the two different perspectives. They verbalized their thoughts to portray attributions, expectations, and reactions associated with each view.

2. *Promotion of an adaptive conception of memory.* This was accomplished through group discussion, in which the leaders presented examples and data that illustrated the credibility of viewing memory as controllable. In addition, participants generated personal examples demonstrating the advantages of this view.

3. *Self-instructional training to implement a view of memory as controllable.* In the context of tackling memory problems, participants learned to identify cognitions related to the two views of memory (e.g., attributions, "strategy-relevant" versus "task-interfering" thoughts). Using modeling, they were taught how to instruct themselves to shift from maladaptive to adaptive cognitions, to foster motivation and task orientation.

Men and women aged 60 to 85 were randomly assigned to one of five treatment groups: (1) cognitive restructuring to promote adaptive beliefs about memory, (2) memory skills training, (3) combined cognitive restructuring and memory skills training, (4) practice on memory tasks, and (5) a no-contact control group. Beliefs about memory (ability and control) and memory performance (working memory, recall of text materials, categorizable word list, and names and faces) were assessed at a pretest and two posttests.

As predicted, those receiving the combined treatment showed the greatest increases in their sense of control and perceived ability to improve memory. Contrary to predictions, all groups improved equally on the memory tasks, although those who had received memory training were more likely to report at the second posttest that they had begun using new strategies for remembering things.

Through the use of a cognitive behavioral intervention, older adults' beliefs about memory controllability were improved. The cognitive restructuring was most effective when it was combined with the self-generated memory strategy training. Older adults in the combined condition developed more favorable beliefs about their ability to improve, the contribution of effort to memory performance, and the inevitability of memory loss. Thus, the combined group increased their sense of control, in terms of viewing memory functioning as controllable through their own efforts rather than as the result of uncontrollable aging.

One important lesson for older adults to learn is that what used to be relatively effortless (e.g., remembering appointments) now may require more effort. The cognitive restructuring intervention informed them that the investment of effort would pay off. Although this research is in the early stages, thus far the cognitive restructuring has been successful in changing beliefs. The implications of changing beliefs for memory performance needs to be explored in future research.

Conclusions

Clearly, the sense of control is a central concern among many older adults. Maintaining a sense of control is an important key to both psychological well-being and to physical health, and, therefore, to quality of life. The sense of control does decline in some domains, but it is possible to hold both internal and external control beliefs at the same time. One can maintain a sense of personal mastery despite a growing recognition that some changes are not within one's control.

In some domains it may be adaptive to relinquish control or to accept a lack of control. Control may not always be possible or desirable. Persistent attempts to control the uncontrollable will be ineffective and lead to feelings of failure (Brim, 1992; Thompson,

Cheek, & Graham, 1988). Older adults, however, are likely to err in the other direction and to assume control is not possible when it is.

A weak sense of control may not necessarily lead to poor outcomes if other key psychosocial factors, such as social support, are strong. Research indicates that social support may serve a buffering function for the ill effects of a declining sense of internal control (Ziff, Spiro, & Lachman, 1993).

One effective approach to optimize functioning is to directly target control beliefs with cognitive restructuring interventions such as the one described above. Good performance requires not only the requisite skills but also adaptive self-conceptions that foster effective use of these skills. Interventions that target beliefs about efficacy and control and motivation in conjunction with teaching problem-solving strategies and other skills are currently being refined. Further work is needed to examine the long-term maintenance and benefits of these interventions for the quality of older adults' lives.

Acknowledgments

The research reported in this paper was supported by grants AG06038 and AG07790 from the National Institute on Aging (MEL), by training grant T32 AG00204 from the National Institute on Aging (MAZ), and by the Health Services Research and Development Service of the Department of Veterans Affairs (ASIII).

References

Abeles, R.P. (1991). Sense of control, quality of life, and frail older people. In J.E. Birren, D.E. Deutchman, J. Lubben, & J. Rowe (Eds.), *The concept and measurement of quality of life in the later years* (pp. 297–314). New York: Academic Press.

Abramson, L.Y., Seligman, M.E. P., & Teasdale, J.D. (1978). Learned helplessness: Critique and reformulation. *Journal of Abnormal Psychology, 87,* 49–74.

Baltes, M.M., & Baltes, P.B. (Eds.) (1986). *The psychology of control and aging.* Hillsdale, NJ: Lawrence Erlbaum.

Baltes, P. B., & Baltes, M. M. (1990). Psychological perspectives on successful aging: The model of selective optimization with compensation. In P. B. Baltes & M. M. Baltes (Eds.), *Successful aging: Perspectives from the behavioral sciences* (pp. 1–34). New York: Cambridge University Press.

Bandura, A. (1977). Self-efficacy: Toward a unifying theory of behavioral change. *Psychological Review, 85*, 191–215.
Boston Globe. (1991, November 18). Associated Press, p. 3.
Bosse', R., Ekerdt, D., & Silbert, J. (1984). The Veterans Administration Normative Aging Study. In S.A. Mednick, M. Harway, & K.M. Finello (Eds.), *Handbook of longitudinal research (vol. 2): Teenage and adult cohorts* (pp. 273–89). New York: Praeger.
Brandtstädter, J., & Renner, G. (1990). Tenacious goal pursuit and flexible goal adjustment. Explication and age-related analysis of assimilative and accommodative strategies of coping. *Psychology and Aging, 5*, 58–67.
Brim, G. (1992). *Ambition: How we manage success and failure throughout our lives*. New York: Basic Books.
Dittmann-Kohli, F., Lachman, M. E., Kliegl, R., & Baltes, P. B. (1991). Effects of cognitive training and testing on intellectual efficacy beliefs in elderly adults. *Journal of Gerontology: Psychological Sciences, 46*, P162–P164.
Elliott, E., & Lachman, M. E. (1989). Enhancing memory by modifying control beliefs, attributions, and performance goals in the elderly. In P. S. Fry (Ed.), *Psychology of helplessness and control and attributions of helplessness and control in the aged* (pp. 339–367). Amsterdam: North Holland.
Gurin, G., & Gurin, P. (1976). Personal efficacy and the ideology of individual responsibility. In B. Strumpel (Ed.), *Economic means for human needs* (pp. 131–157). Ann Arbor, MI: Institute for Social Research.
Kuypers, J.A., & Bengtson, V.L. (1973). Social breakdown and competence: A model of normal aging. *Human Development, 16*, 181–201.
Lachman, M.E. (1985). Personal efficacy in middle and old age: Differential and normative patterns of change. In G.H. Elder, Jr. (Ed.), *Life-course dynamics: Trajectories and transitions, 1968–1980* (pp. 188–213). Ithaca, NY: Cornell University Press.
Lachman, M. E. (1986). Locus of control in aging research: A case for multidimensional and domain-specific assessment. *Psychology and Aging, 1*, 34–40.
Lachman, M.E. (1991). Perceived control over memory aging: Developmental and intervention perspectives. *Journal of Social Issues, 47*, 159–175.
Lachman, M. E., & Leff, R. (1989). Beliefs about intellectual efficacy and control in the elderly: A five-year longitudinal study. *Developmental Psychology, 25*, 722–728.
Lachman, M. E., & Lewkowicz, C. (in preparation). Locus of control and the Big Five personality factors: Convergent and discriminant relations.
Lachman, M.E., Weaver, S.L., Bandura, M., Elliott, E., & Lewkowicz, C. (1992). Improving memory and control beliefs through cognitive restructuring

and self-generated strategies. *Journal of Gerontology: Psychological Sciences, 47,* 293-299.

Levenson, H. (1981). Differentiating among internality, powerful others, and chance. In H. M. Lefcourt (Ed.), *Research with the locus of control construct: Assessment methods* (Vol. 1, pp. 15-63). New York: Academic Press.

Paulhus, D., & Christie, R. (1981). Spheres of control: An interactionist approach to assessment of perceived control. In H. M. Lefcourt (Ed.), *Research with the locus of control construct: Assessment methods* (Vol. 1, pp. 161-188). New York: Academic Press.

Perlmuter, L.C., Monty, R.A., & Chan, F. (1986). Choice, control, and cognitive functioning. In M.M. Baltes & P.B. Baltes (Eds.), *The psychology of control and aging.* (pp. 91-118). Hillsdale, NJ: Lawrence Erlbaum.

Rodin, J. (1983). Behavioral medicine: Beneficial effects of self-control training in aging. *International Review of Applied Psychology, 32,* 153-181.

Rodin, J. (1986). Aging and health: Effects of the sense of control. *Science, 233,* 1271-1276.

Rodin, J., Timko, C., & Harris, S. (1985). The construct of control: Biological and psychosocial correlates. In C. Eisdorfer, M. P. Lawton & G. L. Maddox (Eds.), *Annual review of gerontology and geriatrics* (pp. 3-55). New York: Springer Publishing Co.

Rotter, J.B. (1966). Generalized expectancies for internal versus external control of reinforcement. *Psychological Monographs, 80* (1, Whole No. 609).

Rowe, J.W., & Kahn, R.L. (1987). Human aging: Usual and successful. *Science, 237,* 143-149.

Sale, K. (1990). *The conquest of paradise: Christopher Columbus and the Columbian legacy.* New York: Knopf.

Schulz, R., Heckhausen, J., & Locher, J.L. (1991). Adult development, control, and adaptive functioning. *Journal of Social Issues, 47,* 177-196.

Taylor, S.E. (1989). *Positive illusions: Creative self-deception and the healthy mind.* New York: Basic Books.

Thompson, S. C., Cheek, P. R., & Graham, M. A. (1988). The other side of perceived control: Disadvantages and negative effects. In S. Spacapan & S. Oskamp (Eds.), *The social psychology of health.* (pp. 69-93). Newbury Park: Sage.

Wallston, K. A., & Wallston, B. S. (1981). Health related locus of control scales. In H. M. Lefcourt (Ed.), *Research with the locus of control construct: Assessment methods* (Vol. I, pp. 189-243). New York: Academic Press.

Ware, J.E., & Sherbourne, C.D. (1992). The MOS 36-item short-form health survey (SF-36): I. Conceptual framework and item selection. *Medical Care, 30*, 473–83.

Weisz, J.R. (1983). Can I control it? The pursuit of veridical answers across the life span. In P.B. Baltes & O.G. Brim (Eds.), *Life-span development and behavior* (Vol. 5, pp. 233–300). New York: Academic Press.

Willis, S.L. (1990). Current issues in cognitive training research. In E.A. Lovelace (Ed.), *Aging and cognition: Mental processes, self-awareness and interventions.* (pp. 263–280). Amsterdam: Elsevier.

Yesavage, J. A. (1985). Nonpharmacologic treatments for memory losses with normal aging. *American Journal of Psychiatry, 142*, 600–605.

Ziff, M.A., & Lachman, M.E. (November, 1992). *Sense of control and health: Mediators and moderators.* Presented at the 45th meeting of the Gerontological Society of America, Washington, DC.

Ziff, M.A., Lachman, M.E., & Lewkowicz, C. (1993). Lifestyle not luck: Perceived control, healthy lifestyle, and health.

Ziff, M. A., Spiro, A, & Lachman, M. E. (1993, in preparation). Protective resources for healthy aging: Social support buffers the effects of a lower sense of control.

PART V

Social Structures, Quality of Life, and Aging

Chapter 13

The Changing Structure of Work Opportunities: Toward an Age-integrated Society*

Matilda White Riley and Karyn A. Loscocco

Work structures are gradually changing, providing more opportunity for older people to participate in and contribute to social life. This emerging structural revolution will improve the quality of aging and the productivity of older people. If that were the only societal benefit of such change, it would be significant indeed. Yet in an age-integrated society, the changes made to bring older people back into the social mainstream will simultaneously help to solve the work–family "crunch" felt by many in the middle years of life.

---

*This chapter is one component of Program Age and Structural Change (PASC), conducted by Matilda White Riley at the National Institute on Aging.

Changing Lives

In most developed societies, this century has wrought sweeping changes in people's lives, yet social structures have remained largely fixed.

The Later Years

Perhaps most unfortunate is the fact that American society has little place for older people. Instead, it continues to be structured as if there were still few older people, and precious few who are well enough to be productive. Essentially, older people are living well beyond the point that society has come to expect or to support.

In fact, as shown repeatedly throughout this book, the over-65 population is growing at a much faster rate than the global population growth rate. More and more people are living, and even more will live in the future, in societies in which the majority survive to old age. As the age of leaving the workforce continues to decline, nearly one-third of adult life is now spent in what has become "modern" retirement. To be sure, some older people are so frail or incapacitated that they cannot be productive, but this is not true of the majority. Indeed, most older people have no serious physical disability (Manton, Stallard, & Singer, 1992). The large numbers of the healthy far outweigh those who are disabled or institutionalized. This trend is expected to continue to the year 2000 and at least through 2020.

Moreover, most older people have dramatically greater strengths and potential capacities than society's stereotypic images of "the elderly" allow (See Riley & Abeles, 1990). Studies of social interventions have shown that, with the right support, even the "oldest old" can improve their functioning (Suzman, Willis, & Manton, 1992). For example, given incentives and training, very old people whose performance on intelligence tests has deteriorated can be brought back to their performance level of 20 years earlier (Willis, 1990). Or, given a leg-strengthening regimen, nonagenarians can double their muscle strength, walking faster and farther (Fiatarone, Marks, Meredith, Lipsitz, & Evans, 1990).

The Middle Years

People in their middle years are now juggling more role responsibilities than they did in the past. Fewer and fewer have someone attending full time to family and children. Yet society continues blithely on as though nothing has changed.

Meanwhile, the influx of middle-class mothers into the labor force has set in motion dramatic changes for people in the middle years of life. No longer is the ideology of separate spheres, with work roles for men and family roles for women, consonant with the actual experience of the majority. Even the last bastion of female reserve—mothers of young children—participate actively in paid work. The labor force participation rates of mothers of young children has increased fourfold since 1950. This rate is especially high among African-American women, with nearly 2 out 3 in the labor force, compared to 1 out of 2 white women and 2 out of 5 women of Hispanic origin (U.S. Bureau of the Census, 1992). Furthermore, over half of new mothers are working for pay soon after giving birth. By the time their youngest child reaches 4 years of age, two-thirds of mothers are in the paid labor force. Thus, prior to old age, family and work are now intricately intertwined for a majority of families.

Structural Lag and Age Integration

Structural Lag

These developments constitute "structural lag" (Riley, 1988; Riley, Kahn, & Foner, 1994): structures and norms in work, family, and other social institutions have failed to adjust to the metamorphoses in people's lives. The concept of structural lag rests on a basic principle from the sociology of age (Riley, Foner, & Waring, 1988): Changing lives and changing social structures are distinct but interdependent dynamisms. In a continuing interplay, each influences the other.

For the past several decades in modern societies, the dynamism of changing lives has been outstripping the dynamism of structural change. Social structures have lagged behind the myriad changes in the ways people grow up and grow old. The result of this structural lag is tremendous strain on both individuals and society. Without broad structural changes, individuals and families are forced to find their own ways to adapt to life course realities very different from those for which the social structure was put in place. Further, without structural change, heavy burdens are placed on the economy and the polity. The continuing interplay between lives and structures now presses for such structural change.

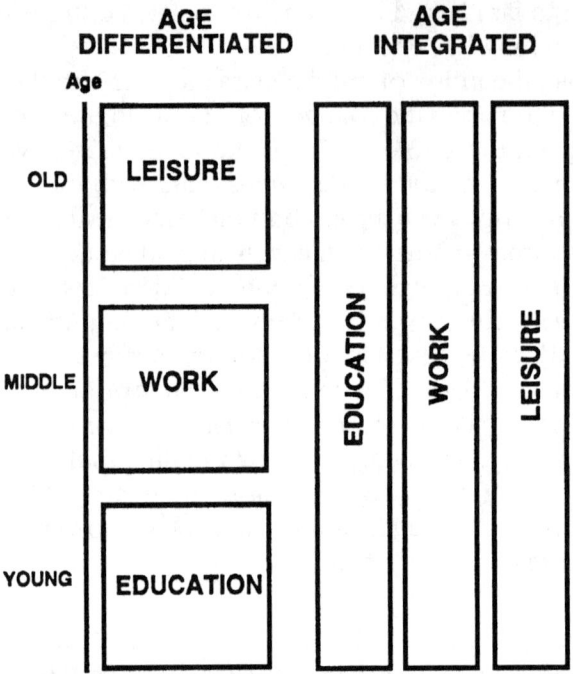

FIGURE 13.1 Types of social structures.

One solution to the problem of structural lag is a movement away from "age differentiated" structures toward "age-integrated" structures (cf. Riley & Riley, 1991). These two "ideal types" are shown in Figure 13.1. The key elements of the first type are reflective of the reality of the past and the key elements of the other portend a very different emergent reality.

Age Differentiated Structures

At one extreme, age-differentiated structures divide societal roles into three well-known boxes: retirement or leisure for older people; work roles for those in the long span of the middle years when family burdens are heaviest; and roles in school, vocational centers, or university reserved for the young. This type of structure is commonplace today. It appears convenient and comfortable, because it is so familiar. Yet these age-based structures and norms are vestigial remains of an earlier era when most people had died before their work was finished or their last child had left home. Such structures emerged in societies where work was the predominant role, achievement or material "success" the predominant value, and paid work the nearly exclusive province of men. (Of course, women at the bottom of the socioeconomic ladder have always participated in the labor force.) These age-based sequences of education, work and retirement have been bolstered by "ageism," the incorrect but persistent belief in inevitable and universal decline in health and capabilities because of aging.

Clearly these traditional age-differentiated structures are failing to accommodate the important changes in people's lives. In the continuing interplay between people who are aging and structures that are changing, trends in one direction simply cannot persist indefinitely. A German scholar (Kohli, 1988; p. 15) notes the absurd outcome of pushing age differentiation too far: "If we extrapolate the trend of the last two decades, we shall, somewhere in the second half of the twenty-first century, reach the point where at the age of about 38, people move from the university directly into retirement." Americans, having accepted the ideology of consumption, find themselves tied to work through mortgages, car payments ,and credit card bills. The liberal vacation policies of western Europe are perhaps enviable, but incomprehensible, to many American workers. Yet there is no guarantee that overlong hours of work result in greater productivity, to say nothing of the ill effects on the quality of life (Schor, 1992).

Age-Integrated Structures

At the opposite extreme from age differentiated structures, Figure 13.1 shows the ideal type of age-integrated structures. Here role opportunities in *all* structures—education, work, and leisure—are open to people of *every* age. Age loses its power to determine when and how people should perform these roles. Neither teen-agers nor retirees are excluded from worksites because of age. There are nursery schools for the very young, and universities open to adults of all ages, including the very old. Extended opportunities for leisure and freedom from work are available even to the middle aged. Ideally, such age-integrated structures lead to a new, *flexible* life course, allowing people to intersperse periods of work with periods of education and of leisure over their entire lives. Throughout society, people of all ages are brought together, leading to a breakdown of ageist bias and rigid age-based norms.

Tendencies Toward Age-Integration

Because the age-differentiated model continues to be the dominant organizing principle for modern society, age-integration may seem nothing more than an unobtainable ideal. Yet there is emerging evidence that elements of the age-integrated model are becoming a reality. Some traditional age barriers are breaking down, and deliberate interventions to offset structural lag seem increasingly feasible.

Apparently spurred by the need to find an alternative market for their services, educational institutions began to open up to older or "nontraditional" students a few decades ago. The women's movement had created tremendous pent-up demand among middle class housewives (Friedan, 1991; p. 262). The next step was to offer education to that growing segment of older people who have the time, finances, and inclination to learn new things. The "University of the Third Age" movement sprang up in Europe; and in the United States, nearly 1,000 colleges are reported to make places for students over age 65. As young and old share college campuses, the structural interventions in education integrate people of all ages. Equally important, these changes have wrought an educational system that is becoming more effective as preparation for productivity and active participation in both work and leisure over a long lifetime.

Similarly, productive opportunities for paid work are no longer confined to the middle years. The long-term shift away from lifetime to "contingent" careers (Henretta, 1992), with the accompanying increase in part-time jobs, has been a boon for many older workers, despite lowered levels of pay and benefits. In fact, men over 65 have among the highest rates of part-time employment (Voydanoff, 1987). Flexible scheduling, "unretirement programs," and job sharing are all programs that bring older people into the labor force. At the same time, these programs give younger people trying to juggle work and family a chance to mold work to family responsibilities, rather than subordinating family to the powerful demands of work, as in the age-differentiated model. These structural changes address the different role "problems" of these two age strata simultaneously: The elderly gain a rewarding productive role, and the role overload of those in their middle years is lessened. Of course, employers too benefit from current trends as, for example, they save by hiring workers part-time and often without benefits.

There are also signs of structural interventions that bring together people of all ages in the three domains of education, work, and leisure. Even with the ups and downs of the United States economy, attempts have been made to allow people to move early from school to work, and later from work back again to school. People in the middle years have greater opportunity to include more leisure activities, rather than concentrating nearly all the "optional time" in retirement. It is becoming both easier and more necessary to change jobs or even careers, rather than remaining in the same position for one's entire work life. For instance, a model of portable pensions has been tested to eliminate a major obstacle to changing jobs; and there have been experiments with provisions for educational leaves from work, for retraining older employees, or for allowing employees to choose several years of leave to be spent over their work lives in education, self-fulfillment, or family care. In the late 1980s reports were that 44% of all United States employers have programs for part-time work, 14% sponsor sabbatical leaves, and 40% make flextime available (Dychtwald, 1989). One-fourth of male and female wage and salary earners and half of the self-employed either take a new postretirement job or remain in their career part-time (Quinn, Burkhauser, & Myers, 1990).

Pressures Toward Age Integration

Underlying these overt changes are latent pressures toward age integration. One strong pressure stems from the rapid technological advances that change the nature of work. Paradoxically, although the typical life course becomes *longer*, the half-life of most occupations has become *shorter*. Because of the fast pace of change in many occupations and professions, many people find themselves out-of-date in a matter of years. In fact, the licensing requirements of states and professional organizations increasingly require that people go back for refresher education every 5 or 10 years (Friedan, 1991; p. 262). This fits the age-integrated model, in which people intersperse periods of work with periods of relearning. In the 1990s the downturn in the economy has curtailed the half-life of more jobs and eliminated others altogether. This calls attention to the strong underlying pressures toward the kinds of structural adjustments that foster age integration—in this case occupational training over the entire course of life, rather than just at the beginning.

These pressures exist in other countries as well (cf., Kohli, Rein, Guillemard, & VanGusteren, 1991). In Eastern Europe, low productivity is requiring a restructuring of the labor force, and older workers are often retained. In Hungary, older workers "retire" from primary employment in the state-controlled economy to reemployment in the private sector, resulting in gains in worker autonomy and income. A similar structure is found in Japan, where many male workers enter a second job after "retirement" from their primary employment.

Thus, in some places and under some conditions, strong pressures are already at work to alter societal structures in the age-integrated direction. It remains to be seen how the private sector will respond to such pressures, and how governments will play their part.

Implications of Change

As scientists concerned with understanding not only the source but also the implications of structural change, let us return to the two dynamisms of changing lives and changing social structures, and the reciprocal influence between them (Riley, 1978; Riley et al., 1988). Figure 13.2 schematizes these dynamisms in a social space bounded on its vertical axis by age (in years) and on its horizontal axis by dates that trace history.

The diagonals correspond to changes in the life patterns of successive cohorts of people, and the verticals correspond to changes in age-related social structures. The intersection of the bars calls attention to the continuing interplay between these dynamisms, as each influences the other. At any given historical moment, people of different ages in all the co-existing cohorts (the diagonal bars) are passing through the age-related structures (one of the vertical bars). As they age, people encounter the role opportunities and norms associated with family, school, work, and community. These people both influence, and are influenced by these structures. Collectively, people are shaping these roles as they act in their everyday lives, and as they exert pressure on public policy.

Implications for Individual Lives

In one direction of the interplay are the implications for the lives of successive cohorts of people who, as they grow older, move through

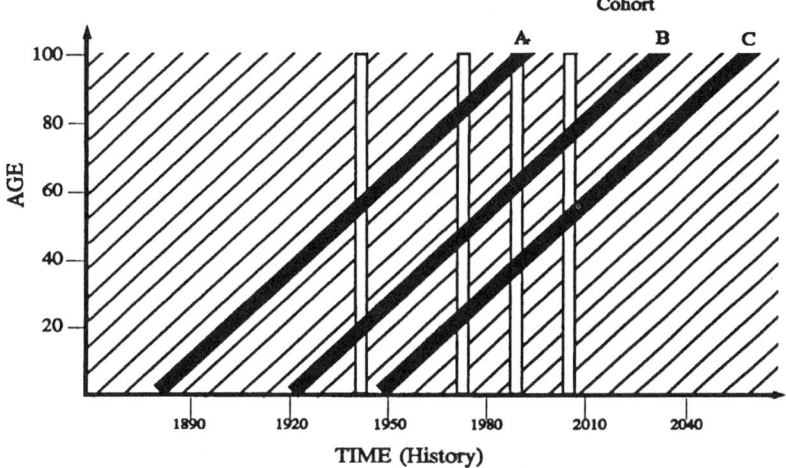

FIGURE 13.2. Changing lives and structural changes.

the structures of the total society. People's lives will certainly be shaped differently by age-integrated as opposed to age-differentiated structures (the polar types depicted in Figure 13.1 above).

In the recent era of age differentiated structures, people were socialized to schedule their lives, at the appropriate ages, within the three rigid stages. In the emerging era of age integration, the rigid structures will give way to new and more flexible roles. At every stage of their lives people will have wider options to be productive in not only the three domains of education, work, and retirement, but the family domain as well.

Given such options, many in the middle years will scale back their work in order to engage in other activities. A Gallup Poll has shown that more than half of all absenteeism among two-income couples with children under 12 was for family-related reasons (reported in Dynerman & Hayes, 1991). Among older people, some will choose to remain in the economic mainstream of society; one U.S. study showed that over a million early retirees would prefer to continue paid work if part-time opportunities were available (McNaught, Barth, & Henderson, 1991). Other older people will contribute to productivity through volunteer roles and by helping other older people (cf. Chapter 5 by deFriese in this volume).

Social Implications

In the reciprocal direction of the interplay, people in different co-existing cohorts are actively pressing for changes in these structures. Within the cohorts of those who are young today, many are dissatisfied with the necessity to finish more and more schooling (due to "educational inflation"). Many of those now reaching the middle years are calling for day care for their children or elderly parents, and for other forms of help with the multiple stresses of combined work and family roles. Many from cohorts now in old age are restive in the prolonged "roleless role" of retirement.

Pressures for wider opportunities are particularly strong among workers at the bottom of the occupational ladder, now all too often locked into deadend or unfulfilling jobs. One study of factory workers found that many felt obliged to stay in the well-paying though alienating jobs they had secured right out of high school: their families depended on it (Loscocco, 1989). Ideally, in an age-integrated system, early occupational choices would not preclude later opportunities for upward mobility, or for jobs that would use people's talents and abilities.

Obstacles to Change

Given the overt and latent pressures toward age integration, it might seem that such a restructuring of society is imminent. Yet important obstacles must be overcome if age integration is to reach its potential for liberating individuals and improving society. Two of the most formidable vestiges of the age-differentiated model are the material values of capitalist society and the persistent elements of the earlier gender division of labor.

Values

The age-integrated society requires movement away from material values that are the hallmark of competitive capitalism and best exemplified by the ideology of individual consumption in the United States. After all, age flexibility in market work cannot guarantee sustained material success. Interrupted work careers generally decrease income (Blau & Ferber, 1986), and few part-time jobs carry full benefits. Family-oriented policies often require financial sacrifice. For example, the long-awaited Family Leave Bill made it possible for employees of large companies to take *unpaid* time off to care for newborns or ill family members. Yet, it remains to be seen how many will feel able or willing to "take advantage" of this loss of income. In fact, as recently as the 1980s, the vast majority of women took less parental leave than was available to them (Kamerman & Kahn, 1987). Because many family-oriented policies lack a monetary component they are inaccessible to those at the bottom of the socioeconomic ladder (Ford Foundation, 1989); and racial-ethnic minorities and female-headed families are hampered disproportionately.

Moreover, the work institutions called for in an age-integrated society must meet worker demands for multiple career paths, unpaid and paid leaves, rewards for life experience, jobs they can share, and opportunities to commit themselves to a company part-time. These are radical changes in a society that continues to organize work on the assumption that employees have a full-time helpmate in the home, a premise no longer true of the majority.

Yet what incentives do companies have to make such changes in a society geared toward maximum profit? Companies make the kinds of changes that benefit employees when it is in their economic interests to do so. Thus, flextime and part-time work are the most commonly available "family-friendly" policies largely because they serve corporate needs. Flextime was originally developed to keep businesses staffed for longer periods of time, to conserve energy and increase workers' productive time (e.g. Voydanoff, 1987). Part-time work saves companies money in a variety of ways, most notably the savings in fringe benefits to which few part-time workers are entitled.

Thus, the sweeping changes of an age-integrated system require a change in corporate as well as consumer values. To date, the calls for workplace flexibility remain couched in the traditional business rhetoric of profit, with little challenge to societal values about work and family. It is, therefore, difficult to envision how a change in values might come about.

Family needs continue to be subordinate to the demands of work institutions, and scholars accept this premise as they make predictions about the future of families. Huber (1986) has written of the "growing disincentives of childbearing," citing the opportunity cost of the mother's time, the expense of raising children, and the negative impact of children on parents' marital satisfaction. Over a decade ago, Hunt and Hunt (1982) cautioned that there may be a polarization of dual career couples: between those with children, who cannot play the corporate career game, and those without children, who are free to devote themselves more fully to the workplace. Until societal values change, flexible work options are in danger of creating such a two-tiered track. From interviews with "careerists" who had changed their work hours, Dynerman and Hayes (1991) conclude that part-time workers are not taken as seriously as their full-time counterparts. No matter how strong the actual commitment to work among those who have scaled down their hours, others treat them as less committed.

Gender Roles

The age-integrated model proposes similar life pathways for men and women. Gender roles will have to change drastically for this to become a reality, however. Women's well-documented responsibility for domestic work and childcare (e.g., Hartmann, 1981; Fox & Nichols, 1983; Pleck, 1985) is an impediment to the age-integrated model of the life course. This is paradoxical, as the century-long rise in women's commitment to paid work represents one of the greatest historical pressures for structural change (Riley, 1992). As long as the work–family strain remains a "women's issue," any changes are likely to be surface accommodations, rather than the fundamental restructuring required to provide equal opportunities for women and men.

The basic problem is that "asymmetrically permeable boundaries" between work and family (Pleck, 1977) continue to be an accurate image of gender roles. Among women, family is still expected to intrude on work, but among men it is quite the reverse. Thus, the new work options are often geared toward women rather than men. Moreover, as many family-oriented company policies are deemed appropriate for women, but not for men, both subtle and overt pressures hinder men from taking advantage of these options. Evidence from Sweden, where parental leave for men as well as women has been available for some time, underscores the need for a change in gender roles (Blau & Ferber, 1986). Swedish men have been slow to take advantage of this opportunity to meet family needs, partly because of men's (and to some extent women's) belief in the role of man as breadwinner, and partly because of tendencies by both supervisors and employers to discount men's family role (Ford Foundation, 1989).

Without attention to the implications for gender inequality, then, many of the more flexible work options may seem deceptively positive. If among married couples it is the wives who take the economically inferior part-time jobs, then the pay imbalance between husbands and wives will continue to widen, with deleterious consequences for power relations and for women's lives in the event of divorce. Moreover, wives working part-time may have even greater difficulty than wives working full-time in getting help with housework from their husbands. Dynerman and Hayes (1991; p. 176) quote a career woman whose husband had taken his share of responsibility for household tasks until she reduced her work schedule, "It all came to a screeching halt when I cut back my hours. Suddenly he thought he had a *wife*."

Overcoming the Obstacles

Powerful as these obstacles to age integration are, past and current trends suggest at least four ways in which they may, in the future, be gradually reduced.

First, corporations and small businesses may become readier to accept both older workers and family-oriented policies. Just as educators have discovered the benefits of older students, many employers, by "taking a chance" on older workers, have been discovering the special benefits to be gained from their accumulated wisdom and expertise (Schrank & Waring, 1983). In addition, more and more employers have begun to recognize, albeit slowly, that family-oriented policies are useful ways to attract and retain topnotch employees. Even though the best family benefit packages are typically afforded by the largest companies, some smaller companies and government agencies that cannot offer lavish salaries have learned to compete for good workers by providing the flexibilities desired by people in both the middle and the later years. As more companies recognize the advantages of openly acknowledging the work–family interface, pressures toward family-oriented company "strategies" will predictably expand.

Second, the long-term changes in demography and family structure may tend to reduce the work–family "crunch." The proportion of the life course during which people have dependent children has long been decreasing (Riley, 1992). Thus the many years with adult offspring may well compensate for the comparatively few years with small children who require care. In the meantime, demands for care of frail elderly parents are being postponed, as longevity and independence of the older generations improve. If such tendencies persist, most people will have only a brief share of the lifetime during which the acute strains of family roles exacerbate the middle-aged stresses from work roles.

Third, as the advantages of age integration become more apparent, men may become readier to transcend the "gender asymmetry in permeable boundaries" and to adopt the flexible life pathways already pioneered by women. The widely publicized "men's movement" has called attention to the importance of men's connection to family, friends, and community. Emerging research suggests that having an enlarged family role is good for men's mental health (Pleck, 1989). If people heed the feminist calls (by both women and men) for a social movement in which the sexes join together to push for more balance in their lives (Brod, 1986; Friedan, 1991), social structures may well bow to the collective pressure. Hopefully this new feminist agenda will include enlarged opportunities for women and men in their later, as well as their earlier, years.

Fourth, and perhaps hardest to imagine for the future, is a scenario in which Americans are willing to sacrifice the goal of full-time, high-paying jobs for more leisure and family time, and for a more equitable allocation by age and gender of whatever jobs are available. Yet palpable evidence that changes in underlying values and structural boundaries are possible comes from the "gender revolution"—the remarkable twentieth-century shift in women's work roles (Riley, 1992). In cohorts of women born early in the century, comparatively few—mainly the economically disadvantaged—engaged in a lifetime of paid work. In each more recent cohort, however, larger and larger proportions of women have spent their adult lives in the labor force until, in the most recent cohorts, women no longer tend to drop out of work even when their children are little. From generation to generation, with the changes in women's lives, more and more work roles have opened up for them, and norms as well as structures have changed. First it became acceptable for women to work. Now it is often expected, even required, that women at all socioeconomic levels, including young mothers, *should* work for pay—at least up to the still rigid age boundary for retirement.

Whether or not, in a future age-integrated society, less exclusive emphasis will in fact be placed on the materialistic values of capitalism is still moot. It is not inconceivable, however, that the broad shift away from lifetime to "contingent" and part-time jobs, and the drastic restructuring of firms, will have far-reaching consequences for people's behaviors and attitudes. Workers may well become accustomed to a degree of austerity. We hope societal values will include increased emphasis on economic support for the disadvantaged—whatever their age, gender, race, ethnic background, or social class. At the same time, there may well be a shift away from exclusive emphasis on consumerism and upward mobility to new emphases on nonmonetary rewards: affection and response from family and friends, recognition for cultural pursuits, pleasure in new adventures. Such release from the stress of over-work is likely to enhance the productivity of the redefined hours and conditions of work.

Toward Future Scientific Advances

There is every advantage in continuing now—before the baby boom cohorts overwhelm the social order—to ask the questions and search for the answers that are raised by the vision of an age-integrated society. Among the current scientific efforts, one is Program Age and Structural Change (PASC) at the National Institute on Aging. Involving a network of scholars (including the authors of this chapter), PASC addresses the widely neglected dynamism of structural changes as they influence human lives. The program aims toward deeper understanding of how age-related changes occur in work, families, and other structures.

Scholars in PASC and elsewhere are gradually building a science base that can serve as a guide for public policy and professional practice. Planning ahead for people's long lives requires a systematically designed overhaul of educational programs, for example, and a carefully studied redirection of health care toward prevention and rehabilitation. It requires assessment of the outcomes of proposed interventions. Moreover, developments toward age integration already underway require continual monitoring if they are to avoid sharpening the other major bases of potential societal cleavage: gender, social class, and race-ethnicity. Also needed are protections against abuses—such as exploiting the labor of the very old and the very young, or failing to protect the resources that can assure an adequate life style for that minority of older people who require support.

Of major concern to PASC is how age barriers to change can be broken down, and how structural opportunities can enhance the quality of aging from birth to death. Here the vision of an age-integrated society provides a useful blueprint. In this society, retirement as it is known today gives way to periods of leisure interspersed throughout the life course with periods of education and work. The lockstep of traditional education is replaced with lifelong learning. This society allows time for family and for children, especially when they are young. Whatever the supply of available jobs at any particular time, these jobs are distributed more evenly across the age range; and work is valued as much for its intrinsic meaning as for its economic returns. Older people have responsibilities as well as rights: they have become less a burden than a productive asset. An age-integrated society has the potential to enhance the quality of individual lives and to help solve the societal problems wrought by structural lag.

As scientific understanding advances, this vision need not remain entirely visionary. Within the realm of possibility, a future society can be glimpsed in which there will in fact be new and more balanced relationships between changing social structures and people's changing lives, and in which opportunities for productive work and for leisure will be distributed more equitably across all ages.

References

Blau, F. D., & Ferber, M.A. (1986). *The economics of women, men and work.* Englewood Cliffs, NJ: Prentice-Hall.

Brod, H. (1992). Fraternity, equality, liberty. In M. Kimmel and M. Messner (Eds.), *Men's lives*, 2nd ed. (pp. 554–566). New York: MacMillan.

Dychtwald, K. (1989). *Age wave: The challenges and opportunities of an aging America.* Los Angeles: Jeremy P. Tarcher.

Dynerman, S. B., & Hayes, L.O. (1991). *The best jobs in America for parents.* New York: Ballantine Books.

Fiatarone, M. A., Marks, E. C., Meredith, C. N., Lipsitz, L. A., & Evans, W. J. (1990). High intensity strength training in nonagenarians: Effects on skeletal muscle. *Journal of the American Medical Association, 263,* 3029–34.

Ford Foundation (1989). *Work and family responsibilities: Achieving a balance.* New York: The Ford Foundation.

Fox, K. D., & Nickols, S. Y. (1983). The time crunch: Wife's employment and family work. *Journal of Family Issues, 4,* 61–82.

Friedan, B. (1991). *The second stage*, 3rd ed. New York: Dell Publishing.

Hartmann, H. (1981). The family as the locus of gender, class and political struggle. *Signs, 6,* 366–394.

Henretta, J. C. (1992). Uniformity and diversity: Life Course Institutionalization and late-life work exit. *The Sociological Quarterly, 33,* 265–279.

Huber, J. (1986). Trends in gender stratification, 1970–1985. *Sociological Forum, 1,* 476–495.

Hunt, L. & Hunt, J. (1982). Dualities of careers and families: New integrations or new polarizations? *Social Problems, 29,* 499–510.

Johnston, W. B., & Packer, A. E. (1987). *Workforce 2000.* Indianapolis.

Kamerman, S. B., & Kahn, A. J. (1987). *The responsive workplace.* New York: Columbia University Press.

Kohli, M. (1988). *New patterns of transition to retirement in West Germany.* Tampa, FL: International Exchange Center on Gerontology, University of South Florida.

Kohli, M., Rein, M. Guillemard, A. M., & VanGusteren, H. (Eds.), (1991). *Time for retirement.* New York: Cambridge University Press.

Loscocco, K. A. (1989). The instrumentally oriented factory worker: Myth or reality? *Work and Occupations, 16,* 3–25.

McNaught, W., Barth, M. C., & Henderson, P. H. (1991). Older Americans: Willing and able to work. In A. H. Munnell (ed.), *Retirement and public policy* (pp. 101–114). Dubuque, IA: Kendall/Hunt Publishing Company.

Manton, K. G., Stallard, E., & Singer, B. H. (1992). Projecting the future size and health status of the U.S. elderly population. *International Journal of Forecasting, 8,* pp. 433–458.

Moen, P. (1992). *Women's roles: A contemporary dilemma.* New York: Auburn House (Greenwood Press).

Pleck, J. H. (1977). The work–family role system. *Social Problems, 24,* 417–427.

Pleck, J. H. (1985). *Working wives, working husbands.* Beverly Hills, CA: Sage.

Pleck, J. H. (1989). The contemporary man. In M. Kimmel & M. Messner (Eds.), *Men's lives,* 1st ed. (pp. 591–596). New York: MacMillan.

Quinn, J. F., Burkhauser, R. V., & Myers, D. A. (1990). *Passing the torch: The influence of economic incentives of work and retirement.* Kalamazoo, Michigan: W.E. Upjohn Institute.

Riley, M. W. (1978). Aging, social change, and the power of ideas. *Daedalus, 107,* 39–52.

Riley, M. W. (1988). The aging society: Problems and prospects. *Proceedings of the American Philosophical Society. 132,* (2), 148–153. Philadelphia, PA: American Philosophical Society.

Riley, M. W. (1992). Age, gender, and the problem of structural lag. Speech delivered to honor the opening of the Life Course Institute, Cornell University, Ithaca, NY, April 27.

Riley, M. W., & Abeles, R. P. (1990). *The behavioral and social research program at the National Institute on Aging: history of a decade.* Working

Document. Bethesda, MD: Behavioral and Social Research, National Institutes of Health.

Riley, M. W., Foner, A., & Waring, J. (1988). Sociology of age. In N. Smelser (Ed.), *Handbook of sociology* (pp. 143-290). Newbury Park, CA: Sage.

Riley, M. W., Kahn, R. L., & Foner, A. (Eds.). (1994). *Age and structural lag.* New York: Wiley.

Riley, M. W., & Riley, J. W., Jr. (1991). Vieillesse et changement des roles sociaux. *Gerontologie et Societie, 56,* 6-14.

Schor, J. B. (1992). *The overworked American: The unexpected decline of leisure.* New York: Basic Books.

Schrank, H. T., & Waring, J. (1983). Aging and work organizations. In M. W. Riley, B. B. Hess, & K. Bond (Eds.), *Aging in society,* (pp. 53-70). Hillsdale, NJ: Lawrence Erlbaum.

Suzman, R. M., Willis, D. P., & Manton, K. G. (Eds.), (1992). *The oldest old.* New York: Oxford University Press.

U.S. Bureau of the Census. (1992). *Current Population Survey,* Washington, DC; U.S. Government Printing Office.

Voydanoff, P. (1987). *Work and family life.* Beverly Hills, CA: Sage.

Willis, S. L. (1990). Current issues in cognitive training research. In Eugene A. Lovelace (Ed.), *Aging and cognition, mental processes, self-awareness, and interventions.* New York: Elsevier.

Chapter 14

Socioeconomic Status and Health over the Life Course

Stephanie A. Robert and James S. House

Promoting health, preventing disease, and reducing expenditures on health care have become national goals, important in their own right and important to efforts to revive a lagging American economy. In an aging society, adults of middle and older age are increasingly the focus of such efforts, because the leading causes of mortality, morbidity, and disability affect primarily this portion of the population. Concern and debate are increasing about whether the continued rise in life expectancy will result in Americans living longer, healthier lives with significant morbidity occurring during only a brief period at the end of life (Fries, 1980, 1984), or whether extended life means an extended period of debilitation such that Americans will live longer, sicker lives (Schneider & Brody, 1983; Manton, 1982; Verbrugge, 1984).

It is unclear which of these scenarios is now occurring and whether potential future changes in life expectancy and maximal life span make one or the other more likely. Clearly a basic goal of research on aging is to extend the relatively healthy, vigorous, and productive years of life and reduce time in illness and disability. This requires moving beyond looking at trends in the total population to identifying factors that predict and promote maintenance of health and effective functioning in middle and later life and increase the "rectangularization" of the mortality, morbidity, and disability curves.

Among the factors affecting the maintenance of health and quality of life in middle and older age, socioeconomic status (SES) seems especially promising and surprisingly understudied in recent years, at least in the United States[1]. Research repeatedly indicates that those with low SES have higher morbidity and mortality rates than those with high SES. An extensive literature review (Antonovsky, 1967) showed that a strong inverse association between SES and mortality was consistently reported despite the use of a variety of different research methods. Kitigawa and Hauser (1973) subsequently found mortality strongly associated with income and education, and recent research continues to find strong SES differentials in mortality in the U.S. (Williams, 1990). Various measures of morbidity (including prevalence of acute or chronic diseases, activity limitations, bed disability days, and self-rated health) are also inversely related to SES (House et al., 1990; Newacheck, Butler, Harper, Piontkowski, & Franks, 1980; Satariano, 1986; Syme & Berkman, 1976). These SES differentials in morbidity and mortality have persisted in the U.S. despite the elimination or control of many infectious diseases; improvements in nutrition, housing, and sanitation, and increased access to medical care for the elderly and the poor through Medicare and Medicaid (Williams, 1990).

Surprisingly, little research on SES differentials in health focuses on the elderly or investigates how these patterns vary by age. The elderly are often left out of such studies altogether (Markides, 1989; Victor, 1989), or they are combined into one large age category such as "60+" without any attention paid to intraelderly age differences (Rowe & Kahn, 1987). Research on SES differentials in health can be criticized for not paying attention to age distinctions, but research on aging and health can similarly be criticized for not considering SES differentials (House et al., 1992; Markides, 1989). In the middle and late 1980s, SES was not even considered in overviews of government statistics on aging and health (e.g. Brody, Brock, & Williams, 1987; National Center for Health Statistics, 1987), and was treated only cursorily in major reviews of the literature on aging and health (e.g., Shanas & Maddox, 1985).

Only recently have the issues of aging, health, and SES been considered together. A limited but growing body of theory and research suggests that the process by which health changes with age may be stratified by SES. Much research has shown that SES differentials in adult mortality seem to be minimal during young adulthood, large in middle age, and then smaller again in old age (Antonovsky, 1967; Haan, Kaplan, & Camacho, 1987; Kaplan, Seeman, Cohen, Knudsen, & Guralnik, 1987; Kitigawa & Hauser, 1973; Wilkins, Adams, & Brancker, 1989). More recent work has considered various measures of health and confirmed this pattern for morbidity and functional status (House et al., 1990; Longino, 1990). House and colleagues (1990) suggest that individuals with higher SES are able to postpone not only mortality but also significant morbidity and disability until relatively late in life, whereas lower SES people experience significant levels of mortality, morbidity, and disability beginning relatively early in midlife (see Figures 14.1 and 14.2).

Therefore, successful efforts to maintain the health of people as they age need to be based on an understanding of why health is stratified by SES. Similarly, efforts to reduce SES differentials in health should take into account the mechanisms that produce age variation in how SES relates to health. A theoretical explanation for SES differentials in health needs to explain both the mechanisms accounting for the wide SES differentials in health in middle age and early old age, as well as the apparent minimal differentials seen in early adulthood and advanced old age.

In this chapter, various general explanations for SES differentials in health are evaluated in terms of their success or failure in accounting for the observed variation in the relation of SES to health over the adult life course. The explanations discussed are: (a) selective mobility and selective survival, (b) access to health care, (c) psychosocial, behavioral, and environmental factors, and (d) age stratification.

Also identified are major methodological and theoretical issues for future research aimed at understanding the mechanisms linking SES to health over the life course. The chapter concludes with a discussion of the implications of current knowledge for achieving maintenance or improvements in health in an aging society.

Selective Mobility and Selective Survival

Selective mobility theories suggest that the association between SES and health may flow from health to SES: The healthy in society may move up the socioeconomic scale, whereas the unhealthy move down. One selective mobility argument is that health at early ages

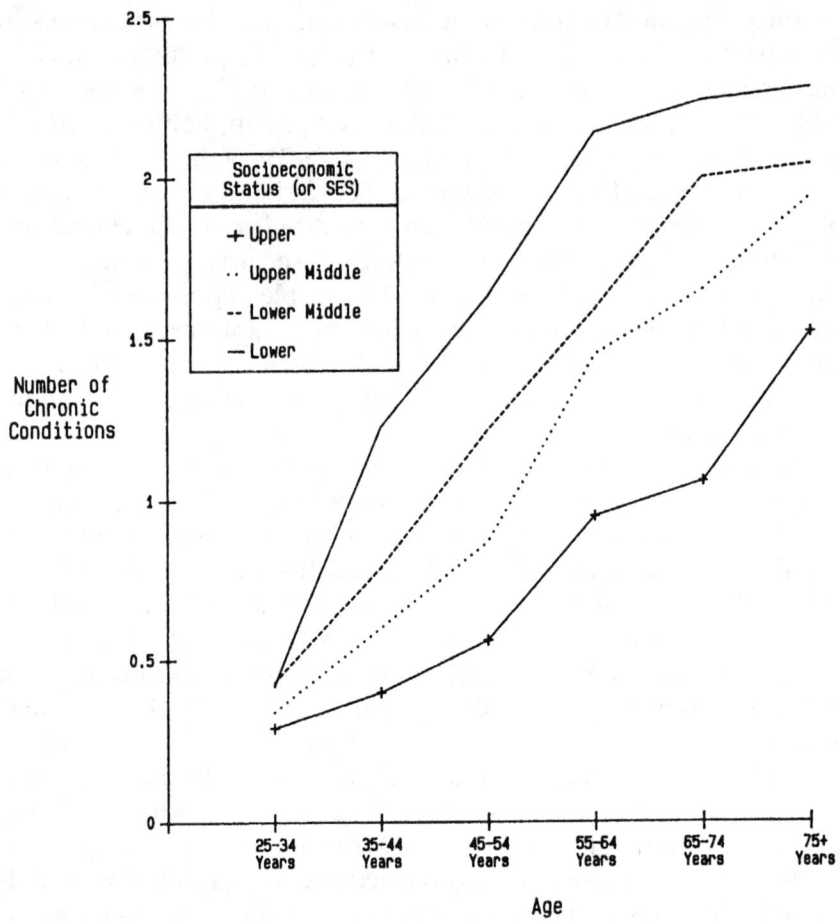

FIGURE 14.1 Age by Number of Chronic Conditions Within Levels of Socioeconomic Status
Source: House et al. (1992). 1986 Americans' Changing Lives Interview Survey Data, n=3,617

plays a role in determining the level of education and later occupation and income that an individual achieves. A second selective mobility argument describes how unhealthy people can "drift" into lower socioeconomic statuses by losing their jobs, moving into less prestigious occupations, or experiencing losses in income. Although the size of these effects cannot be accurately estimated without lifelong longitudinal data (Carr-Hill, 1987), evidence from Great Britain indicates that

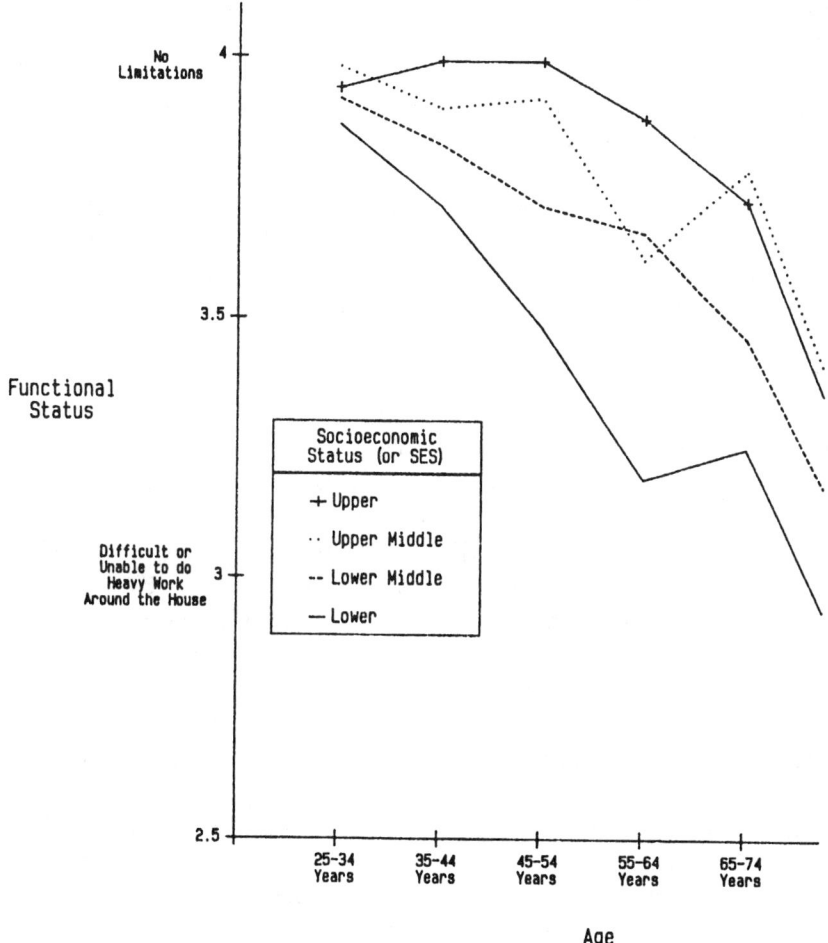

FIGURE 14.2 Age by Functional Status Within Levels of Socioeconomic Status
Source: House et al. (1992). 1986 Americans' Changing Lives Interview Survey Data, n=3,617

selective mobility seems to account for comparatively little of observed SES differentials in mortality (Fox, Goldblatt, & Jones, 1985; Wadsworth, 1986; Wilkinson, 1986, 1989). Moreover, the effects of selective mobility cannot, by themselves, logically account for diminished SES differentials in health either in early adulthood or later old age. Indeed, they would predict increased differentials over the life course.

The *selective survival* thesis does not account for the poorer health and mortality experience of lower SES persons over most of the life course, but rather attempts to account only for the narrowing of SES differences in old age: "disadvantaged high mortality populations appear to experience a greater amount of removal of the least robust persons before old age, so that the surviving elderly in such populations might include a relatively high rate of hardy persons" (Markides, 1989, p. 18). SES differentials in health are expected to be smaller in old age than in middle age because a disproportionate number of low SES people would have died during middle age leaving only more hardy low SES people to survive with the increasingly frail high SES elderly (Markides & Machalek, 1984).

Although the selective survival thesis is not usually invoked to fully explain the diminished relationship between SES and health in later old age, researchers have used it as a partial explanation even if the actual effects were not measured in the analyses (e.g. House et al., 1990; Longino, Warheit, & Green, 1989; Satariano, 1986). The evidence for selective survival effects, however, is largely inferential because such effects are virtually impossible to measure or estimate in cross-sectional studies or in studies with only limited longitudinal data. Measuring or estimating these effects should be included in future longer-term longitudinal research.

Future consideration of the selective survival thesis also needs to explain why some people are hardy and some are not. In order to truly understand the mechanisms of selective survival, more needs to be known about the "successful agers" (Rowe & Kahn, 1987): Those who are healthy survivors in older age despite their low socioeconomic positions. What is it about their past and current biological, psychological, social, and environmental experiences and exposures that allows them to be "hardier" than many of their higher SES peers?

Medical Care

Another explanation for diminished SES differentials in health at older ages may be found in variations in access to medical care over the life course. In old age, Medicare may equalize access to medical care, thereby diminishing the relationship between SES and health in later old age. However, many argue that medical care plays only a minor role in determining health status at any age, and no direct evidence has yet been presented that equalization in access to medical care substantially reduces SES differences in health.

Studies in the U.S. and England suggest that the dramatic declines in mortality in modern times were primarily due to environmental and standard of living improvements rather than advances in medical care (McKeown, 1979; McKinlay & McKinlay, 1977). Although equal access to medical care is recognized as an important goal, most research finds that differential access to and use of medical services explains little of the observed SES differentials in health (Blaxter, 1983; House et al., 1992; Marmot, Kogevinas, & Elston, 1987; Williams, 1990). The Black Report (DHSS, 1980) indicated that increased access to medical care in Britain, resulting from the establishment of the British National Health Service, was not accompanied by improvements in SES differentials in health. In fact, SES differentials in health may even be widening in Britain (Wilkinson, 1986). Similarly, Wilkins and colleagues (1989) found little evidence of decline in SES differentials in mortality in Canada over a period (1971 to 1986) during which national health insurance was introduced. Despite the wide variety of health care systems and varying degrees of access to medical care seen in different countries, strong SES differentials in health are found in most developed and many third-world countries.

There is also no clear evidence that the advent of Medicare or Medicaid in the U.S. altered SES differences in health. Direct controls for brief survey indicators of having health insurance and rate of utilization of medical care have contributed little to explaining variations in health by age and SES (House et al., 1992). Thus, differential access to medical care is an implausible explanation both for the wide SES differences in health in middle or early old age and for the narrowing of such differences in early adulthood and later old age. Two qualifications are in order, however. First, even if medical care has little impact on SES differences in morbidity, disability, activity limitations, and mortality, it can play an important role in improving quality of life, especially for the elderly, by limiting the length and severity of acute and some chronic conditions and by alleviating pain or discomfort. Second, it must be noted that although access to care has not been found to significantly reduce SES differences in health, little attention has been paid to measuring the effects of how access to broader forms of care do or would reduce SES differences in health. The current research focus on medical care has primarily measured the effects of access to treatment of serious acute or chronic conditions. Less attention has been paid to the effects of access to preventive care, nonmedical types of care, or community-based long-term care. The latter forms of health care may be more consequential in explaining and alleviating SES differentials in health, but they are not adequately covered or provided in most health insurance or health care plans, including Medicare and Medicaid. The impact and importance of these broader forms of health care need to be more adequately addressed in future research and policy.

Psychosocial, Behavioral, and Environmental Factors

A social structure and personality perspective may be used to explain how SES is related to health through intermediate mechanisms (Williams, 1990). According to this perspective, various psychosocial, behavioral, and environmental factors are more proximate determinants of health, but the distribution of these factors is determined by social structural factors such as SES. People with lower SES are more likely to be exposed to or characterized by environmental and psychosocial risk factors that are associated with poor health and earlier death, whereas people with higher SES tend to have psychosocial characteristics, health behaviors, and work and community environments that are protective of health.

The major psychosocial, behavioral, and environmental risk factors for poor health and mortality include: (a) lack of a sense of control (Rodin, 1986); (b) lack of social relationships and supports (Berkman & Breslow, 1983; House, Landis, & Umberson, 1988); (c) chronic and acute stress (Pearlin, Lieberman, Menaghan, & Mullan, 1981; Theorell, 1982; Thoits, 1983); (d) health behaviors such as smoking, immoderate eating and drinking, and lack of physical exercise (Berkman & Breslow, 1983); and (e) physical, chemical, biological, and psychosocial hazards and stressors at work (Goldsmith & Hirschberg, 1976; Karasek & Theorell, 1990) and at home or in the community (Devesa & Diamond, 1983; Haan, Kaplan, & Camacho, 1987).

Lower SES groups are disadvantaged on all of these risk factors (House et al., 1992; Williams, 1990) as would be expected if they explain SES differences in health. If these risk factors also account for the diminished relationship between SES and health in early adulthood and advanced old age, SES differences in *exposure* to these risk factors and/or the *impact* of them must differ by age. House and colleagues

(1992) hypothesized that SES differences in exposure to risk factors are greatest in middle and early old age because the effects of SES accumulate over the life course, but are mitigated at older ages by U.S. social welfare policies (such as retirement, Social Security, and Medicare). Further, the impact of most risk factors increases with age because of greater biological and perhaps also psychological vulnerability. Thus, House and colleagues (1992) predict:

> On average, we should see the largest socioeconomic differentials in health in middle and early old age because these age groups are most likely to be characterized by both sizable SES differentials in exposure to risk factors and substantial impact of the risk factors. In contrast, in early adulthood, SES differentials in exposure may be sizable but their health impact is muted, whereas in later old age SES differentials in exposure become somewhat muted even if their impact remains strong. (p. 4)

House and colleagues (1992) tested this hypothesis to see if exposure to and impact of psychosocial and behavioral risk factors could account for observed SES differentials in health across adult age groups. They used data from the Americans' Changing Lives survey based on a representative sample of noninstitutionalized adults aged 25 or older living in the 48 contiguous states. They measured SES using an index combining education and income components. Health status variables included a count of chronic conditions, an index of functional status, and a self-rated measure of limitation of daily activities. Risk factors included smoking, relative weight, alcohol consumption, indices of social relationships and supports, indicators of acute and chronic stress, and a self-efficacy index.

Results indicated that lower SES strata were more likely to be in the high risk category or level on all risk factors. For some risk factors this difference by SES was constant across age groups, but for a majority it was greatest in middle age and early old age. Further, the impact of about half of the risk factors tended to increase with age. For each measure of health, the SES differentials across all age groups were reduced by 50%–75% once exposure to and impact of the risk factors were accounted for. The investigators concluded that "the combination of differential exposure to risk factors across SES groups and different impact of the risk factors across age groups substantially explains the social stratification of aging and health" (House et al., 1992, p. 23).

This study provides both theoretical and empirical support for a fairly comprehensive explanation of SES differentials in health throughout the life course. It explains how a number of risk factors may mediate the relationship between SES and health, but the investigators recognize that other risk factors not considered in their analysis should be included in future research. Another set of risk factors that might be considered in future research includes measures of physical, chemical, biological, and psychosocial hazards and stressors located in the work place, at home, or in the community. For example, Haan et al. (1987) found residence in a poverty area to be associated with increased risk of death, even after adjusting for age, gender, race, baseline physical health status, low income, lack of medical care, unemployment, education, health practices, social isolation, and psychologic uncertainty or depression.

Another factor to include in future analyses should be "residues" of early life experience. This would allow for recognition that health status is a reflection of not only current exposure to deprivation, but also of past exposure to deprivation (McLeod & Kessler, 1990). Abeles (1992) emphasizes that the impact of social stratification and aging processes on health status is both contemporaneous and cumulative. Future research could explore the relative effects on health status of contemporaneous, cumulative, and early life exposures to risk factors over the life course. Haan et al. (1989) further suggest that:

> *Given that the health disadvantage associated with lower SES may begin early and may be cumulative over the life span, it is still possible that different risk factors may be responsible for the poor health of lower SES people at different stages of life. It is important for our understanding of this phenomena to examine the pattern of such etiologic risk factors in addition to looking at them singly. (p. 82)*

Therefore, research should test whether different risk factors or combinations thereof are more or less important to health at various stages of the life course (DHSS, 1980).

Age Stratification

Age stratification theory offers two explanations for the diminished relationship between SES and health in advanced old age. Both emphasize the importance of viewing age as an indicator of position in a social stratification system that unequally distributes resources and opportunities based on age. The first explanation is that the effects of SES on health are muted in later old age by the strong effects of age stratification on health. The second explanation is that the true effects of social status on health are masked in old age by the use of inappropriate indicators of social status for people at older ages.

The first explanation recognizes that although SES is an important social structural factor that affects health, other stratification systems such as those based on gender, race, and age also impose constraints and opportunities affecting health (Abeles, 1992). From an age stratification perspective, age is not just a biological factor that affects health, nor is it simply a measure of time that implies accumulation of experiences and behaviors that affect health. Age is also a social factor because of the social meaning attached to different stages of the life course. Matilda White Riley (1978) says "that the meanings we attach to age have power. They become age stereotypes, shaping our personal plans, hopes, and fears. They become age constraints, built into the social structure, molding the course of our lives." (p. 49).

It could be argued that because of the general devaluation of the social status of the elderly in our youth-oriented society (Stahl & Feller, 1990), those in old age are at the bottom of an age hierarchy. Lindheim and Syme (1983) present evidence that those at the bottom of any hierarchy may have decreased resistance to disease because of low self-esteem, little perceived control over their lives, and few opportunities for meaningful participation in society. Being at the bottom of the age hierarchy may also be a source of stressful life conditions (Pearlin, 1989). Therefore, age stereotyping may affect the health of the elderly by damaging self-esteem and perceived control, by limiting opportunities for meaningful roles in old age, and by being a source of stress.

Because the effects of ageism cut across SES groups, ageism may have effects on health in old age that are stronger than the effects of SES differentials, thereby muting SES differentials in health in later old age. Perhaps the status and experiences of individuals as "older persons" become more salient than their socioeconomic positions as determinants of health status.

A second age stratification explanation for the diminished relationship between SES and health in advanced old age is suggested by Berkman (1988):

> *While income, education, and occupation may be good indicators of social class in both the hierarchical sense and in terms of access to goods and resources in middle age, they may not be accurate reflections of social position and its relative advantages in old age. In old age, social position may be determined by where one stands relative to one's peers according to different criteria (e.g., leadership in volun-*

> *tary activities rather than lifetime occupation) or where one is relative to where one was throughout the working years. (p. 45)*

If, as Berkman suggests, income, education, and occupation are not good indicators of the relative socioeconomic status of older persons, then it is little wonder that they predict health less strongly at older ages. Alternative indicators of SES may show greater effects on health in older ages, suggesting that the impact of SES on health is not really diminished in older age, but that SES is a function of different factors in older ages. Berkman suggests two such factors: status in voluntary organizations, or some indicator of status in older age relative to status earlier in life. Similarly, Kaplan and Haan (1989) also argue that *dynamics* of income may be more important than *level* of income when predicting health outcomes among the elderly, and find some supporting evidence: Using 1965–1974 data from an Alameda County study, they found that changes in income were more predictive of mortality than baseline income measures. Elderly respondents who reported a decrease in income of at least $10,000 during the previous 9 years had 1.2 times the risk of death over those 9 years compared with those with no change in income.

Although focusing on change in status is possible using measures of change in income, this approach will not work with measures of education level because education level usually does not change in old age. Similarly, it would be difficult to look at changes in occupational status in old age given the variety of occupational changes that are possible. Perhaps rather than looking at specific occupational changes in old age, research and theory should consider broader role changes in older ages and their effects on health status. In any case, if patterns of change and continuity of status are important to the health of those in advanced old age, static measures of SES used in most research might mask true SES differentials in health in advanced old ages (cf., Abeles, 1992).

Berkman also suggested that there could be entirely different criteria by which socioeconomic status should be measured in older ages. Although she gave "leadership in voluntary activities" as an example of a potential measure of social status, participation in such activities is a way of adjusting to role changes in old age for only a small group of people. More universally relevant may be indicators of assets or wealth instead of or in addition to income.

Age stratification explanations for why SES differentials in health are smaller in later old age are still theoretically underdeveloped, much less empirically investigated. They raise issues that should be addressed in future research on social stratification and health, however. An age stratification approach emphasizes that changes in social status as well as current and past social status may all have an impact on health. It also suggests a broadening of conceptualizations of social status to include new indicators beyond education, income, and occupation that might measure other important aspects of social status or ranking—particularly in old age.

Future Research Issues

This review suggests that the changing relationship between SES and health over the life course is not likely to be accounted for with a single overarching explanation. Therefore, future research should attempt to assess the effects of multiple and interacting factors. Currently, the social structure and personality framework seems most theoretically and empirically plausible. It posits that the relationship between SES and health is mediated by psychosocial, behavioral, and environmental factors. *Exposure* to these risk factors increases on average through late middle or early old age, but decreases after that, whereas the *impact* of these risk factors increases with age. Research based on this framework not only accounts for much of the overall SES differentials in health, but it explains why the pattern of differentials changes over the life course. This framework also has the ability to integrate the individual and interactive effects of other stratification systems (such as race or gender) on health, although this potential has not yet been fully realized.

Although the effects of selective mobility and selective survival need to be recognized and measured, these factors seem to play only a minor role in explaining the persistent pattern of SES differentials in health over the life course, over time, and across countries. Focusing on these explanations alone obscures the idea that inequality in society has a real impact on health (Carr-Hill, 1987). Finally, although equal access to health care may be an appropriate goal, it alone has not and will not lead to significant decreases in SES differentials in health over the life course.

Future research needs to determine whether observed cross-sectional patterns in SES differentials in health reflect cohort effects or changes within individuals as they age. House et al. (1992) used two waves of the Americans' Changing Lives (ACL) data to perform a short-term (2.5 year) longitudinal analysis to begin answering this question. Their analysis indicated that the observed cross-sectional pattern of SES differentials in health among different age groups may be interpreted as representing how the relationship changes as individuals age, but the results are quite partial and preliminary. Researchers need to perform similar studies covering longer periods of time to verify these findings and to measure the effects of selective mobility and selective survival on SES differentials in health throughout the life course. Similarly, research on the impact of *changes* in social status on the health of Americans can best be performed using longitudinal, multiwave data.

Researchers must also be challenged to reevaluate the measures used in most studies. The discussion of the age stratification perspective raised the issue of testing different measures of social status—particularly when studying the elderly. Also discussed was how at the intervening level, the independent, interactive, and combined effects of various psychosocial, behavioral, and environmental factors on health status throughout the life course need to be measured. For example, are some risk factors more important than others at different ages? Do certain combinations of risk factors have effects on health status greater than the sum of their individual risks? Finally, a variety of different health outcome measures need to be used—including self-reported physical, functional, psychological, and emotional health, biological indicators of physical health, and clinical evaluations of health status. The impact of social stratification on health may vary depending on the measures of social status, intervening mechanisms, and health status used.

Policy Implications

The importance of research on social stratification and health lies in its potential for informing social action or policy to improve health. This can occur by simply describing patterns of differential health status by SES, age, race, and gender. Such patterns help target health improvement efforts to groups where differentials in health are greatest. For example, because SES differentials in health seem to be largest in middle age and early old age, efforts to improve health should be targeted at low SES people of middle and early old ages.

Another route to informing health policy is to explain *why* differentials exist so that approaches to improving health can be designed to attack the underlying *causes* of the differentials. As such, the explanations of SES differentials in health discussed in this chapter suggest three approaches to improving or maintaining health: (1) changing individual behavior and lifestyles, (2) improving socioeconomic conditions, and (3) changing how society views and treats older people.

Individual Behavior Change

As mentioned earlier, some research finds that psychosocial and behavioral risk factors mediate the relationship between SES and health throughout the life course. Therefore, changing psychosocial and behavioral risk factors is one approach to improving health. Various health promotion and disease prevention efforts have focused on changing individual behaviors such as smoking, diet, and exercise as well as improving psychosocial factors such as stress, coping abilities, sense of control, and social supports.

Despite the proliferation of various health promotion efforts targeting unhealthy lifestyles and behaviors, such programs to this date have had limited effectiveness for people with low SES (Wilkinson, 1986; Williams, 1990). In fact, some health promotion efforts have exacerbated SES differentials in health by improving further the health of people with high SES, but not improving the health of people with low SES (Vågerö, 1991; Wilkinson, 1989). In general, people of higher SES are more likely to participate in individual health promotion interventions (Mettlin, Cummings, & Walsh, 1985; Wilkinson, 1989) and are more likely to succeed at changing risky health behaviors through these programs (Wilcox et al., 1985). Research is needed to understand why this is so, and what can make health promotion more effective among lower SES groups.

Similarly, little research examines the success of health promotion interventions among people of different age groups. The elderly are often not included in general health promotion and disease prevention studies because it is thought that there would be few measurable health benefits at older ages (Hickey & Stilwell, 1991). Some evidence indicates, however, that health promotion interventions can improve health outcomes for the elderly (Hickey & Stilwell, 1991; Kaplan & Haan, 1989) and many people advocate health promotion efforts throughout old age (Fried and Bush, 1988; Hickey and Stilwell, 1991; Rowe and Kahn, 1987). Successful models for younger ages should not be assumed to be equally effective for older persons; yet interventions designed specifically for older persons need to be evaluated to see if they are, in fact, more appropriate and successful for the elderly.

Improving Socioeconomic Conditions

Although some believe that health policy should primarily focus on promoting individual responsibility for health and on individual change of lifestyles and behaviors (Knowles, 1990), others believe that this focus leads to a "blaming the victim" mentality (Crawford, 1990). By focusing on an individual's responsibility for health, the social structural factors that cause the differential health behavior patterns are ignored (Crawford, 1990). The social structure and personality framework suggests that unhealthy lifestyles and behaviors are only the more proximate causes of poor health. Low SES and the social, economic, and environmental conditions associated with it are the more fundamental causes of both unhealthy lifestyles and poor health (House et al., 1990; Williams, 1990).

As such, many argue that improvements in health are best achieved by attacking these root causes of poor health (Carr-Hill, 1987; Dutton & Levine, 1989; Williams, 1990). House and colleagues (1992) suggest that "theory, research, and policy aimed at eliminating extreme socioeconomic deprivation and moderating socioeconomic inequality may be important and necessary complements to the direct reduction of psychosocial risk factors" (p. 28). Focusing on improving socioeconomic deprivation and inequality may be necessary because there is reason to believe that the relation of SES to health might persist even if current psychosocial, behavioral, and environmental factors were ameliorated. Williams (1990) argues that:

> *The pathogenic factors determining health status have not been static over the course of this century. The intervening mechanisms have changed but the SES gradient in health persists. Earlier explanations that focused on overcrowded housing, inadequate sanitation, poor hygiene, and malnutrition probably were correct at that time (cf. McKeown, 1979). They are less important now because other features similarly linked to the structure of society have taken their place.* (p. 91)

Currently in the U.S., members of higher SES groups are ridding themselves of risky health lifestyles and behaviors whereas those in lower SES groups are not. For example, health risk factors such as smoking, poor diet, and lack of exercise, which used to be more prevalent in higher SES groups, are now more prevalent among lower SES groups (House et al., 1990; Williams, 1990). A diffusion of innovations theory might view health promotion efforts as resources that are adopted first by higher SES groups before diffusing more slowly to lower SES groups (Blaxter, 1983). By the time current health promotion innovations diffuse to lower SES groups, however, new intervening factors may link SES to health, and the higher SES groups will be the first to have the knowledge and resources to adapt to these changes. Therefore, although health programs and policies that focus on improving access to medical care and on getting people to change their lifestyles and behaviors will improve the overall health of people in our society, they will not succeed in eliminating or significantly reducing inequalities in health unless accompanied by improvements in socioeconomic conditions and inequality.

Changes in Societal Views and Treatment of the Elderly

The discussion of the impact of age stratification on the health of the elderly suggests that in order to improve the health of the elderly, it may be necessary to go beyond improving their lifestyles and behaviors and even go beyond improving the socioeconomic conditions of their lives. Although at the individual level efforts can be made to help the elderly cope with and adjust to changes in roles and status that they may face, such a focus ignores the structural factors that limit the roles available to the elderly in the first place (see Riley and Loscocco, Chapter 13, this volume). At the social structural level, improving the socioeconomic conditions of the elderly may improve their health, but will not eliminate all health effects deriving from the age stratification system. Changing ageist views and treatment of the elderly may also be important to improving the health of the elderly. Such changes include being open to new age norm formations (Riley, 1978) so that old age can be seen by the nonelderly and the elderly alike not as a time of necessary decrement and decline, but as a time of continued positive and productive roles in society. Matilda White Riley (1978) says that: "We have an opportunity too to act upon the broadening knowledge base, to exert control over life course definitions as they develop. The meanings of age are not unchangeable" (p. 50). What is important here is the recognition that society has the ability to improve the health of its citizens not only by changing lifestyles and behaviors or by improving the material conditions of life, but also by changing the various social hierarchies that interact to shape and constrain lives.

Acknowledgments

The writing of this chapter was partially supported by a fellowship to the first author from the National Institute on Aging, grant #2-T32-AG 00117-06, for Social Research Training on Applied Issues of Aging (Ruth Dunkle, Principal Investigator), and by National Institute on Aging Grant #P01AG05561 to the second author.

Notes

[1] In this chapter, SES refers to an inequality in ranking characterized by differential access to a variety of resources and opportunities. SES is usually measured by occupation, income, education, or some combination thereof. Because various indicators of SES may influence health in different ways, most research appropriately refers to the specific indicators of SES (such as income or education). For ease and economy of presentation, we will use the term SES to refer to the broad range of indicators, but will often specify particular indicators of SES (e.g., education or income) when discussing specific research studies.

References

Abeles, R. P. (1992). Social stratification and aging: Contemporaneous and cumulative effects. In K. W. Schaie, D. Blazer, & J. S. House (Eds.), *Aging, health behaviors, and health outcomes* (pp. 33–37). Hillsdale, NJ: Lawrence Erlbaum Associates.

Antonovsky, A. (1967). Social class, life expectancy and overall mortality. *The Milbank Memorial Fund Quarterly, 45*, 31–73.

Berkman, L. F. (1988). The changing and heterogeneous nature of aging and longevity: A social and biomedical perspective. In G. L. Maddox & M. P. Lawton (Eds.), *Annual Review of Gerontology and Geriatrics* (pp. 37–68). New York: Springer Publsihing Co.

Berkman, L. F., & Breslow, L. (1983). *Health and ways of living*. New York: Oxford University Press.

Blaxter, M. (1983). Health services as a defence against the consequences of poverty in industrialized societies. *Social Science and Medicine, 17*, 1139–1148.

Brody, J. A., Brock, D. B., & Williams, T. F. (1987). Trends in the health of the elderly population. *Annual Review of Public Health*, *8*, 211–234.
Carr-Hill, R. (1987). The inequalities in health debate: A critical review of the issues. *Journal of Social Policy*, *16*, 509–542.
Crawford, R. (1990). Individual responsibility and health politics. In P. Conrad & R. Kern (Eds.), *The sociology of health and illness: Critical perspectives* (pp. 387–395). New York: St. Martin's Press.
Department of Health and Social Security (1980). *Inequalities in health: Report of a research working group (The Black Report)*. London: Department of Health and Social Security.
Devesa, S. S., & Diamond, E. L. (1983). Socioeconomic and racial differences in lung cancer incidence. *American Journal of Epidemiology*, *118*, 818–831.
Dutton, D. B., & Levine, S. (1989). Socioeconomic status and health: Overview, methodological critique, and reformulation. In J. P. Bunker, D. S. Gomby, & B. H. Kehrer (Eds.), *Pathways to health: The role of social factors* (pp. 29–69). Menlo Park, CA: The Henry J. Kaiser Family Foundation.
Fox, A. J., Goldblatt, P. O., & Jones, D. R. (1985). Social class mortality differentials: artefact, selection or life circumstances? *Journal of Epidemiology and Community Health*, *39*, 1–8.
Fried, L. P., & Bush, T. L. (1988). Morbidity as a focus of preventive health care in the elderly. *Epidemiologic Reviews*, *10*, 48–64.
Fries, J. F. (1980). Aging, natural death, and the compression of morbidity. *New England Journal of Medicine*, *303*, 130–135.
Fries, J. F. (1984). The compression of morbidity: Miscellaneous comments about a theme. *The Gerontologist*, *24*, 354–359.
Goldsmith, J. R., & Hirschberg, D. A. (1976). Mortality and industrial employment. *Journal of Occupational Medicine*, *18*, 161–164.
Haan, M., Kaplan, G. A., & Camacho, T. (1987). Poverty and health: Prospective evidence from the Alameda County study. *American Journal of Epidemiology*, *125*, 989–998.
Haan, M. N., Kaplan, G. A., & Syme, S. L. (1989). Socioeconomic status and health: Old observations and new thoughts. In J. P. Bunker, D. S. Gomby, & B. H. Kehrer (Eds.), *Pathways to health: The role of social factors* (pp. 76–117). Menlo Park, CA: The Henry J. Kaiser Family Foundation.
Hickey, T., & Stilwell, D. L. (1991). Health promotion for older people: All is not well. *The Gerontologist*, *31*, 822–829.
House, J. S., Kessler, R. C., Herzog, A. R., Mero, R. P., Kinney, A. M., &

Breslow, M. J. (1990). Age, socioeconomic status, and health. *The Milbank Quarterly, 68,* 383–411.

House, J. S., Kessler, R. C., Herzog, A. R., Mero, R. P., Kinney, A. M., & Breslow, M. J. (1992). Social stratification, age, and health. In K. W. Schaie, D. Blazer, & J. S. House (Eds.), *Aging, health behaviors, and health outcomes* (pp. 1–32). Hillsdale, NJ: Lawrence Erlbaum Associates.

House, J. S., Landis, K., & Umberson, D. (1988). Social relationships and health. *Science, 241,* 540–545.

Kaplan, G. A., & Haan, M. N. (1989). Is there a role for prevention among the elderly? Epidemiological evidence from the Alameda County study. In M. G. Ory & K. Bond (Eds.), *Aging and health care: Social science and policy perspectives* (pp. 27–51). New York: Routledge.

Kaplan, G. A., Seeman, T. E., Cohen, R. D., Knudsen, L. P., & Guralnik, J. (1987). Mortality among the elderly in the Alameda County study: Behavioral and demographic risk factors. *American Journal of Public Health, 77*(3), 307–312.

Karasek, R. A., & Theorell, T. (1990). *Healthy work.* New York: Basic Books.

Kitagawa, E. M., & Hauser, P. M. (1973). *Differential mortality in the United States: A study in socioeconomic epidemiology.* Cambridge, MA: Harvard University Press.

Knowles, J. H. (1990). The responsibility of the individual. In P. Conrad & R. Kern (Eds.), *The sociology of health and illness: Critical perspectives* (pp. 376–386). New York: St. Martin's Press.

Lindheim, R., & Syme, S. L. (1983). Environments, people, and health. *Annual Review of Public Health, 4,* 335–359.

Longino, C. F. (1990). The relative contributions of gender, social class, and advancing age to health. In S. M. Stahl (Eds.), *The legacy of longevity* (pp. 79–92). London: Sage Publications.

Longino, C. F., Warheit, G. J., & Green, J. A. (1989). Class, aging, and health. In K. S. Markides (Eds.), *Aging and health: Perspectives on gender, race, ethnicity, and class* (pp. 79–110). London: Sage Publications.

Manton, K. G. (1982). Changing concepts of morbidity and mortality in the elderly population. *Milbank Memorial Fund Quarterly, 60*(2), 183–244.

Markides, K. S. (1989). Aging, gender, race/ethnicity, class, and health: A conceptual overview. In K. S. Markides (Ed.), *Aging and health: Perspectives on gender, race, ethnicity, and class* (pp. 9–22). London: Sage Publications.

Markides, K. S., & Machalek, R. (1984). Selective survival, aging and society. *Archives of Gerontology and Geriatrics, 3,* 207–222.

Marmot, M. G., Kogevinas, M., & Elston, M. A. (1987). Social/economic status and disease. *Annual Review of Public Health, 8,* 111–135.

McKeown, T. J. (1979). *The role of medicine: Dream, mirage, or nemesis*. Princeton, NJ: Princeton University Press.

McKinlay, J. B., & McKinlay, S. J. (1977). The questionable contribution of medical measures to the decline of mortality in the U.S. in the twentieth century. *Milbank Memorial Fund Quarterly, 55*, 405–428.

McLeod, J. D., & Kessler, R. C. (1990). Socioeconomic status differences in vulnerability to undesirable life events. *Journal of Health and Social Behavior, 31*, 162–172.

Mettlin, C., Cummings, K. M., & Walsh, D. (1985). Risk factor and behavioral correlates of willingness to participate in cancer prevention trials. *Nutrition and Cancer, 7*(4), 189–198.

National Center for Health Statistics (1987). *Health statistics on older persons: United States, 1986—Vital and Health Statistics* (Series 3, No. 25. Public Health Service. DHHS No. (PHS) 87-1409) Washington DC: U.S. Government Printing Office.

Newacheck, P. W., Butler, L. H., Harper, A. K., Piontkowski, D. L., & Franks, P. E. (1980). Income and illness. *Medical Care, 18*, 1165–1176.

Pearlin, L. I. (1989). The sociological study of stress. *Journal of Health and Social Behavior, 30*, 241–256.

Pearlin, L. I., Lieberman, M. A., Menaghan, E. G., & Mullan, J. T. (1981). The stress process. *Journal of Health and Social Behavior, 22*, 337–356.

Riley, M. W. (1978). Aging, social change, and the power of ideas. *Daedalus, Fall, 107*, 39–52.

Rodin, J. (1986). Aging and health: Effects of the sense of control. *Science, 233*, 1271–1276.

Rowe, J. W., & Kahn, R. L. (1987). Human aging: Usual and successful. *Science, 237*, 143–149.

Satariano, W. A. (1986). Race, socioeconomic status, and health: A study of age differences in a depressed area. *American Journal of Preventive Medicine, 2*, 1–5.

Schneider, E. L., & Brody, J. A. (1983). Aging, natural death and the compression of morbidity: Another view. *New England Journal of Medicine, 309*, 854–857.

Shanas, E., & Maddox, G. L. (1985). Health, health resources, and the utilization of care. In R. H. Binstock & E. Shanas (Eds.), *Handbook of aging and the social sciences* (pp. 697–726). New York: Van Nostrand Reinhold.

Stahl, S. M., & Feller, J. R. (1990). Old equals sick: An ontogenetic fallacy. In S. M. Stahl (Ed.), *The legacy of longevity* (pp. 21–34). London: Sage Publications.

Syme, L. S., & Berkman, L. F. (1976). Social class, susceptibility, and sickness. *The American Journal of Epidemiology, 104,* 1–8.

Theorell, T. G. T. (1982). Review of research on life events and cardiovascular illness. *American Journal of Epidemiology, 104,* 1–8.

Thoits, P. (1983). Dimensions of life events as influences upon the genesis of psychological distress and associated conditions: An evaluation and synthesis of the literature. In H. Kaplan (Eds.), *Psychosocial stress: Trends in theory and research* (pp. 33–103). New York: Academic Press.

Vågerö, D. (1991). Inequality in health—some theoretical and empirical problems. *Social Science and Medicine, 32,* 367–371.

Verbrugge, L. M. (1984). Longer life but worsening health? Trends in health and mortality of middle-aged and older persons. *Milbank Memorial Fund Quarterly, 62*(3), 475–519.

Victor, C. R. (1989). Inequalities in health in later life. *Age and Ageing, 18,* 387–391.

Wadsworth, M. E. (1986). Serious illness in childhood and its association with later-life achievement. In R. G. Wilkinson (Eds.), *Class and health: Research and longitudinal data* (pp. 50–74). London: Tavistock Publications.

Wilcox, N. S., Prochaska, J. O., Velicer, W. F., & DiClemente, C. C. (1985). Subject characteristics as predictors of self-change in smoking. *Addictive Behaviors, 10,* 407–412.

Wilkins, R., Adams, O., & Brancker, A. (1989). Changes in mortality by income in urban Canada from 1971 to 1986. *Health Reports* (Statistics Canada catalogue 82-003), *1*(2), 137–174.

Wilkinson, R. G. (1986). Socio-economic differences in mortality: Interpreting the data on their size and trends. In R. G. Wilkinson (Eds.), *Class and health: Research and longitudinal data* (pp. 1–20). London: Tavistock Publications.

Wilkinson, R. G. (1989). Class mortality differentials, income distribution and trends in poverty 1921–1981. *Journal of Social Policy, 18,* 307–335.

Williams, D. R. (1990). Socioeconomic differentials in health: A review and redirection. *Social Psychology Quarterly, 53*(2), 81–99.

Chapter 15

New Directions in Socioeconomic Research on Aging

James P. Smith

Every so often, an area becomes poised for major new breakthroughs in knowledge. Socioeconomic research on aging is at just such a threshold. An obvious reason is that the questions are so compelling. The tilt of the population's age structure toward the old dictates what the important public policy issues of the moment and of the next decades will be—the ability to provide adequate health and income for the largest growing segment of our population, and whether any control can be exercised over the two major items in the federal budget—social security and medical care.

This chapter is organized around these three fundamental changes—new findings in research on aging, the emergence of important new data sets, and the growing transnational character of aging research. In the first section, some exciting new research findings that impact on older people's ability to age successfully are briefly highlighted. The second section focuses on three new surveys that will eventually transform socioeconomic research on aging—two RAND supplements to the Panel Study of Income Dynamics, the new Health and Retirement Survey, and the Health and Asset Survey of the Oldest Old. The final section of the chapter deals with how well these new directions in research on aging will transfer to other cultural settings, especially those in the developing world.

Socioeconomic Research on Aging

During the last decade, important new economic research has been conducted in four areas that speak to older Americans' ability to age successfully. These four areas are their labor force transition into retirement, their ability to sustain adequate income, the importance of family members to help out in times of poor health, and, finally, the impact of poor health on the elderly's hard-earned but vulnerable wealth positions. In this section, some illustrative examples of that research are briefly highlighted.

Transition to Retirement

The first area in which significant progress was made concerns the labor force transition into retirement. Dramatic shifts in labor force behavior, especially among older men, have occurred over the last three decades. As indicated in Figure 15.1, their labor force involvement uniformly fell during this period. The largest changes took place among men in their early 60s, whose participation rates fell by almost 25 percentage points.

Why are older men so less likely to work now than in the past, and what is likely to happen in the future? The reasons are mainly financial, built into the way social security and private pensions are currently structured. A decade ago, such a conclusion would have been met with widespread skepticism. Retirement was widely viewed as influenced principally by institutional customs and laws (e.g., mandatory retirement laws) and the ability of workers to continue on the job as dictated by their health.

Figure 15.2 based on the work of Ward (1984) demonstrates this point about the central role of social security. The upper half of this figure plots the probability of retiring at each age, conditional on still working. The bottom part plots the implicit subsidy or tax on work inherent in the structure of social security benefits. The correspondence between these charts is striking. Male retirement has two distinct spikes at ages 62 and 65. Note that these are the very ages when the social security program switches from a subsidy to working for another year to a tax on work which takes place at age 62, and when

NEW DIRECTIONS IN SOCIOECONOMIC RESEARCH

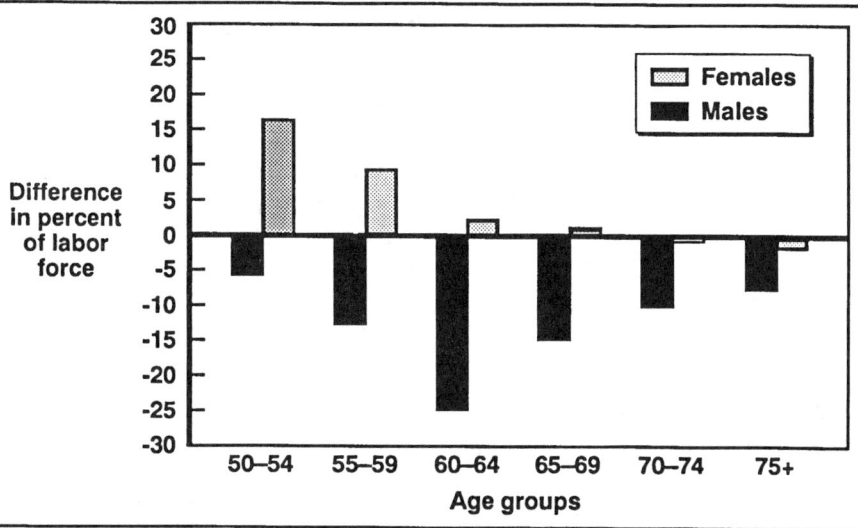

FIGURE 15.1 Changes in Labor Force Participation 1963–1990.

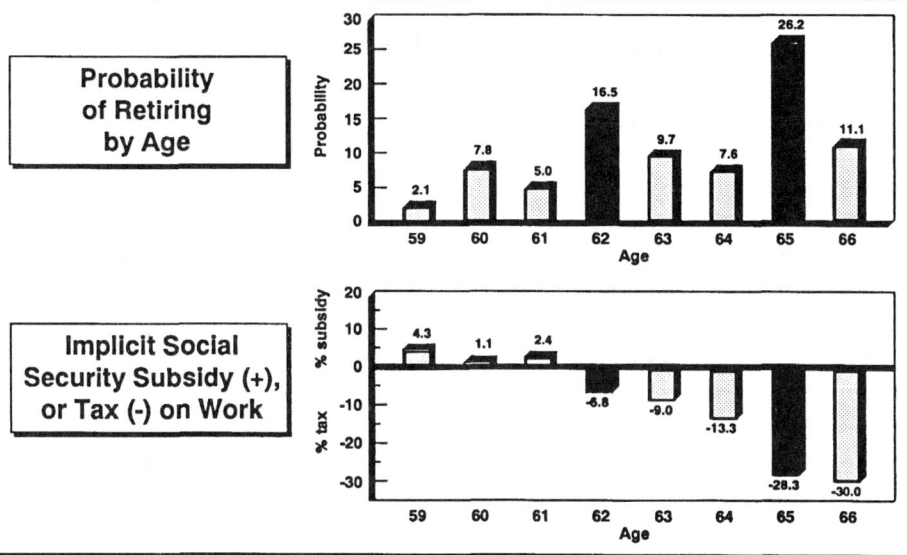

FIGURE 15.2 Role of Social Security in retirement.

TABLE 15.1
Percent of Persons in Poverty by Definition of Income (1990)

	Age Group				
	65-74	75+	Under 18	25-44	All
Conventional Money Income	9.7	16.0	20.6	10.4	13.5
Minus Taxes Plus Transfers	7.3	12.9	15.1	8.6	11.0
Plus Imputed Return on Housing	4.9	8.2	14.2	8.1	9.8

the size of that tax increases dramatically (at age 65). Ward estimates that at least half of the increased retirement at age 62 and at ages 65 and beyond is due to the social security program.

Much of the remainder is due largely to similar financial incentives present in private pensions and to mandatory retirement. A body of research, by scholars associated with the National Bureau of Economic Research under the leadership of David Wise, has documented the key role played by private pension plans (Wise, 1989). Private pensions have grown rapidly in recent decades, covering more than half of the private sector workers. Using data from private sector firms, Wise and his associates have shown that the structure of private sector pension plans contains large financial incentives and disincentives to working for another year. The precise age at which the incentive to retire kicks in varies depending on the structure of the firm's pension plan. Yet, in spite of how complicated these pension plans typically are, the research at the National Bureau leaves little doubt that workers respond to these financial carrots and sticks.

The central role that financial incentives in pensions and social security play in shaping retirement decisions offers some hope for the ability to adjust to a daunting future—the retirement of the large baby-boom cohorts in the next century. The implicit formulas in these programs can be manipulated to alter their incentives. Currently retired cohorts received large wealth subsidies from social security—receiving far more in benefits than they paid in taxes. The demographic reality is that this happy situation cannot continue when today's workforce retires. Indeed, future cohorts' benefits are most likely to fall because next century's smaller workforce will not be willing or able to pay for them. The least painful way of making that adjustment may be to alter the structure of social security and pension programs so that they encourage rather than discourage work for those well enough to work.

Adequate Income

When the changing economic status of the elderly is addressed, there is some good news to tell. This is one of the real success stories of American public policy. Over the past three decades, the economic status of older Americans improved dramatically and did so more rapidly than for any other age group. To illustrate this good news, Figure 15.3 plots poverty rates for the elderly population alongside the pov-

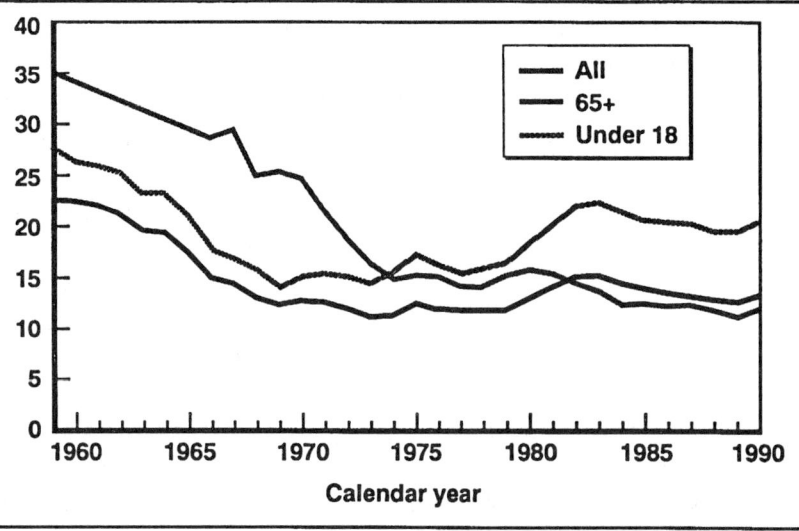

FIGURE 15.3 Poverty rates by age.

erty rate for all Americans. In addition, the poverty rate for those at the other end of the life cycle—America's children—is charted.

When John Kennedy was elected president, more than one in every three Americans were poor, echoing a percentage invoked by his New Deal predecessor 30 years earlier. Today, only one in every eight older persons is poor. Across these years, poverty declined twice as fast among the elderly as it did for all Americans. The contrast at the different ends of the life-cycle is especially stark. When we first started talking about the war on poverty, the image that entered our mind was that of an older person. Today, it is a child. Even if we take 1970 as our starting point, poverty among the elderly has been cut in half, whereas that of children has risen by a third.

Even these positive trends understate the good news for older people, because the real poverty rate of the elderly is probably much lower (see Table 15.1). If taxes paid are excluded, but the value of noncash benefits that the poor received (food stamps, Medicaid, Medicare) are added in, the poverty rate of those aged 65–74 would fall by another 2 ½ points. If the implicit rental value of housing is also included, the highlighted numbers in the final row remain. It is these numbers that most economists believe more accurately reflect real economic welfare. This means that instead of one in every ten older persons in poverty, only one in twenty of the elderly are. As can be seen from these tables, the effects of these adjustments are much larger on the elderly than they are for other age groups.

The preponderance of good news should not obscure the equal reality that many older people remain economically vulnerable. This vulnerability is triggered by certain demographic transitions, particularly those into extreme poor health and the death of a spouse. Figure 15.4 measures poverty among the most susceptible population—single elderly women. One in every four nonmarried older women is poor, more than twice the rate for all older people. Among widows, poverty rates now run as high as 40% in this age range. The prospects for older black nonmarried women are particularly bleak, where seven in every ten live below the poverty line. Treating the elderly as a single homogeneous group has lost whatever meaning it may have had either analytically or politically. It is an equally valid description of life among older Americans to claim that only one in every 20 older Americans is poor as it is to point out that seven of every ten single elderly black women is mired in poverty.

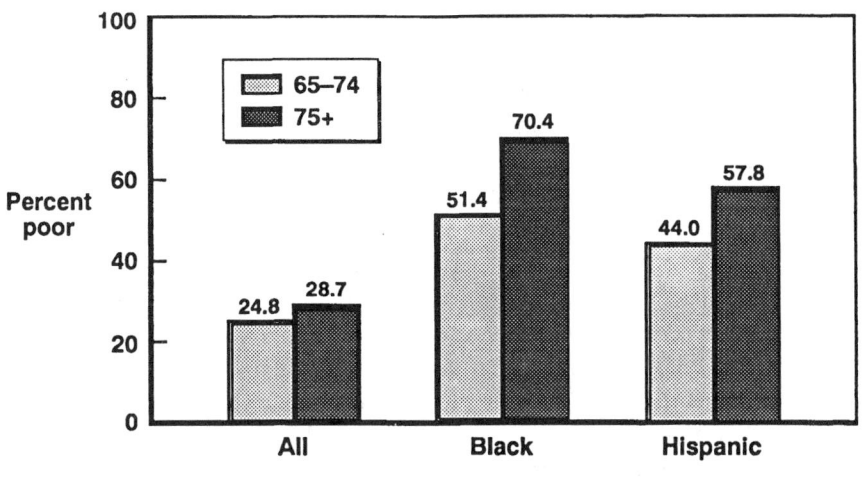

FIGURE 15.4 Who are the elderly poor? 1990 poverty rates for non-married women.

Health and Wealth Among the Elderly

These income data suggest that the key risks to successful aging rest in the complex two-way interactions between wealth and good health and the social and financial support networks set up within families. Debates about the direction of causation have made conclusions about the relation of health and wealth of older populations difficult to pin down. Although healthier households are also wealthier ones, is that simply because higher incomes lead to better health? Or does poor health restrict a family's ability to accumulate assets because of their limited ability to work or through their rising medical expenses? Or perhaps neither direction of influence is important, and the association merely reflects some observed third factor, which makes some people healthier and wealthier. To answer this question requires panel data (to average out these individual differences) and good health and wealth information to isolate the reasons for the association. Unfortunately, research on these questions is only just beginning so that this summary must be tentative and suggestive.

Data provided by Hurd, indicates that the association between health and wealth may not be trivial. For example, among all households aged 65–69, those in very good or excellent health have more than twice as many assets as those with at least one household member in poor health. But that is not the full story, because these differences in initial assets expanded in the future. Over the subsequent years, assets grow by almost 6% among households in excellent health. In sharp contrast, households in poor health saw their already low asset levels diminish further.

The most straightforward mechanism for this association is that wealthier people enjoy better health and live longer and healthier lives. Increased wealth can improve health and lengthen longevity for a number of reasons—better access to medical care, reduced risk behaviors, and a better diet and nutrition to name just a few. In research that is part of the RAND Center for Aging Research, Lillard and Weiss (1992) estimate that even after they control for the reverse effect of health on wealth, greater economic resources still reduce mortality risks. But does poor health also threaten the wealth accumulated by the elderly over their lifetimes? This research by Lillard and Weiss indicates that even after one accounts for the influence of wealth or health and eliminates other factors that might influence both, poor health has a direct and quantitatively large impact on the economic resources of the elderly. For many couples, when one of the spouses becomes ill, wealth growth ceases as the couple must use all the subsequent wealth increases to compensate for their lost sources of income and to finance their increased medical needs. To put it another way, an episode of poor health essentially wiped out the entire future growth in assets of a couple over the next 10 years.

Some reasons why widows are so vulnerable is more apparent from Figure 15.5, which contrasts the wealth of couples who remain together with that of another family in which the woman became a widow. This figure, based on the important work of Hurd and Wise (1989), suggests that the increased poverty of widows reflects three forces. First, the widowed women were less well off even before their husbands died. Second, less wealthy families are more likely to experience a death of a spouse and transit into widowhood. Finally, a large fraction of the assets of an older family vanishes when the husband dies. This includes part of his social security wealth, but also, for many families, his pension wealth or the annuity income associated with it disappears when the husband dies.

These behaviors are even more complex, since work at RAND indicates that marriage and mortality themselves are closely intertwined. The observed relation between marriage and mortality may reflect

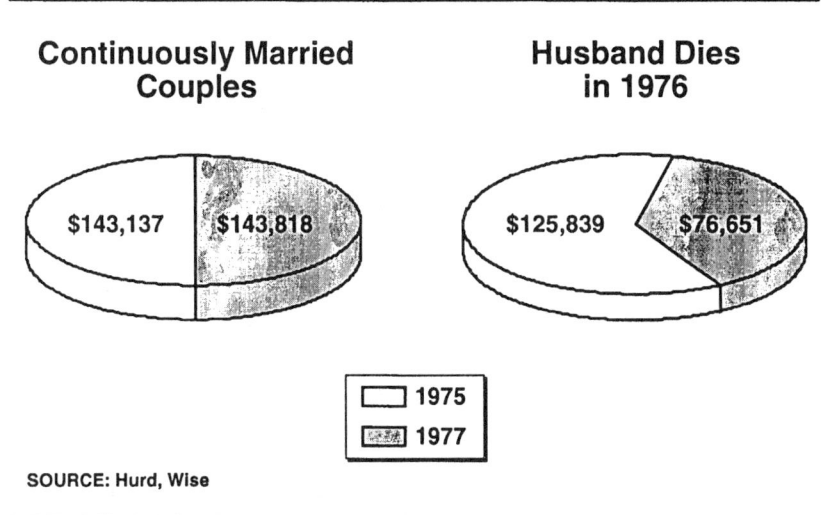

FIGURE 15.5 Effect of widowhood on health. Husband dies in 1976.

two distinct effects—a selective effect where those least likely to die marry, and a productive effect where marriage itself (through the combination of financial resources or the care of a spouse) enhances longevity. Similarly, the end of a marriage through divorce, separation, or death (with its accompanying stress and financial depreciation) may shorten life.

For example, according to recent research by Lillard and Waite (1992), continuously married men have the highest probability of surviving and never-married men have the highest mortality risks. This disparity with married men rises continuously over ages, strongly suggestive of a productive effect of marriage. Additional evidence in support of the productive effect of marriage comes from their finding that married men can mitigate the risks by living with another adult. These transitions out of marriage are important because they speak directly to the role of marriage in affecting subsequent health.

These new research findings are just a start in the collective attempt to unravel the complexities of the interactions between economic well-being and health functioning among older Americans. One constraint on further progress has been the quality of the underlying data. In the past, datasets with state-of-the-art health measurement typically had very limited economic information, whereas those surveys that were known for the quality of their economic information were dismissed as inferior in their health data. In the next section, some potentially important new data collection efforts, which will go a long way toward solving this problem, are discussed.

New Data Collection Efforts

The research just summarized was largely based on the best data sets on aging available during the 1980s; in particular, the original Retirement History Survey, the Survey of Income and Program Participation (SIPP) and Panel Study of Income Dynamics (PSID). In recent years, concerns about these data have been raised because of their timeliness, the quality of much of their noneconomic data, and what was left out of these surveys. Fortunately, there are three new surveys on the horizon that will eventually transform scientific and policy work on aging. These new surveys combine state-of-the-art health and economic information. Because they are longitudinal panels, they also allow for the joint modeling of health and retirement as the dynamic processes they truly are. To link individual behavior to public policy instruments, respondents were matched to key administrative records such as social security and Medicare. Finally, the generations were connected and the complete end of the life-cycle is spanned by the new surveys.

Three new surveys will eventually transform scientific and policy work on aging. The first of these are two Rand supplements to the Panel Study of Income Dynamics (PSID). The PSID is the premier longitudinal economic data set in the United States. Each year for the last 24 years, it has collected high-quality and detailed information on each respondent's income and labor force behavior. At irregular intervals, health and wealth modules (of somewhat lesser quality) were fielded. Now, almost a quarter century of complete economic and labor force history for the 7000 families (and 35,000 individuals) is currently available in the survey.

Equally important, PSID has followed all relatives of the original respondents and folded them into its longitudinal design. Thus, a 12-year-old child of a 45-year-old parent in 1968 would now both be members of the panel at ages 36 and 69, respectively. Because this panel is ongoing, it offers an unprecedented opportunity to understand transfers and interactions of the extended American family as the original parents age. In the last few years, RAND staff developed two important supplements to the PSID. The 1990 supplement concentrating on the health of older respondents had three parts. The first was a self-administered questionnaire to all respondents 50 and over. They were asked detailed questions on their physical and mental health functioning and status, the existence of chronic conditions, and their health risk behaviors. The second part was a telephone survey for all individuals 65 and over. They were asked about health care utilization and expenditures, nursing home and hospital admissions, and all sources of time and money support in times of poor health from their families. Finally, PSID records were linked to Medicare files. This data, which will be released in the public domain in the next year or two, represent a quantum leap in research possibilities.

The 1991 RAND supplement focused on the 7,200 parents of the PSID respondents. Panel members were asked about the health status, chronic conditions, and disabilities of all parents of both the husband and wife. All nursing home and hospitalization episodes were recorded, as well as all time and financial support given. The unique feature of this supplement is the extensive reliance on proxy responses to document the lives of the elderly population. Fortunately, the unique design of the PSID allows for a detailed evaluation of accuracy of these proxy responses. Many of the elderly parents for whom their adult children were asked to describe their parents' health and economic conditions are also PSID respondents themselves. For this subsample, their own assessments can be checked against the proxy answers of their adult children. The value of this RAND PSID supplement is potentially quite large. For example, it is one of the few data sets that provides sufficient sample size to analyze the determinants of nursing home entry. It also links the generations in a unique way. Mature adult children may often make the critical decisions about the living arrangements, health, and economic well-being of their frail elderly parents.

The second new initiative is the Health and Retirement Survey (HRS), the first round of which went into the field in the fall of 1992. HRS is a national panel of 8000 households in their preretirement years (ages 51–61). Because of their increasing importance in the policy debate, both blacks and Mexican Americans are over sampled. Given its focus on the preretirement years, not surprisingly the principal objective of HRS is to monitor the causes and consequences of retirement. Health functioning has been raised to equal status, however. This is not simply because health is an important conditioner of retirement. Rather, this dual status of health and economics results from a conviction that these outcomes are closely intertwined and by a desire to monitor future health transitions, especially as respondents eventually enter their post-retirement years. The eventual hope is that this sample will serve as the basis for a long-term epidemiological assessment—one that would have unprecedented background information.

HRS instruments will span the spectrum of behaviors of interest—on the economic side, work, income, and wealth; on the functional side, health and cognitive status, disability, and mental well-being. The household survey will also be linked with the major administrative records—social security and eventually, as the respondents age, with Medicare files.

The major gap of people left from these first two initiatives are the oldest-old. There are too few such people in the PSID, and it will be the better part of two decades before the HRS sample ages into this subpopulation. This leads to the third of the recently proposed NIA initiatives—the health and asset dynamics of the oldest old (AHEAD). This sample, derived from the same screen as the HRS, includes 7,000 respondents 70 and older, a large number of whom will be over 85. Currently, an oversample of the black population will be conducted.

Given the different age span, the objectives of this survey shifts toward the key concerns in this segment of the life cycle. To what extent are the transitions in physical and cognitive functioning related to economic resources and intergenerational transfers? Who are the people vulnerable to Medicaid spend-down and how does that spend-down take place—through the sale or transfer of assets or through consumption? Finally, what are the key early markers of successful aging and how can they be sustained and enlarged? They survey instruments here will monitor the key outcomes—objective and subjective measures of health and economic status. Time and money transfers between the generations will be captured, and those who move into nursing homes will be followed. Finally, as with the other two initiatives, AHEAD will be linked to key administrative files—including Medicare, Medicaid, and the National Death Index.

Cross-National Research on Aging

The final section of this chapter deals with how well new directions in aging research will transfer to other cultural settings, especially those in the developing countries. Reservations about the ability to transfer span the complete spectrum—the questions that are important to ask, the theoretical and modeling approaches to be explored, and the kind of data to be collected. Although it is always a bit misleading and unfair to summarize a wide diversity of views as if they fall neatly into bipolar camps, it does sharpen the issues.

At one end of the spectrum are "research globalists" (including this author), analytical models in hand ready and willing to export them to all parts of the globe. At the other extreme are "cultural isolationists." To them, each country and setting is unique with a distinct mosaic of history, culture, and institutions. In their view, it produces more harm than insight to force onto developing countries behavioral models derived from and more suited to the United States.

We may well have been too cautious on this issue of transference. Institutions in developing countries indeed are quite distinct, and they need to be understood before deciding how they should be incorporated into any analytical structure. Similarly, some survey questions in the form that they are asked in the United States may be simply absurd in many other parts of the world. But, with all that said, people are people—they have similar goals and needs and face constraints in achieving those objectives. To put it most simply, they try to strive for what is desirable and avoid what is costly.

One point that should not be controversial is that aging and health is the emerging issue in the third world. The demands placed on health care systems in the developing countries will grow dramatically in the coming decades. Not only will the capacity of their systems have to expand dramatically, but the type and mix of services will have to change to serve an older population with a markedly different pattern of diseases.

The Indonesian Example

This point can be illustrated with one developing country, Indonesia, that RAND is currently studying intensively. One reason for their increased concern about the elderly is purely demographic. As in many other developing countries, Indonesian birth rates have been declining rapidly and will continue to do so for the foreseeable future. At the same time, mortality risks at all ages have been falling rapidly. The demographic consequence is certain—a dramatic tilt in the age structure toward the old. In Indonesia, the size of the population of those age 60 and over will quadruple over the next 30 years, whereas that of younger people will stabilize. These shifts in Indonesia's age structure combined with other likely demographic trends—increased urbanization and rising incomes—foretell a need for a very different public health system than the one that exists there today. As demonstrated in Figure 15.6a, health risks will shift dramatically from the acute infectious diseases of the young—diarrhea, respiratory infections, and measles—toward the more chronic noninfectious diseases of the old—heart disease and cancer.

Figure 15.7 highlights the pressures that are being placed on the Indonesian medical system by the aging of their population. Inpatient admissions will almost quadruple among those age 60 and over. With this dramatic shift in patient mix, the Indonesian health system may well have to be revamped from top to bottom. Both the existing personnel and the physical facilities are geared for a much different population of patients than that which will exist tomorrow. Moreover, this tomorrow is not in some distant future, a problem safely put aside for the next generation. As we can see from 15.6b, these changes are already well underway. Mortality rates for acute infectious diseases fell by a third between 1985 and 1990, and by 1995 chronic disease mortality may well outrank deaths due to infectious diseases.

Cross-National Similarities in Behaviors

One objection often raised against the globalist view is that the underlying behaviors are fundamentally different across diverse national settings. Evidence is accumulating indicating that this objection is not based on a solid empirical footing. For example, data from three quite diverse countries (see Gertler, Rahman, Strauss, Ashley, & Fox, 1992) illustrate across-national similarities in health behaviors of older people. The three countries are the United States, Malaysia, and Jamaica. The outcomes they highlight are the effect of economic resources (as measured by education) and health and gender differences in health functioning. As shown earlier, more schooling improves health status and reduces mortality in the United States. But does the association transfer to other nations—nations with very different levels of economic development and with quite distinct health problems?

In both of these developing countries, education has a strong persistence and positive impact on health status and functioning. Although education levels are lower in these countries than in the United States, Gertler et al. show that in each case more schooling improves health for both men and women. The positive effect of school-

NEW DIRECTIONS IN SOCIOECONOMIC RESEARCH • 289

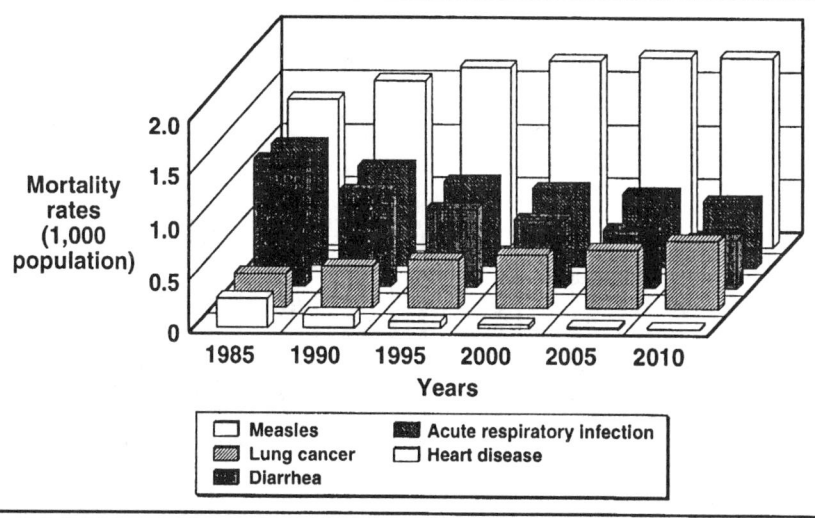

FIGURE 15.6a Specific causes of mortality: Present and projected.

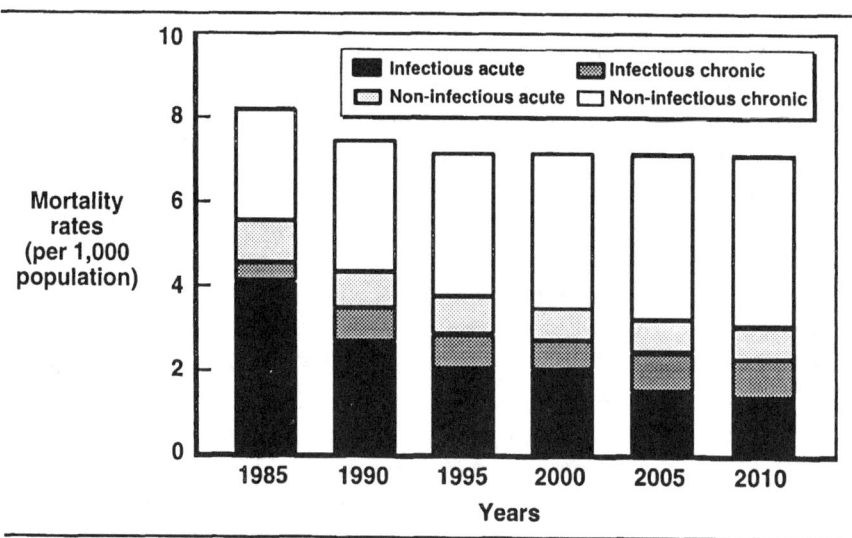

FIGURE 15.6b Types of mortality: Present and projected.

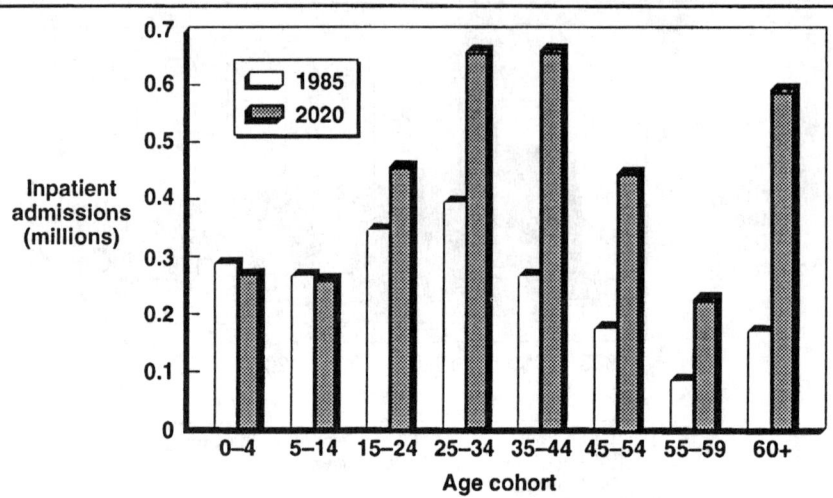

FIGURE 15.7 Inpatient admissions by age cohort: Indonesia, 1985 versus now.

ing on health persists across the components included in the standard activities of daily living (ADLs). Whether ADLs measure difficulty with vigorous activities, with walking up stairs, or bending, schooling improves health. Rising schooling levels and the higher economic wealth that flows from it are one of the underlying reasons why health levels have been improving in many developing countries.

Another research finding that persists across many diverse cultural settings is the gender difference in health. Probably the most often repeated gender health statistic is that virtually throughout the world, male life expectancies fall short of those experienced by women. With this as their basis, unfortunately some have jumped to the conclusion that health status is persistently better for women than for men. This conventional wisdom may well be wrong. In virtually all other dimensions of health that Gertler and his colleagues examine (that is, excluding mortality), the gender bias in health favors men.

For example, Jamaican women at all points in the life course are significantly more likely to be in fair or poor health than are Jamaican men. In addition, if poor health is used as a marker of onset, aging takes place at a much younger age than it does in the United States. More than 15% of men in their fifties report themselves in fair or poor health in Jamaica, and one in every three women in that age range do so. The situation in Malaysia is quite similar. As all the age groups show, Malaysian women are in poorer health than Malaysian men. In addition, the fraction of the youngest old in poor health is extremely large.

If this world tour is completed with a return ticket to the United States, these gender differences in reported health are not simply a by-product of the lower living standards in developing countries. Nor are these differences a result of a single unrepresentative measure of health outcomes. These gender differences persist throughout all the activities of daily living and in all three countries.

A final example is the important dual relationship between health and income that was noted earlier for the United States. In this case, the research is from yet another setting—Sierra Leone. There the interest centered on the same question—does poor health, in this case moderate malnutrition, lower incomes and productivity of adult farm labor? If anything, the potential impact of health on income is even more direct and immediate in such settings. When physical labor is the most important production input, poor health means that energy levels are difficult to sustain, bouts of sickness are more frequent and crop output falls. But as discussed in the research survey for the United States, causation may well run in the other direction. Better-off farmers have better diets, and their nutrition levels are lower.

In Strauss' research (1986), he estimated the impact of adult nutrition levels on farm output. As was the case in the United States, Strauss found that both directions of influence between economic status and health were important in Sierra Leone. Increases in income had a significant and large impact on nutrients available, and subsequently on health states. In addition, he estimated that the lack of nutrients significantly reduced farm output. A 10% rise in calories raises output by 3%. Not surprisingly, these effects were much larger for the poorly nourished. The effects themselves are quite important. In order to achieve the same impact by manipulating agricultural prices, it would be equivalent to a drop in stable prices by almost half.

The New International Surveys

The similarity of research questions on aging issues across national boundaries has been matched by common research constraints. Even more so than in the United States, inadequate data has been the major limitation on research on aging in developing countries. In most third world countries, research and data collection has focused on the other end of the life-cycle—fertility and family planning or infant nutrition and mortality. The major multinational surveys—the World Fertility Surveys and the Demographic and Health Surveys—give little information about what life is like for older people in these countries. Unfortunately, the policy issues of the next decades will reflect a very different demographic time bomb than the one for which policymakers have been preparing. The loud ticking they should now be hearing is the count of the aging of their populations. They now have little data to prepare themselves for that certain demographic reality, however.

In light of this reality, a growing number of researchers have been involved in significant new data collection efforts in many developing countries. Although these efforts are unrelated administratively, they are linked by a common set of themes and concerns. First, they all strive to have adequate samples of the elderly population. More importantly, they have learned the painful lessons of the earlier U.S. surveys of the elderly by integrating health, social support and economic modules into a single survey design. Finally, they do not repeat another earlier mistake by recognizing that the elderly do not live in isolation and that the generalizations must be linked.

Although there a number of such efforts, the character of these new surveys can be illustrated by the Indonesian Family Life Survey (IFLS), currently being conducted by RAND. The IFLS sample includes over 7,000 households across geographic areas spanning over 94% of the Indonesian population. The unique feature of its sample design for research on the elderly is that the IFLS contains two related samples. The first subsample is well within the mainstay of the traditional demographic surveys by sampling all ever married women less than 50 years old. The innovation is that all seniors in those households (those over 50 years old) are also given a full set of survey instruments. In addition, a separate sample of individuals over 50 who are not co-resident with a married woman less than 50 is conducted. In combination, these two samples constitute a random sample of the senior population in Indonesia. By linking with the ever married women's sample, generations have been effectively linked.

This linkage is important because the well-being of many older persons in these countries depends critically on their interactions with their kin. In many instances, older parents will live with their adult children when their own work careers end and their health deteriorates. Even when they live apart, transfers of time and money between the generations of the extended family are frequent and quantitatively large. In such situations, analyzing the well-being of the elderly by sampling only the elderly makes little sense. In the IFLS, respondents were queried about their health status (using a culturally adapted set of ADLs), and their health care utilization. Rich and detailed data are also available on the underlying determinants of these outcomes, including retrospective information on income and wealth, social support networks, and the quality and quantity of health care facilities with which the respondents interact. Detailed recording of all the transfers of time and money between the generations in the year before the survey are also available.

Optimism about the future stems from the fact that the IFLS is but one example of many such innovative surveys that are springing up around the world. Just as the new U. S.-based surveys will revitalize aging research in this country, these new international surveys will revolutionize transnational research on aging.

The first area with new research findings concerns the retirement transition where a number of economic studies demonstrated that the sharp drop in employment among older men was largely due to financial incentives implicit in private pension plans and social security. The second substantive area concerns the ability of older Americans to sustain adequate income, an ability that has increased significantly over time. In spite of the general improvement in the economic status of the elderly population, many older people are economically vulnerable. This vulnerability is related to key demographic transitions, particularly those with poor health and the death of a spouse. Finally, an important new research area involving social scientists is beginning to have some success in unraveling the two-way causality involving the dual relation of health and wealth.

Conclusions

This chapter argues that socioeconomic research on aging is poised for significant new scientific breakthroughs. These advances will start with important new substantive insights about the determinants of healthy aging among older Americans. The insights will be made possible in part by some new multipurpose surveys that will in time have a revolutionary impact on socioeconomic research on aging.

One important departure from the past is that these new advances in theory, method, and data are rapidly moving across national boundaries. Because of their rapidly changing age structure, aging is fast becoming the emerging policy issue in developing countries.

These countries will have even less time than was available in the United States to adapt their institutional structures toward the health and income problems of the elderly. Fortunately, they will be able to learn from the U. S. experience. Recent research has shown that in contrast to the expectations many of the underlying behaviors of the elderly are quite similar across quite different countries. To cite one example, the empirically strong association of education with health status apparently persists across cultural settings as distinct as the United States, Malaysia, and Jamaica. Soon it will be possible to determine whether these similarities persist across more complex modeling of behavior, because a powerful new group of surveys of older populations are emerging in many developing countries that parallel the best new U. S. surveys.

References

Gertler, P., Rahman, O., Strauss, J., Ashley, D., & Fox, K. (1992). *Gender differences in adult health: An international comparison.* Santa Monica, CA: RAND.

Hurd, O. D., (1990). Research on the elderly: Economic status, retirement, and consumption and savings. *Journal of Economic Literature, 28*(2), 565–637.

Hurd, M. D., & Wise, D. A. (1989). The wealth and poverty of widows: Assets before and after the husband's death. In D. Wise (Ed.), *The economics of aging.* Chicago: University of Chicago Press.

Lillard, L. A., & Weiss, Y. (1992). *Uncertain Health and survival: Effects on end of life consumption.* Santa Monica, CA: RAND, Center for Aging Studies.

Lillard, L. A., & Waite, L. J. (1992). *Till death do us part: Disruption and mortality in later adulthood.* RAND Center for Aging Studies.

Recommendations to the NIA Extramural Program on Priorities for Data Collection in Health and Retirement Economics. (1988, May). Report of the Ad Hoc Advisory Panel to the Behavioral and Social Research Program, National Institute on Aging.

Strauss, J. (1986). Does better nutrition raise farm productivity? *Journal of Political Economy, 94,* 297–320.

Ward, M. P. (1984, June). The effect of Social Security on male retirement behavior. Santa Monica, CA: RAND, June 1984.

Wise, D. A. (Ed.). (1989). *The economics of aging.* Chicago: University of Chicago Press.

Chapter 16

Minority and Socioeconomic Status: Impact on Quality of Life in Aging

H. Asuman Kiyak and Nancy R. Hooyman

This chapter examines both the objective and subjective quality of life of older minorities, focusing on the socioeconomic status, health and psychological well-being of older people of color who are defined by the federal government as protected groups: African American, Hispanic Americans, Pacific Asian Americans, and Native Americans. The disproportionately high rates of poverty among older persons of color are both a determinant and a component of their quality of life. Indicators of objective quality of life such as rates of disability, morbidity and mortality, and living environment, as well as subjective indicators such as psychological well-being, are all influenced by socioeconomic status. These components will be briefly reviewed along with structural factors that affect quality of life. For many older minorities, greater risk of poor quality of life is not unique to old age, but the result of historical and lifelong structural conditions, such as discrimination, unemployment and underemployment, and barriers to adequate health care. In some instances, social and cultural factors, such as the social support of family, friends, community and church, and cultural and spiritual values and beliefs, may partially mitigate the negative effects of poverty, enhancing their quality of life. The chapter concludes by suggesting interventions to improve the quality of life of older ethnic minorities.

Definitions

For purposes of this chapter, ethnic minority elderly includes older people belonging to groups whose language and/or physical and cultural characteristics make them visible and identifiable, who have experienced differential and unequal treatment, and who have regarded themselves as objects of collective discrimination and oppression by reason of their race (Markides, Liang, & Jackson, 1990). Although our focus is on people of color who have experienced economic and racial discrimination throughout their lives, we also consider how ethnicity or cultural homogeneity, especially in terms of values related to family and community, influences quality of life.

Minorities represent only 9.8% of the U. S. population over age 65, with 8% of African Americans, 5% of Hispanics, and 6% each of Pacific Asian Americans and Native Americans (including American Indians, Eskimos, and Aleuts) in that age group (U. S. Bureau of the Census, 1991). Differences in birth and mortality rates and in immigration patterns are primarily responsible for the lower percentage of elderly within these ethnic minority groups as compared to the Caucasian population. A general trend is the growing presence of females who are more likely than older men to be widowed or divorced in each of these populations (U. S. Senate Special Committee on Aging, 1992). Because women among all older populations are more likely to be poor than their male counterparts, the combination of ethnic minority status, gender, and marital status increases the risk of poverty in old age.

Although small in size, ethnic minority populations are of increasing concern to gerontologists, because of the disproportionately greater number of socioeconomic and health problems they face that impair their quality of life relative to whites. In addition, their proportion is expected to increase at a higher rate than for Caucasians by the twenty-first century. Because of the large proportion of children today in these minority groups, many of whom, unlike previous generations, will reach old age, 15% of the older population is expected to be people of color in 2020, increasing to 21.3% in 2050, compared with less than 10% in 1990 (Taeuber, 1992; U. S. Bureau of the Census,

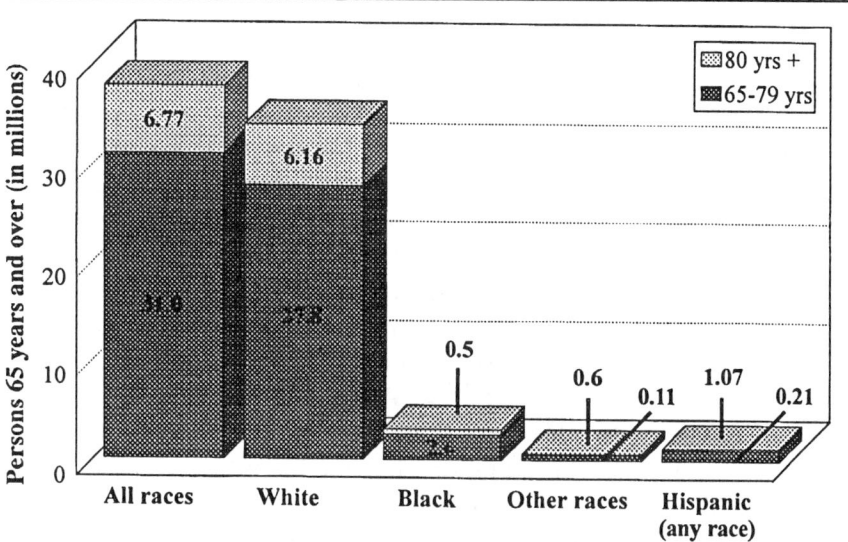

FIGURE 16.1 Persons 65 years and over: 1990 (numbers in millions). SOURCE: U.S. Bureau of the Census (1991).

1989). In fact, it has been predicted that the immigrant groups of the twentieth century—Hispanics, Asian, and Pacific Islanders—will redefine American culture in the twenty-first century (Torres-Gil, 1986). During that transition, an aging society will need to grapple with the cultural homogeneity and generally lower quality of life of elderly minority populations and the cultural diversity of its younger minority populations, and the implications of this for the quality of life of future cohorts of ethnic minority elderly.

Two distinct issues should be kept in mind in this discussion of ethnic minority elderly: the unique historical calendar of life events and culture and their impact on lifestyles, many of which are positive; and the consequences of racism, ageism, discrimination, and prolonged poverty, most of which are negative. In fact, the "multiple hierarchy stratification" perspective views ethnic minority status as another source of inequality along with class, gender, and age that puts ethnic minorities at greater risk of lower quality of life in old age (Markides, Liang, & Jackson, 1990).

Although there are some recurring themes in analyses of ethnic minority status and older people, variations within as well as among these groups must also be considered. Differences in immigration patterns, birthrates, region, social class, rural or urban location, gender and acculturation level add to the intragroup variations, making generalizations about quality of life of each of these ethnic groups difficult. As examples of this within-group diversity, African Americans include blacks from the Caribbean, Africa, and native born to the U. S., and differ from one another in terms of cultural background, socioeconomic status, and geographic location. Hispanics, who are defined by the U. S. Bureau of the Census as Spanish-speaking persons in the United States, incorporate many groups, each with its own distinct national/cultural heritage, history and dialect: Mexicans, Puerto Ricans, Cubans, Central or South Americans, including the growing number of recent immigrants from El Salvador, Nicaragua, and Columbia, and the native Mexican American or Chicano population. Although bonded by a common language, these groups differ substantially in terms of geographic distribution, education and socioeconomic status. Mexican Americans, many of whom are recent immigrants, are the largest group, constituting 64% of the Hispanic population (U. S. Bureau of the Census, 1991). Cubans, the wealthiest and best educated, have the largest proportion of foreign-born elderly among the three major Hispanic groups.

Pacific Asian elderly are also diverse in terms of language, culture, acculturation to the U. S., and socioeconomic status. They consist of three main groups with markedly different experiences with discrimination, isolation, and occupational and educational opportunities. These include immigrants, often Japanese American and Chinese American, who arrived as young adults during the turn of the century and often lived in ethnic ghettos; children born to those immigrants, many of whom have experienced geographic and occupational mobility; and elderly immigrants from Vietnam, Cambodia, and other Southeast Asian countries who came after the Vietnam War, often as parents or grandparents of younger immigrants. For this reason, they are generally less acculturated and have lower incomes than earlier immigrants. Recent immigrants from Laos, Cambodia, and Vietnam also have a higher proportion of older persons than do other Pacific Asian groups.

The Native American population includes Indians, Eskimos and Aleuts; there are over 250 federally recognized tribes (65 communities have not received federal recognition, but have been assigned tribal status by the states); many urban Indians do not live on reservations; and over 200 distinct languages are spoken. More Native American elderly live in rural areas than do other minority elderly, with nearly 25% on reservations or in Alaskan Native villages.

Although tremendous diversity exists between and within these groups of ethnic minority elderly, a common pattern is lower socioeconomic status, oftentimes throughout their lives, increasing the risk of physical and mental health problems in old age.

Poverty as a Risk Factor for Quality of Life

Despite the dramatic improvements in the economic well-being of the older population as a whole since the mid-1960s, pockets of poverty persist, particularly among white women and elderly persons and men and women of color. Although African Americans form only about 8% of the population age 65 and over, they represent 36% of the low-income elderly. In 1990s, 34% of the African American families headed by persons aged 65 and over fell below the poverty line, more than three times the proportion of older white families (19.3%) who were poor (U. S. Bureau of the Census, 1991). Among Hispanic Americans, 27% are poor. Another 33% compared to 18% of older whites, are at the "near poverty" threshold with incomes below 125% of poverty (Bass, Kutza, & Torres-Gil, 1990). Three out of every five dollars of retirement income comes from Social Security or Supplemental Security Income for Hispanic elderly, compared to two out of every five dollars for older whites (Miranda, 1990). Fourteen percent of Pacific Asian elderly live below the poverty level, although there is a tremendous variation among them, with Japanese American elderly economically better off than other ethnic minority groups (Gould, 1989). The poverty rate for Pacific Asian elderly may be higher than official statistics indicate, however, as the number of employed adults, often self-employed as farmers or in small business, is greater than in other groups, thereby inflating "family" income. In fact, for Chinese and Filipino men over age 75 who live alone, the poverty rate is 41% compared to 31% among their male peers in the general population (Kim, 1983; Liu, 1986). Native Americans appear to be the poorest of these four ethnic minority groups, with their average income approximately 75% that of all other elderly groups (National Indian Council on Aging, 1984). The poverty rate increases in rural areas, with 32% of Native Americans having incomes below federal poverty levels compared with 10% of whites (Gould, 1989). Native American families headed by an elderly person in rural communities are twice as likely to live below the poverty line than their urban counterparts (Manson & Callaway, 1990). By age 45, incomes have usually peaked among male Native Americans, and decline thereafter.

Being female and living alone increases the risk of poverty. The income of African Americans and Hispanics who live alone is about 33% lower than that of older whites living alone. And older minority women who live alone form the poorest group in our society (Kasper, 1988). For example, 66% of older African American women and 61% of Hispanic older women living alone fall below the poverty line compared to 25% among their white counterparts (Taeuber, 1990; U. S. Senate Special Committee on Aging, 1992). Accordingly, the incidence of poverty increases dramatically among households composed of unrelated African American individuals, especially women age 65 and over. The median income of African American women is 66% that of white women; in fact, the proportion of older African-American female-headed families in poverty has increased in the past decade, at the same time that the rate of poverty among the elderly as a whole has decreased (U. S. Senate Special Committee on Aging, 1992). Differences in education do not explain the income gap between older African American and older white women; for example, poverty is almost as high among African American women who attended high school as among those with less than 6 years of schooling (Jackson, 1985).

Older minority women are more likely than their male counterparts to be poor and living alone, because of their longer life expectancy and lower remarriage rates. The exception to this gender pattern is among the older Pacific Asian population, where men living alone constitute a larger percentage of the population. This is not due to men's greater life expectancy, however, but to the continuing influence of disproportionate male immigration in the early part of the century and past restrictions on female immigration. Despite the fact that older Pacific Asian women are more likely to be married than their white counterparts, among female heads of households over age 75, the poverty rate increases, ranging from 31.1%-40.4% (Kim, 1983; Liu, 1986).

Structural Factors Underlying Poverty

Structural factors underlie these high rates of poverty. These include: lifelong discrimination in education and employment, resulting in low levels of education and high levels of unemployment and underemployment; barriers to social and health programs and policies; and language differences. As examples of such structural conditions, 57% of older African Americans and 64% of Hispanics today have had only eight years or less of schooling compared with only 30% of white elders (Taeuber, 1992). The primary reason for older African Americans' lower socioeconomic status is their pattern of limited employment opportunities and periods of unemployment throughout their lives, as well as their concentration in low-paying, sporadic jobs with few benefits, many of which were not covered by Social Security prior to the 1950s. African American elderly are also more likely to leave the workforce earlier than their white counterparts, often because of health problems. Out of economic necessity, however, they often return to work after retirement, creating the phenomenon of the "unretired/retired" (Gibson, 1989; Harper & Alexander, 1990). This movement in and out of the work force reduces not only their lifetime earnings, but also their retirement benefits. As a result, they are more likely to receive only the minimum Social Security benefits and to rely on Supplemental Security Income (SSI) and less likely to receive pension income than are whites.

Limited education and language differences underlie the poor economic status of Hispanics. Mexican Americans and Puerto Ricans are the most educationally deprived group in our society, with 16% of those 65 and older having had no education (U. S. Senate Special Committee on Aging, 1988). More than any other group, both young and old Hispanics have retained their native language. In fact, it has been estimated that more than 60% of older Hispanics are not proficient in English, which, while preserving their cultural identity, is a barrier to their education, employment, and utilization of social and health services (Cuellar, 1990; Torres-Gil, 1986).

Lifetime patterns of low-paying jobs, often in self-employment, garment factories, service or farming work not covered by Social Security or other pensions, underlie the poverty of Pacific Asians, particularly Chinese and Filipino elderly. Older Filipino males, in particular, were often concentrated in domestic, migrant, agricultural or other unstable work, often living in homogeneous male camps and failing both to gain any retirement benefits and to develop close ties with family and neighborhood. In addition, patterns of immigration markedly affect the occupational and educational background and, in turn, the socioeconomic status of Pacific Asians. For example, because of denial of property rights and employment discrimination, most Asian elderly who immigrated prior to 1984 are less educated and more economically deprived than their white counterparts. Older Pacific Asians have, on the average, only 6 years of school, with the exception of Japanese Americans, who average 8.5 years. Many still speak only their native language, with only 1.4% of the foreign-born Chinese elderly and less than 1% of the Japanese elderly speaking English (Kim, 1983).

Similar to other ethnic minority populations, the poverty of older Native Americans tends to reflect lifelong patterns of unemployment, employment in jobs, especially on reservations, that were not covered by Social Security, and poor working conditions. An additional factor, however, is that historical circumstances and federal policies toward tribes have intensified the pattern of economic underdevelopment and impoverished in these communities. Congress and the Bureau of Indian Affairs, not the individual states, largely determine daily practices on the reservations. Although the Bureau's regulations are intended to ensure basic support, the Bureau is criticized for its inflexibility and for spending 90% of its budget on maintaining and supporting the bureaucracy, with only 10% actually going to services for Indian people (Cook, 1990).

Both older Hispanics and Pacific Asians often qualify for public financial supports such as SSI, but do not apply. After years of living under discrimination and fear of deportation, they may resist seeking help from government agencies. Hispanics who entered the country illegally have been unable to apply for Social Security, Medicare, or Medicaid. This legal barrier to eligibility, however, has recently been altered by changes in immigration laws for those who entered prior to 1982.

Health Status as a Component of Quality of Life

Because lower income, particularly lifelong poverty, tends to be associated with poorer health outcomes at all ages, income level is one of the major factors influencing quality of life. As an example, data from the National Health Interview Survey reveal that 44% of older people with low incomes, compared with 22% of those with higher incomes, report chronic diseases and greater limitations in activities of daily living (NCHS, 1987). Given the high proportions of ethnic minorities who are living in poverty, their risk of chronic disease, disability, and mortality is greater than that of Caucasians. Accordingly, "early aging," whereby physiological aging tends to precede chronological aging, with those in their late forties experiencing health disabilities typical of 65-year-old whites, is an example of poorer quality of life among ethnic minority elderly.

A clear indicator of poorer health status, and therefore of quality of life, is the lower life expectancy among ethnic minorities: 66 years for African American men and 74.5 years for African American women; compared with 72.6 and 79.3 years respectively for Caucasian men and women (NCHS, 1992). Survival to old age is least likely among African Americans; 66% can expect to reach age 65, compared with 80% of whites and Hispanics and 71% of American Indians (Taeuber, 1990). This dramatic difference reflects African Americans' greater vulnerability to social and economic conditions across the life span, including the dramatically increasing homicide rate and other traumas among African American males in young adulthood and middle age.

The prevalence of chronic diseases is twice as high among African Americans as among whites (Harper & Alexander, 1990). They experience hypertension more frequently and at an earlier age than their white peers. As a result, deaths due to stroke as well as nonfatal strokes that can disrupt the older person's activities of daily living are more common among African Americans aged 35 to 74 than in whites. Obesity is also a health problem among 60% of African American women over age 45, which can lead to complications of hypertension and diabetes (Waller, 1989). Kidney failure, which may result from hypertension and diabetes, is more common in older African Americans with the rate of diabetes mellitus among African American women 50% higher than white women and 16% higher in African American men than their white counterparts, resulting in twice the rate of amputations as in whites (Lieberman, 1988). African Americans also have higher death rates from cancers of the lungs, prostate, and cervix than do whites, even though the incidence of these cancers is not necessarily greater among blacks. Similarly, their 5-year survival rate for cancer of the cervix, uterus, and esophagus is lower than for any other segment of the population (National Cancer Institute, 1986).

Given the higher incidence of chronic conditions, it is not surprising that African Americans experience more days of functional and bed disability and at earlier ages than whites. In the Charleston Heart Study, 56% of older African women and 39% of African American men were disabled, compared to 43% of white women and 26% of white men. Proportionately more African American elderly are completely incapacitated and unable to carry on any major activity, although still residing in the community (Harper & Alexander, 1990).

Similarly, the poverty of Hispanic Americans is a major factor in their generally poor health, with 85% of older Hispanics reporting at least one chronic condition and 45% reporting some limitation in activities of daily living (Cuellar, 1990). Arthritis, hypertension, circulatory disorders, diabetes, cataracts, glaucoma, and heart disease are the most common health problems. Hispanic women have higher mortality rates from cervical cancer and cancer of the uterus, and at an earlier age than do white women. The greater proportion of older Hispanic men compared to the white population is due to the higher mortality rate of Hispanic women at earlier ages, not to greater longevity among Hispanic men.

Native American elderly appear to have the poorest health of all elderly, with a higher incidence than whites of accidents, tuberculosis, diabetes, heart disease, liver and kidney disease, hypertension, strokes, hearing and visual impairments, and problems stemming from obesity, gall bladder or arthritis. In fact, 71% suffer limitations in their ability to perform activities of daily living (Manson, 1989). Although liver and kidney problems often result from lifelong drinking, alcoholism, generally takes its toll before old age. The death rate from alcoholism among American Indians is seven times higher than that of the general population, but alcohol-related deaths drop sharply among those who have reached age 55 (Rhoades, 1990).

An exception to the pattern of poorer health than their white counterparts appears to occur among Japanese and Chinese elderly, although health statistics are limited for these groups. Their apparent greater life expectancy may be due to the lower incidence of most diseases, especially heart disease, hypertension, and strokes in these two groups compared to whites, although the rate of digestive system cancer is higher in Japanese Americans (Kii, 1984; Park, Yokoyama, & Tokuyama, 1991). The relatively better health status of these two Pacific Asian groups may be due to their diet, with lower fat and higher carbohydrate intakes compared with whites (Choi et al., 1990). Less comparative research has been conducted on the health status of other Pacific Asian groups.

Other structural factors in addition to low socioeconomic status underlie the higher incidence of chronic disease and "early aging" among elderly people of color, as well as greater rates of disability and mortality. A primary factor is the barrier to health care, with ethnic minorities having less access to health care, although they may use hospital emergency rooms more than their white counterparts. Because African Americans have limited access to specialists, they are less likely to receive specialized procedures, such as electrocardiograms (EKGs) or bypass surgery, and more likely to die from a myocardial infarct (Feller, 1983). As another example of structural causes, the higher risk of cancer among African Americans appears to be due to inadequate access to and discontinuity of health care (especially preventive care); higher occupational and residential exposure to cancer-causing substances; higher rates of obesity; higher prevalence of smoking, which has increased since 1990, compared to a decrease among whites; and less knowledge about cancer and its prevention (Baquet, 1988). Among all groups of elderly, Hispanics are the least likely to have a regular physician, to use hospitals, and to seek preventive care or dental care (Miranda, 1990). Use of Western health services tends to be low across all Pacific Asian groups; approximately 33% of Pacific Asian elderly have never seen a Western doctor or dentist (Kim, 1990). The majority of Native American elderly rarely see a physician, often because of living in isolated areas and lacking transportation. The Indian Health Service provides health care to those on reservations, but very few urban elderly seek out such care, generally because of the cost, transportation difficulties, or professionals' lack of sensitivity to Indians' ritual folk healing or cultural definitions of disease (Rhoades, 1990). Another structural barrier to health care is that the Indian Health Service emphasizes services to youth and families and acute care rather than long-term care, such as skilled and intermediate care facilities (Manson, 1989).

A critical aspect of these barriers is less access to health insurance, especially private insurance, among older ethnic minorities. Although 94% of whites have Medicare and 73% have private insurance, the corresponding proportion of African Americans is 87% and 42% respectively (Harper & Alexander, 1990; Manuel, 1988). Eighty-three percent of Hispanics receive Medicare benefits (Miranda, 1990), whereas only about 50% of American Indian elders receive Social Security and medicare benefits, and less than 40% receive Medicaid (Cook, 1990). A pattern across all ethnic minority groups is the small proportion who are in nursing homes compared to their white counterparts. Although it can be argued that these lower rates are due to family care, other reasons are lack of finances and discriminatory practices on the part of some long-term care institutions.

Cultural factors also underlie lower utilization of mainstream professional health services, such as mistrust of Caucasian medical providers, reliance on folk medicine and religious healing, and difficulty in comprehending English. As examples, many Native Americans prefer traditional health care from their tribal medicine people. Among Chinese American elderly who value traditional healing practices, hospitals are seen as places to die, not to get well (Baker, 1990). Southeast Asian refugees' belief in the supernatural powers of ancestral and natural spirits may be a cause of their low utilization of health care. Such belief systems are often a barrier to utilization of mental health services, particularly when mental illness is defined as stigma (Kim, 1990). Language may be a greater barrier than cultural or religious beliefs, however, as bilingual and bicultural personnel within service programs appear to reduce some of the resistance to the use of Western health services (Yip, 1981). Another barrier has been the myth held by some services providers that Pacific Asian elderly do not have problems and "take care of their own."

Living Arrangements and Quality of Life

Where one lies also affects one's quality of life and tends to be associated with socioeconomic status. Older African Americans in metropolitan areas are more likely to live in the central city (69.1%), whereas their white counterparts are equally distributed between central and suburban communities (39% and 40%, respectively)(Manuel, 1988). Central-city residence results in greater vulnerability to crime; for example, 13% of African American elderly are victims of violent crime and 9% of theft with bodily contact, compared with 7% and 2%, respectively among their white counterparts (Gibson, 1983). Accordingly, deaths in late life, due to lifestyle and environmental hazards, including accidents and homicides among men, are much higher than among whites, except for those over age 80. In contrast, Pacific Asian elderly have tended to live in ethnic enclaves in larger cities. These tightly knit communities tended to provide a center for leisure activities and for service delivery, reducing vulnerability to strangers.

Social Networks and Quality of Life

Numerous studies over the past 20 years have pointed to the significant role of supportive social networks in enhancing an older person's quality of life (Blazer, 1982; Sarason, Sarason, Potter, & Antoni, 1985). There is some evidence that strong social networks, both within the extended family and the ethnic community (e.g., the Black church) serve as a buffer and compensate, to some extent, for socioeconomic inadequacies and health limitations (Jackson, Chatters, & Neighbors, 1982).

The family is a primary source of social support across all ethnic minority groups, with family relationships strongly influenced by historical and cultural factors. Although most older African Americans do not live in extended families, approximately 20%, as compared to 12% of their white peers, live with some family members other than their spouse. Comparative studies depict older African Americans as having larger extended families, a higher frequency of family-based households, and higher levels of social support from family members than do whites (George, 1988; Taylor, Chatters, & Mays, 1988). Accordingly, older African American women are more likely than white women to have family living with them in their homes. Typically, these are three generational households, with older women providing financial assistance and care for grandchildren as well as children of other family members and friends. Such intergenerational households that develop out of financial necessity illustrate the resourcefulness of African American families whose domestic networks expand and contract according to economic resources (Johnson & Barer, 1990). The creation of "fictive kin," including foster parents or children who function in the absence of blood relatives or when family relationships are unsatisfactory, is another source of loving support for African American elderly (George, 1988).

Historically, the extended family has been a major support to older Hispanics, especially in rural areas. An early study of informal supports found that Hispanic elderly had consistently higher levels of interaction and a greater potential for support from children than did either white or African American elderly, even controlling for gender, social class and levels of functional ability (Cantor, 1979). Older Hispanics, especially widowed women over age 75, are more likely than whites to believe that older persons should be cared for in the community and to live with their adult children (Cuellar, 1990). The percentage of older Hispanics living in multigenerational families has declined recently; however, with their urbanization and greater acculturation, younger Hispanics are increasingly unable to meet their older parents' expectations and to support an extended family in one location. Nevertheless, even when families are living apart, members tend to perform numerous support functions. Although families remain the most important system of support for their older members, a division of labor appears to be emerging between the family, which provides support and personal care, and public agencies, which provide financial assistance and medical care (Cuellar, 1990).

Although Pacific Asians represent tremendous diversity in terms of country of origin, degree of acculturation, and transcending values and religion, they share the common values and reciprocal exchanges between young and old and the prestige of being old, and seek outside help only in desperate circumstances. Nevertheless, there are variations in cultural identification within families and the inevitable clashes that occur when different generations have different languages, values and ethos, with the younger generation experiencing geographic and social mobility and acculturation into the larger society. As examples of this variation, Chinese American elderly generally live with their children only in cases of extreme poverty or poor health, and often depend on them for translation assistance, despite their strong commitment to family and filial responsibility. Korean American elderly accept separation from their children as a way to promote the children's happiness and success. As a result of these differing values, the majority of Pacific Asian elderly live by themselves or with a spouse, not with children, even though the proportion of extended family arrangements is higher than among whites.

"Honoring" and giving respect to elders and sharing family resources are an integral part of the ethos of Native American culture. In many Native American tribes, a deep reverence for nature and belief in a supreme force, the importance of the clan, and a sense of individual autonomy as a key to group cohesiveness and lack of competition underlie their practices toward their elderly. Historically, the old were accorded respect and fulfilled specified useful tribal roles, including that of the "wise elder" who instructs the young and assists with child care, especially for foster children and grandchildren. Elders also maintained responsibility for relating tribal philosophies, myths, and traditions and served as religious and political advisors to tribal leaders. These relationships have changed, however, with the restructuring of Native American life by the Bureau of Indian Affairs and by the increasing urbanization of Native populations. Despite these changes, many Native American elderly, particularly in rural settings, continue to live in an extended family, with approximately 66% living with and financially supporting family members. Some 25% of Indian elderly care for at least one grandchild, and 67% live within five miles of relatives (Manson & Callaway, 1990).

Such strong family ties can enhance quality of life, but they can also serve to result in the underutilization of social and health services. For example, the value placed on family support by many Native Americans, combined with deep mistrust of governmental programs, can put pressure on families to keep their elders at home, even when families lack the resources to do so (Manson, 1989).

The church often provides a support network of spiritual help, companionship, advice encouragement, and financial aid, particularly for African American and Hispanic elderly. The church is also a setting for older ethnic minorities to help others, an important role often lost with illness and disability. A strong spiritual orientation has been found to be related to feelings of well-being, self-esteem, and personal control, characteristics that reflect quality of life. In fact, the religiosity and social support of the church may explain why older African Americans report a greater sense of life satisfaction than do their white counterparts, despite less desirable objective living conditions (Chatters & Taylor, 1989; Krause & Tran, 1989; Taylor & Chatters, 1991).

Community and neighborhood ties can also enhance quality of life despite low socioeconomic status and health problems. Older African Americans tend to draw from a more varied pool of friends, fellow church members and other associational contacts, and to use them interchangeably more than their white counterparts. Such social networks tend to expand as needed to include friends, neighbors, and fellow church members as helpers, especially among widowed African American women (Watson, 1990). For first-generation Japanese or Issei, a value that transcends that of family is group conscience, characterized by cohesiveness, strong pride, and identity through devotion to and sense of mutuality among peer group members. This value has been preserved through residential and occupational isolation from mainstream American culture. As noted earlier, close-knit Pacific Asian enclaves in large urban areas have provided a locus for leisure, service delivery, and support particularly through benevolent societies and clubs. Yet the current cohort of Pacific Asian elderly are often caught between their cultural traditions of group and family honor and the values of their adopted culture that stress independence and self-sufficiency, making them loath to ask others for support. In addition, the social support functions served by the closely knit community will probably not exist for future generations of pacific Asians, who have become more geographically and socially mobile.

Implications for Improving Quality of Life

Given the central role that poverty plays in reducing quality of life among elderly ethnic minorities, it is not sufficient merely to provide more social and health services to minorities in late life. A multifaceted approach that addressees underlying structural conditions such as discrimination against specific minority groups, is needed to prevent poverty and poor health across the life span. Educational and health interventions can begin at an early age, through early childhood education and nutrition programs. Efforts to assist young persons of color to complete high school, college or a vocational program, combined with job training, can reduce historical patterns of sporadic and low-paying employment that result in poverty, and can improve quality of life in old age.

An intergenerational approach may be effective in addressing these issues. An approach that brings together children, young adults, and elderly to provide educational and employment opportunities (e.g., tutoring of school children by minority elders, job training in health or social service agency for elderly as translators or service providers, or in a home repair program) can serve multiple functions. It may reduce the competition for scarce resources among young and old, and encourage the transfer of cultural values to the young. This approach also recognizes the strong kinship ties that are characteristic of many minority populations, as described in the last section. Cross-cultural understanding can be enhanced by pairing ethnic minority elders with white children or young adults in these tutorial and job training programs, and vice versa.

Efforts to enhance quality of life through improved health and social services requires a thorough understanding of health values and beliefs about disease prevention among ethnic minorities. More research is needed on what motivates minority elders to seek preventive medical, dental and, mental health services, including research on how to motivate ethnic minority elders to participate in health promotion *research*! It is important to examine differences between and within ethnic minority groups in health beliefs and practices. For example, differences in health status between Cuban Americans and Mexican Americans may be a function of health beliefs and practices, not just income.

Programs aimed at ethnic minorities must recognize and build into their service delivery system cultural differences between and within these groups. At the simplest level, staff members must reflect the languages and cultures of the ethnic groups that they aim to serve. Service providers must also be sensitive to their clients' cultural values, and recognize traditional medicines and healers. It is incumbent upon health professionals from a particular ethnic group to be aware of their own biases, often in favor of Western medicine and with less tolerance of folk medicine practices of elders from their *own* ethnic group.

Finally, quality of life must be examined multidimensionally. The strength of social networks and spiritual values in mitigating the impact of physical frailty and poverty for many minority elders cannot be denied. Although these personal values are more difficult to quantify, they may in fact represent the key element in well-being that can overcome financial, environmental, and health barriers in old age.

References

American Association of Retired Persons. (1987). *A profile of older Americans*. Washington, DC: AARP.

Baker, F. M. (1990). Ethnic minority issues: Differential diagnosis, medication, treatment and outcomes. In M. S. Harper (Ed.). *Minority aging*. U. S. Department of Health & Human Services. USDHHS Publication Nol. HRS (P-DV-90-4). Washington, DC: U. S. Government Printing Office.

Baquet, C. R. (1988). Cancer prevention and control in the Black population. In J. S. Jackson (Ed.) *The black American elderly*. New York: Springer Publishing Co.

Bass, S. A., Kutza, E. A., & Torres-Gil, F. (1990). Diversity in aging: The challenges facing the White House Conference on Aging. In S. A. Bass, E. A. Kutza & F. Torres-Gil (Eds.), *Diversity in aging*. Glenview, ILL: Scott Foresman & Co.

Blazer, D. (1982). Social support and mortality in an elderly community population. *American Journal of Epidemiology, 115*, 684–694.

Brown, D. (1990). The Black elderly: Implications for the family. In M. S. Harper (Ed.), *Minority aging* USDHHS No. HRS(P-DV-90-4). Washington, DC: U. S. Government Printing Office.

Cantor, M. H. (1979) The informal support system of New York's inner city elderly: Is ethnicity a factor? In D. E. Gelfand & A. J. Kutzik (Eds.), *Ethnicity and aging: Theory, research and policy*. New York: Springer Publishing Co.

Chatters, L., & Taylor, R. J. (1989). Age differences in religious participation among Black adults. *Journal of Gerontology, 44*, S183–S189.

Choi, E. S., McGandy, R. B., Dallal, G. E., Russell, K. M., Jacob, R. A., Schaefer, E. J. & Sadowski, J. A. (1990). Prevalence of cardiovascular risk factors among elderly Chinese Americans. *Archives of Internal Medicine, 150*, 413–418.

Cook, C. D. (1990). American Indian elderly and public policy issues. In M. S. Harper (Ed.), *Minority aging*. USDHHS No. HRS(P-DV-90-4). Washington, DC: U. S. Government Printing Office.

Cuellar, J. (1990). Hispanic American aging: Geriatric educational curriculum development for selected health professions. In M. S. Harper (Ed.) *Minority aging*. USDHHS No. HRS(P-DV-90-4). Washington, DC: U. S. Government Printing Office.

Feller, B. (1983). Americans needing help to function at home. *Advance data from Vital and Health Statistics*, National Center for Health Statistics, Washington, DC: U. S. Government Printing Office.

George, L. K. (1988). Social participation in late life: Black-white differences. In J. S. Jackson (Ed.), *The black American elderly*. New York: Springer Publishing Co.

Gibson, R. (1983). Special social needs of the Black elderly: Recent research findings from the panel study of income dynamics and the National Survey of Black Americans. Paper presented at annual conference of the National Assoc of Area Agencies on Aging, Washington, D. C.

Gibson, R. (1986). Outlook for the Black family. In A. Pifer & L. Bronte (Eds.), *Our aging society*. New York: W. W. Norton, 1986.

Gibson, R. (1989). Minority aging research: Opportunity and challenge. *Journal of Gerontology 44*, S52–S53.

Gould, K. H. (1989). A minority-feminist perspective on women and aging. *Journal of Women and Aging, 1, 195–216*.

Harper, M., & Alexander, C. (1990). Profile of the Black elderly. In M. S. Harper (Ed.), *Minority aging*. USDHHS No. HRS(P-DV-90-4). Washington, DC: U. S. Government Printing Office.

Jackson, J. (1985). Race, national origin, ethnicity and aging. In E. Shanas and R. Binstock (Eds.), *Handbook of aging and the social sciences*. New York: Van Nostrand Reinhold.

Jackson, J. S., Chatters, L. M., & Neighbors, H. W. (1982). The mental health status of older Black Americans. *The Black Scholar, 13*, 21–35.

Johnson, C., & Barer, B. (1990). Families and networks among older inner-city Blacks. *The Gerontologist 30*, 726–733.

Kasper, J. (1988). *Aging alone: Profiles and projections*. Baltimore: The Commonwealth Fund Commission.

Kii, T. (1984). Asians. In E. Palmore (Ed.), *Handbook on the aged in the United States*. Westport, CT: Greenwood Press.

Kim, P. (1990). Asian American families and the elderly. In M. S. Harper (Ed.),*Minority aging*. USDHHS No. HRS(P-DV-90-4). Washington, DC: U. S. Government Printing Office.

Kim, P. (1983). Demography of the Asian-Pacific elderly: Selected problems and implications. In R. L. McNeely and J. L. Colen (Eds.), *Aging in minority groups*. Beverly Hills: Sage.

Krause, N. (1987). Stress in racial differences in self-reported health among the elderly. *The Gerontologist, 27*, 72–76.

Krause, N. & Tran, T. V. (1989). Stress and religious involvement among older Blacks. *Journal of Gerontology, 44*, S4-S13.

Lieberman, L. S. (1988). Diabetes and obesity in the elderly Black Americans. In J. S. Jackson (Ed.), *The black American elderly*. New York: Springer Publishing Co.

Liu, W. T. (1986). Health services for the Asian elderly. *Research on aging, 8*, 156–175.

Manson, S. M. (1989). Long-term care in American Indian communities: Issues for planning and research. *Gerontology, 29*, 38–44.

Manson, S. M., & Callaway, D. G. (1990). Health and aging among American Indians. In M. S. Harper (Ed.), *Minority aging*. USDHHS No. HRS(P-DV-90-4). Washington, DC: U. S. Government Printing Office.

Manuel, R. C. (1988). The demography of older blacks in the United States. In J. S. Jackson (Ed.), *The Black American elderly*. New York: Springer Publishing Co.

Markides, K., & Liang, J. L., & Jackson, J. (1990). Race, ethnicity and aging: Conceptual and methodological issues. In R. Binstock and L. George (Eds.) *Handbook of aging and the social sciences* (3rd ed). New York: Academic Press.

Miranda, M. (1990). Hispanic aging: An overview of issues and policy implications. In M. S. Harper (Ed.), *Minority aging*. USDHHS No. HRS(P-DV-90-4). Washington, DC: U. S. Government Printing Office.

National Cancer Institute (1986). *Cancer among Blacks and other minorities: Statistical profiles* (NIH Publication No. 86–2785), March 1986.

National Center for Health Statistics (1987). Health statistics on older persons: United States 1986. *Vital and Health Statistics*, Series 3, No. 25 DHHS Pub. No. 87-1049. Washington, DC: U. S. Government Printing Office.

National Center for Health Statistics (1992). *Health, United States, 1990*. Monthly Vital Statistics Report, *40*, 8(S)2, January 1992.

National Indian Council on Aging (1984). Indians and Alaskan natives. In E.

Palmore (Ed.), *Handbook on the aged in the United States*. Westport, CT: Greenwood Press.

Park, C. B., Yokoyama, E. & Tokuyama, G. H. (1991). Medical conditions at death in Hawaii. *Journal of Clinical Epidemiology, 44*, 519–530.

Reed, W. L. (1984). *Access to services by the urban elderly*. NTIS Publications, No. PB-84-245364. Baltimore: Institute for Urban Research.

Rhoades, E. (1990). Profile of American Indians and Alaska natives. In M. S. Harper (Ed.), *Minority aging*. USDHHS No. HRS(P-DV-90-4). Washington, DC: U. S. Government Printing Office.

Sarason, I. G., Sarason, B. R., Potter, E. H. & Antoni, M. H. (1985). Life events, social support and illness. *Psychosomatic Medicine, 47*, 156–163.

Soldo, B., & Agree, E. (1988). America's elderly. *Population Bulletin, 43*, 1–46.

Taeuber, C. M. (1990). Diversity: The dramatic reality. In S. A. Bass, E. A. Kutza, & F. Torres-Gil (Eds.), *Diversity and aging*. Glenview, IL: Scott Foresman.

Taeuber, C. M. (1992). *Sixty-five plus in America*. Current population reports: Special studies (Series P-23, No. 178). Washington, DC: U. S. Department of Commerce.

Taylor, R. J. & Chatters, L. M. (1991). Nonorganizational religious participation among elderly Black adults. *Journal of Gerontology, 46*, S103–S110.

Taylor, R. J., Chatters, L. M., & Mays, J. M. (1988). Parents, siblings, in-laws and non-kin as a source of emergency assistance to Black Americans. *Family Relations, 37*, 298–304.

Torres-Gil, F. (1986). Hispanics: A special challenge. In A. Pifer & L. Bronte (Eds.), *Our aging society*. New York: W. W. Norton.

U. S. Bureau of the Census. (1991). Consumer income. *Current population reports*. (Seriers P-60, No. 175). Washington DC: U. S. Department of Commerce.

U. S. Bureau of the Census. (1989). Projections of the population of the U. S. by age, sex and race: 1988–2080. *Current population reports*. Washington, DC: U. S. Department of Commerce.

U. S. Bureau of the Census. (1990). *Poverty in the United States: 1990* (Series P-60, No. 175). Washington DC: U. S. Department of Commerce.

U. S. Bureau of the Census. (1991). Age, sex, race and Hispanic origin information from the 1990 census. *Current population reports*. Washington DC: U. S. Department of Commerce.

U. S. Senate Special Committee on Aging. (1988). *Aging America: Trends and Projections,* 1987–1988. Washington, DC: U. S. Government Printing Office.

U. S. Senate Special Committee on Aging. (1992). *Aging America: Trends and projections: 1990–1991*. Washington, DC: U. S. Department of Health and Human Services.

Waller, J. B. (1989). Challenges to the provision of health care to minority aged. *First annual summer symposium: Geriatric Education Center of Michigan*. Ann Arbor, MI, June 1989.

Watson, W. H. (1990). Family care, economics and health. In Z. Harel, E. A. McKinney, & M. Williams, (Eds), *Black aged*. Newbury Park, CA: Sage.

Wing, S., Manton, K. G., Stallard, E., Hames, C. G., and Tyroler, H. A. (1985). The Black/white mortality crossover: Investigation in a community-based study. *Journal of Gerontology, 40*, 78–84.

Yeo, G. W. (1993). Ethnicity and nursing homes: Factors affecting use and successful components for culturally sensitive care. In C. M. Barresi & D. E. Stull (Eds.), *Ethnic elderly and long-term care*, New York: Springer Publishing Co.

Yip, B. (1981) Accessibility of services for Pan-Asian elderly: Fact or fiction? In E. P. Stanford (Ed.), *Minority aging: Policy issues for the 80s*. San Diego, CA: Campanile Press.

PART VI

Policy Implications

Chapter 17
Public Policy and Long-Term Care

Carroll L. Estes and Liz Close

The research agenda concerning health status, health promotion, and disease prevention in the elderly is well documented (IOM, 1991). In contrast, there is a dearth of empirical work on the effects on older and disabled persons of public policy concerning the organization, financing, and delivery of long-term care (LTC). The growing health care burden of the disabled and socially dependent older population (Kunkel & Applebaum, 1992; Manton & Suzman, 1992) emphasizes the urgency of addressing this issue despite the recent finding that the magnitude of disability rates among the elderly decreased slightly in the last decade (Manton, Corder, & Stallard, 1993).

Within the existing social structure, inequities in access to health care occur across the lifespan (Estes & Rundall, 1992). The complex and dynamic relationships between the need for and utilization of formal and informal long-term care are not yet clearly explicated. It has been argued that public policy tends to reflect and preserve existing inequalities in the social structure, particularly the relative positions of advantage and disadvantage that are structured along racial, ethnic, gender, and class lines (Estes, 1979). The existence and effects of such potential policy bias will neither be illuminated by research, nor eliminated by social policy unless scientific inquiry focuses sharply on understanding the social structures and social processes that impede access to a quality life.

Science continues to identify, analyze, and suggest remedies for specific organic diseases as well as some behavioral ills. Much less research attention, however, has been given to explicating the societal mechanisms and sociocultural forces that might explain the origin, manifestation, acceleration, and prevention of specific diseases and chronic conditions endemic to certain population groups. Many of these "individual" diseases and chronic conditions may be mediated more by life course experience associated with sociostructural location than by genetic, biological, or even behavioral factors. Thus the capacity of science to inform public policy is contingent on well-designed research that explicitly addresses the sociostructural dimensions of health and the effects of differential access to resources (including health and long-term care) across the life course.

This chapter briefly reviews the interplay of major societal forces shaping public policy and long-term care, highlights current knowledge about selected social issues, and suggests specific knowledge that is needed to assist in the design of long-term care policy with special focus on a research agenda that will address policy considerations attentive to racial, ethnic, gender, and social class differences.

Societal Forces Shaping Public Policy

Public policy and long-term care are shaped by the confluence of four societal forces: sociodemographic changes, the biomedicalization of aging, unresolved problems concerning health care access and costs, and dependency (Estes, Swan, & Associates, 1993).

Demographic changes reviewed in earlier chapters indicate several trends relevant to the influences of population dynamics on policy decisions concerning long-term care in the United States. By the mid-twenty-first century, as a result of the rapidly increasing over-65 (and particularly over-85) population group, the need for long-term care (for both home care and nursing home care) will at least triple and associated costs will increase ten-fold (Rice, 1986; Taeuber, 1992). There will no doubt be absolute increases in the need for long-term care since even the most optimistic declines in disability rates "do not wholly compensate for population aging" (Manton et al., 1993, p. 5164). Notably, increasing "population frailty" (Verbrugge, 1989) and increasing life expectancy but worsening health (Brody, Brock, & Williams, 1987; McKinlay, McKinlay, & Beaglehole, 1989; Verbrugge, 1991) combine to place an extraordinary demand on the long-term care system in the future. Regardless of the specific forecasting model used, the predicted increase in the elderly population raises ominous issues (Kunkel & Applebaum, 1992).

The biomedicalization of aging has significantly influenced research and the development of a knowledge base in the field of aging (Estes, 1979; Estes & Binney, 1989; Estes et al., 1993). The tendency to focus on individual organic pathology amenable to medical intervention has resulted in the conceptualization of old age as a disease, aging as a medical problem, and palliation of the aging process as a venerable goal.

The unrelenting issues of health care costs and access—compounded by gaps in private insurance protection and negligible long-term care insurance coverage—render quality of life for elderly in the future increasingly problematic (Estes et al., 1993). Out-of-pocket expenses for health care consume increasingly larger proportions of the elderly's disposable retirement income because Medicare currently covers less than one-half of the cost of their health care. Recent Congressional budget agreements add more than $10 billion to out-of-pocket Medicare beneficiary costs by 1996 (U.S. Senate Special Committee on Aging, 1991). Health care costs have become particularly burdensome to older women who pay as much as 42% of their annual income for medical expenses not covered by Medicare (Families, USA, 1992; ICF, 1985).

The life chances of elders (mortality, disability, chronic illness, and self-reported health) are strongly influenced by gender, race, ethnic status, and social class (Estes & Rundall, 1992). Recent research indicates that age related-disease and disability among the elderly is related to cumulative exposure to risk rather than simply to aging per se (Manton & Suzman, 1992). Long-term care policy and associated research should be informed by and attentive to the nature, extent, and effects of persistent risk exposure associated with the sociostructural characteristics of populations. Dependency and the contribution of social policy and practice (e.g., age discrimination) induce more dependency, which reflects a major potential problem. The medical and high-tech approach to care of older persons, as well as declining access to health care, further exacerbate the sense of loss of personal control and elder dependency.

As a result of multiple changes occurring in the past decade, the system of community-based services has been challenged, weakened, and transformed (Estes et al., 1993). Public policy simultaneously financed the medicalization of care (Estes & Binney, 1989), challenged the charitable impulse in nonprofit service delivery through cost containment and competition, and indirectly fostered the dependency of elders through its major long-term care policy—the impoverishment and institutionalization of elders who need extensive long-term care and are not covered for it under Medicare.

The research agenda in public policy and long-term care calls for investigation of the continuing interplay of various societal forces in the social production of a dependent elderly population and the attendant challenges to traditional structures of long-term care. The process by which older persons are empowered in their own care involves active participation in decisions concerning their care and the accumulation of knowledge and skills to make informed choices (Estes et al., 1993). Governmental, organizational, and professional structures, as well as societal norms, that facilitate or impede progress toward the goal of empowerment need to be thoroughly explicated. Kunkel and Applebaum (1992) urge a research focus that examines new structural models for the delivery of long-term care; the priority research areas presented in this chapter support and resound this recommendation.

Illustrative Research Problems Related to LTC and Aging

One difficulty for research is that projections of long-term care (LTC) needs in the U.S. are largely based on current patterns of availability and utilization of existing LTC resources. Problems arise from projecting need based on the present service delivery system rather than on theoretically and empirically derived hypothetical models of alternative policies. Examples of problematic assumptions that need to be examined in future research are that the family is the appropriate (and most desirable) LTC provider in the community; that women's labor force participation does not interfere with the informal LTC that women provide; that there will be no erosion in the need for long-term care regardless of scientific advances in aging; and that public opinion is likely to remain stable regardless of the mismatch between chronic care needs and acute care policy. Priority areas of inquiry address these interrelated assumptions and include: research on older women and their health across the lifespan, informal care system costs and benefits, factors determining the need for and utilization of long-term care services, and the effects and effectiveness of various long-term care policy options. Research on the effects of policy intervention needs to investigate questions regarding the role of social policies in alleviating, as well as creating, dependency.

Older Women and Health

Although females are the majority of persons 65 years of age and older and they are the great majority of persons over 85, research on older women and their health issues is underdeveloped. The fact that most research on health has been on males is acknowledged in the recent establishment of the National Institute of Health (NIH) Office of Research on Women's Health (Kirschstein, 1991). Older women are a vulnerable population about whom relatively little is known. For example, little is known about how risk factors vary for older women or how gender roles and life experiences of men and women are associated with different health effects. Rodin and Ickovics (1990) have identified several factors that are likely to differentially affect men's and women's health in old age including sociostructural conditions that promote continuing imbalances in role expectations related to work and family and concomitantly in power, equality, and control. Key issues also pertain to women's patterns of health care access and utilization. These include observations that women account for 70% of all psychoactive drug prescriptions (Lipton & Lee, 1989); two-thirds of all surgical procedures (Travis, 1988); limited use of certain kinds of medical technologies (e.g., cardiac catheterization), yet the high use of others (e.g., reproductive technologies); and relatively restricted access to health insurance (Rodin & Ickovics, 1990).

The differing sociodemographic profiles of older women and men raise additional questions about both health status and access to health care that are extremely important for the formulation of public policy and long-term care. Although women in the United States live an average of 8 years longer than men, evidence strongly suggests they live those years in poorer health due to the high incidence of disability associated with chronic conditions and the higher incidence and prevalence of acute fatal diseases among men (Verbrugge, 1991). Older women also have higher rates of institutionalization than older men. These gender differences become greater after age 75 (Minkler & Stone, 1983; NCHS, 1991; U.S. Senate, 1988). Rodin and Ickovics (1990) observe that these differences are theorized to emanate from biological and social (life-style) explanations. Stress and sociodemographic factors have emerged as important explanatory variables to account for gender differences in physical health. The relationship between social class and health is well established. Older women's vulnerable economic status is also demonstrated. For example, older women have lower incomes from every source including pensions and social security, and three-fourths of elder poverty is female (O'Rand, 1988; Sofaer & Abel, 1990). Much more needs to be understood about the intersection of these gender and social class differences with health in old age.

Gender differences in access to health insurance are well documented, with women generally having more limited access to care. Older women spend a substantial portion of their income on out-of-pocket health care expenses, with Medicare covering on average about one-third of their expenses. Particularly for single older women, the costs exceed one-third of their annual income (ICF, 1985; U.S. House of Representatives, 1990). It is significant that, as a consequence of their socioeconomic status including poverty, widowhood, and care-giving responsibilities, older women are more affected than men by governmental policy changes and particularly program cutbacks (Rodin & Ickovics, 1990).

The research agenda in older women's health is not only large; the research must go beyond simply using gender as a predictor variable, to embrace "gender as a dynamic construct that itself varies across ethnic groups and social classes and works in complex interactions with other psychological and social factors" (Russo, 1987, p. 54).

Informal Care

It is well established that women are the major providers of informal unpaid long-term care for the 80% of LTC given to impaired older persons. Controversy about the relative proportions of women "sandwiched" by caregiving for both younger and older family members (OWL, 1989; Rosenthal, Matthews, & Marshall, 1989; Stone & Kemper, 1989) indicates a continuing need for explication of this contemporary phenomenon. Much more research is needed to further specify the subgroups of older women "in the middle" and to understand associated cohort health and economic risks. In addition, the effects of contending with informal care provision and workplace responsibilities has potentially tremendous influence on both the individual lives of women and the economic well-being of the labor force. Research in this area is challenging in part due to ambiguous definitions of formal and informal care (NRC, 1988), underdeveloped measures of workforce disruption, and minimal knowledge of the long-term health effects of caregiver burden.

Increasing longevity means that caregiving spouses will be older themselves. Adult female children of older persons are likely to be less available as future caretakers as a result of changes in family size, increasing employment among middle-aged women, and physical distance from elderly parents (NRC, 1988). Pressures on the informal caregiving system will grow as caregivers of the future will have informal care responsibilities for not just one, but two, disabled parents. Assuming continuing birthrates, there will be fewer adult children to care for their older parents (Stone & Kemper, 1989). How these changes will ultimately increase the demand for formal health and personal care services has not been investigated.

The movement toward services and systems that promote independent living and support informal caregivers for the elderly cite the preference of most individuals to remain at home as evidence that nursing homes should be an approach of last resort for care delivery to disabled older persons (Harrington et al., 1991). The fact that elders are believed to prefer to live at home does not necessarily mean that their care, by definition, should be provided by family, friends, and other informal caregivers, with or without subsidy.

Knowledge about the use of formal care services to supplement or substitute for informal care is growing. Formal care provision does not appear to substitute for informal care (Tennstedt & McKinlay, 1989) and recent evidence strongly suggests that increases in paid home care will not deter current levels of informal support (Hanley, Wiener, & Harris, 1991). The exclusive use of formal care services is rare among older impaired persons (Commonwealth Fund Commission on Elderly People Living Alone, 1989) and the relationship between formal and informal care appears to be more one of complementarity rather than substitutability (DeFriese & Woomert, 1992). There is also some research indicating that use of formal services to augment in-home care does not reduce or mediate the negative effects of caregiving. It has been suggested that much of the stress suffered by primary informal caregivers involves frustrations related to negotiating home care coordination among a plethora of agencies, regulations, and negatively oriented service providers (McKinlay, Crawford, & Tennstedt, 1993).

On the policy level, the cumulative data on informal care point, rather menacingly, to a significant and potentially unstable (even volatile) "nonsystem" of informal long-term care, staffed to a major degree by economically poor, stressed older women with limited access to resources—many of whom will, themselves, constitute the largest group of LTC consumers in the nation by the year 2020. This situation raises the salience of a research agenda that is attentive to the social policy consequences and effects of informal care, but it must be one that addresses both the caregiver *and* the care recipient perspectives (Barer & Johnson, 1990); the design of systems to effectively link informal and formal care services provided to frail older persons; the economic and environmental realities of informal and formal care patterns across ethnic, racial, gender, and socioeconomic variables; and the questionable stance of public policy promoting informal care by embracing kinship obligation (Collins, 1991; Finch, 1989) as an appropriate social contract for provision of health and social services to older persons (Estes & Rundall, 1992; Phillipson, 1992).

Long-Term Care

Health services research is a relatively new field that has been empirically, rather than theoretically driven. Because the knowledge base is just now emerging, policymakers have had to cope with extremely complex health policy questions without a coherent cumulative body of knowledge elucidating the social behavior of the health field. Although health services research must be responsive to present and future policy needs, the constant pressure to achieve immediate results poses a serious problem for the scientific development of the field. These urgent demands present difficulties in attaining an environment that is committed to the long view that will support the required period of conceptualization and specification, methodological and data-base development, and the rigorous, yet tedious, research process on which the accretion of scientific knowledge must be built.

There is an ever-mounting impatience with health services research because of increasing concern about high and rising costs and deepening problems of access. In addition, the proliferation of new technologies appears to add to health care costs rather than to contain them, in many cases, without improving either quality or outcomes of care (McKinlay et al., 1989). Based on the agenda setting work of several authors and institutions (Greenlick, 1989; IOM, 1991; Rodin &

Ickovics, 1990) important issues in long-term care relate to broader social policy questions yet to be well defined and analyzed.

Medical, Functional, and Social Needs in the LTC Population. It is now well established that there are complex relationships between medical conditions and the use of acute care services on the one side, and chronic disabilities and the use of LTC services on the other. The users of LTC services are also high users of acute care services, and many elders' first need for LTC results from an acute care incident. Cross-sectional studies that have been used to date to explore these dynamics are substantially limited. Research is needed to explore the dynamic relationships over time between the need for medical care and the need for long-term care and the variety of environments in which care is provided (Capitman, 1989; Kane & Kane, 1989; Ory & Duncker, 1992; Weissert, 1991; Weissert, Pawlecek, & Creary, 1988).

Need and Utilization of Formal LTC Services. Caution should be used in interpreting current patterns of LTC utilization as valid indicators of the future need for LTC. Low income among the disabled elderly and the lack of community services in many states and localities retard and distort the extent to which needs are met through the formal service system. Because of these distortions by wealth, service availability, and third party coverage and reimbursement policies, care must be exercised in interpreting utilization data as adequate or accurate measures of need. Factors such as living arrangements, income, preferences, and professional values should be considered in any attempt to predict future needs.

Efficiency and Effectiveness of Services. Knowledge of how to deliver community LTC is less developed than either medical or nursing home care. Because of continuing government and consumer interest in expanded public and private funding for services, this area should be a primary focus of research and demonstration. In addition to traditional organizational efficiency measures such as productivity, longitudinal studies should employ multiple measures to explicate characteristics and health outcomes associated with various components of the service delivery system. Policy research needs to consider the impact of policy (e.g., OBRA 1987, U.S. Congress, House of Representatives) on the quality, outcomes, and costs of analogous care in different care settings.

Financing Arrangements. The role of health insurance in reducing or exacerbating financial barriers to all types of care for older persons has not been sufficiently explored. Even with Medicare one can not assume that there is uniformity of health insurance coverage and risk protection among beneficiaries (PPRC, 1988). In addressing the problem of financial risks of illness and injury, an important and understudied area is the determinants of patterns of public and private health insurance arrangements in the elderly population. Policy discussions about health service financing for the elderly do not often consider the differential effects of proposed changes or alternatives on men and women, although the effects may be different because insurance coverage, income and assets, availability of caregivers, and other variables are mediated over many years by factors that tend to vary by gender. Gender also is important because of the relationship of women's ability to pay to husband's pensions and health insurance entitlements and gender-typed jobs in previous work history, and because of the significance of personal economic resources that could compensate for lower levels of functional capacity.

Financing Disease Prevention and Health Promotion. Medicare and Medicaid are *disease* insurance programs; they pay for services and treatment of medically diagnosed conditions. Preventive services such as health screening and health promotion are generally not covered and must be financed by each beneficiary. A fundamental question for research and policy is whether omission of health screening and preventive services financing leads to underconsumption with consequent increased morbidity, mortality, and health care expenses.

Financing Long-Term Care and Mental Health Services. Financing of LTC services represents a crucial problem in supplying appropriate incentives for providers. Without adequate adjustment for case mix (risk), providers often skim off the lightest care patients, leaving the heavier care patients with substantial barriers to access. Current payment mechanisms do not provide appropriate dynamic incentives. Providers are paid to maintain patients at current or higher levels of dependency and there is little research on the resources required to rehabilitate patients to improve functional levels. Various models of financing health care system elements need to be theoretically and empirically investigated to determine financing mechanisms that support higher levels of independence among care recipients and the associated cost outcomes for LTC and mental health care providers. Scholarly debate (Cohen, Kumar, McGuire, & Wallack, 1992; Harrington et al., 1991) facilitates the conceptualization of these challenges.

Effects of Financial Barriers on Access, Use, and Health Outcomes. The sources of financing of health services for the aged are many and varied, including third-party payments and out-of-pocket payments. The latter include payments for premiums, co-insurance, balance billing, deductibles, uncovered services, and unclaimed coverage. The sources of funds to meet these out-of-pocket liabilities are multiple as well, including current income, savings, gifts from relatives, charity, loans, and debt forgiveness by providers. With the elderly spending 4.3 months of their average annual Social Security checks (18% of their incomes) on medical care, financial barriers remain a real and substantial obstacle for many aged persons, despite Medicare and Medigap coverage. Such barriers are associated with hesitance to seek timely care (PPRC, 1988), which may negatively affect health outcomes. Evaluation is needed in the area of income and price elasticities of demand for health care services by aging populations and effects of financial barriers on access, use, and health status of older persons and their standards of living.

Priority Areas of Research

Principles guiding the design and implementation of and research on public policy and long-term care include attention to: (1) the possibility that specific interventions may generate more rather than less dependency; (2) the multiple levels of intervention needed to promote empowerment, including interventions that deal with everyday lives, professional practice and organization, and social structure (Riley & Riley, 1989); and (3) maximizing personal control, sense of self-efficacy and competence, and control of the elder's environment (Rodin, 1989). The challenge on all three levels is to break the link between aging and dependency (Phillipson & Walker, 1986). Research is a vital and essential element of meeting this challenge.

Priority areas for research on public policy and long-term care based on the three illustrative issues reviewed in this chapter are presented in Table 17.1.

Conclusion

Social, behavioral, and health services research hold great promise for informing policymakers about crucial elements of public policy and long-term care. Without serious, sustained efforts, the development and implementation of policies to maximize active life expec-

TABLE 17.1
Priority Areas for Research on Public Policy and Long-Term Care

Older Women and Health

- the link between social and economic conditions of women and multiple epidemiological dimensions of health and illness across the life span
- the effects on older women of public policy, including policy that directly or indirectly affects labor force participation, retirement, income, and long-term care
- conditions that uniquely or disproportionately affect older women (eg., osteoporosis, breast cancer)
- mechanisms by which racial and ethnic status and social class influence older women's health

Informal Care

- the economic and psycho-social consequences for older caregivers and the relation of these to health and illness and to social policy
- the relationships between the formal and informal provision of care, caregiver and care recipient burden, and socioeconomic class, gender, race, and ethnic status
- documentation of total support process in older life as basis for designing systems which effectively inter-relate formal and informal care systems
- relationship between informal and formal care including outcomes of untargeted formal services

Long-Term Care (Health Services Research)

- longitudinal studies that trace changes in needs, access, and utilization patterns that accompany transitions between acute and chronic care, between forms of acute care, and between forms of chronic care
- the equity, effects, and effectiveness of long-term care policy per se to differentiate LTC policies that exacerbate or create dependency from those that do not
- the determinants of health insurance arrangements by older persons and the relationship of health insurance coverage to health care access and utilization
- cost-effectiveness and net benefits of alternative disease prevention and health promotion strategies and services targeted to aging populations
- determinants of risk of LTC and mental health care expense and the efficacy of innovative rehabilitation strategies for frail and chronically dependent older persons
- relationship of income, social class, and LTC insurance to access and utilization of health care and social services

tancy will not be realized, however (Estes & Rundall, 1992; Katz et al., 1983)

To succeed, social policy and the research on it must attend to an understanding of how health in old age is linked to social factors that shape the entire life course. Health status at age 65 does not come "out of nowhere". Location in the social structure (e.g., gender, social class, racial/ethnic group) mediates lifelong opportunities to engage in healthful behaviors and obtain health care (Estes & Rundall, 1992) as well as to live in health-enhancing environments. The import of adequate income and social opportunities throughout the lifecourse including access to prenatal, primary, and preventive care, should not be underestimated nor continue relatively uninvestigated. Much work remains to be done to understand these relationships and to document the impact of social policy on health and health care in old age.

Social structural change in the direction of universal life course entitlement (Estes & Binney, 1988) would promote the abatement of inequities based on age, gender, race, and class (Estes et al., 1993). The "plasticity" of the aging process represents more than mind-body phenomena—our individual and collective perceptions of the process influence its malleability (Estes, et al., 1993). As scholars we must give as much research attention to the concepts of empowerment and equity as we do to those of efficiency and cost. Research knowledge does not yet exist that would permit the design of long-term care policy that would promote healthy aging throughout the life course for Americans irrespective of racial, ethnic, gender, or social class origins. The health and quality of life of future generations of elders depends on our commitment to the development of research that investigates present gaps and extends our knowledge of the multifaceted experience of aging under defined social structural conditions.

Public policy reform including the elimination of economic obstacles that block access to health care is high on the current federal agenda. The Clinton administration's commitment to health care reform constitutes a signpost announcing that change in the health care system is no longer debatable. Rather, the exact nature and extent of that reform now constitute the discussion. Although costs are a central concern, issues of access to care have been restored to the dialogue on health care. It is expected that there will be universal access to uniform benefits without discrimination with regard to preconditions or preselection screening. Long-term care is a unifying force; it is an issue that binds families and generations through the universality of caregiving, women's roles, and the children's stake. A long-term care system, however designed and financed, relies heavily on the body of scientific knowledge generated in the social and behavioral sciences to adequately address the structural conditions necessary to ensure a high quality of life for older and disabled persons.

References

Barer, B. M., & Johnson, C. L. (1990). A critique of the caregiving literature. *The Gerontologist, 30*, 26–29.

Brody, J. A., Brock, D. B., & Williams, T. F. (1987). Trends in the health of the elderly population. In J. E. Fielding & L. B. Lave (Eds.), *Annual review of public health*, Vol. 8 (pp. 211–234). Palo Alto, CA: Annual Reviews.

Capitman, J. A. (1989). Policy and program options in community-based long-term care. *Annual Review of Gerontology and Geriatrics, 9*, 357–388.

Cohen, M. A., Kumar, N., McGuire, T., & Wallack, S. S. (1992). Financing long-term care: A practical mix of public and private. *Journal of Health, Politics, Policy and Law, 17*(3), 403–423.

Collins, J. (1991). Power and local community activity. *Journal of Aging Studies, 5*(2), 209–218.

Commonwealth Fund Commission on Elderly People Living Alone. (1989). *Help at home: Long-term care assistance for impaired elderly people*. Report prepared by Diane Rowland. Baltimore, MD.

DeFriese, G. H., & Woomert, A. (1992). Informal and formal health care systems serving older persons. In M. G. Ory, R. P. Abeles, and P. D. Lipman, (Eds.) *Aging, health, and behavior* (pp. 57–82). Newbury Park, CA: Sage.

Estes, C. L. (1979). *The aging enterprise*. San Francisco, CA: Jossey-Bass.

Estes, C. L., & Binney, E. A. (1989). The biomedicalization of aging: Dangers and dilemmas. *The Gerontologist, 29*(5), 587–596.

Estes, C. L., & Rundall, T. G. (1992). Social characteristics, social structure, and health in the aging population. In M. G. Ory, R. P. Abeles, & P. D. Lipman (Eds.), *Aging, health, and behavior* (pp. 299–326). Newbury Park, CA: Sage.

Estes, C.E., Swan, J.H., & Associates. (1993). *The long-term care crisis: Elders trapped in the no care zone*. Newbury Park, CA: Sage.

Families USA Foundation. (1992). *The health cost squeeze of older Americans*. Washington, DC: Families USA Foundation.

Finch, J. (1989). *Family obligations and social change*. London: Polity Press and Basil Blackwell.

Greenlick, M. R. (1989). *Health services research on aging*. Draft report. Liaison Team for Health Services Delivery Research, Institute of Medicine Committee on a National Research Agenda on Aging.

Hanley, R. J., Wiener, J. M., & Harris, K. M. (1991). Will paid care erode informal support? *Journal of Health Politics, Policy, and Law, 16*(3), 507–521.

Harrington, C., Cassell, C., Estes, C. L., Woolhandler, S., Himmelstein, D. U., & The Working Group on Long-Term Care Program Design, Physicians for a National Health Program. (1991). A national long-term care program for the United States: A caring vision. *Journal of the American Medical Association, 266*(21), 3023–3029.

ICF, Inc. (1985). *Medicare's role in financing the health care of older women.* Paper submitted to the American Association of Retired Persons (AARP). Washington, DC: ICF.

Institute of Medicine (IOM). E. T. Lonergan (Ed.) (1991). *Extending life, enhancing life: National research agenda on aging.* Washington, DC: National Academy Press.

Kane, R. A., & Kane, R. L. (1989). Transitions in long-term care. In M. G. Ory & K. Bond (Eds.), *Aging and health care: Social science and policy perspectives* (pp. 217–243). London: Routledge.

Katz, S., Branch, L., Bronson, M., Papsidero, J., Beck, J. & Greer, D. (1983). Active life expectancy. *New England Journal of Medicine, 309*(20), 1218–1224.

Kirchstein, R. L. (1991). Research on women's health. *American Journal of Public Health, 81*, 291–293.

Kunkel, S. R., & Applebaum, R. A. (1992). Estimating the prevalence of long-term disability for an aging society. *The Journal of Gerontology: Social Sciences, 47*, s253–s260.

Lipton, H. P., & Lee, P. R. (1988). *Drugs and the elderly: Clinical, social, and policy perspectives*. Stanford, CA: Stanford University Press.

Manton, K.G., Corder, L.S., & Stallard, E. (1993). Estimates of change in chronic disability and institutional incidence and prevalence rates in the U.S. elderly population from the 1982, 1984, and 1989 National Long-term Care Survey. *Journal of Gerontology: Social Sciences, 48*(4), S153–S166.

Manton, K. G., & Suzman, R. (1992). Forecasting health and functioning in aging societies: Implications for health care and staffing needs. In M. G. Ory, R. P. Abeles, & P. D. Lipman (Eds.), *Aging, health, and behavior* (pp. 327–357). Newbury Park, CA: Sage.

McKinlay, J. B., Crawford, S., & Tennstedt, S. (1993). Everyday social and physical impact of providing informal care to dependent elders. *Milbank Memorial Fund Quarterly*.

McKinlay, J. B., McKinlay, S. M., & Beaglehole, R. (1989). Trends in death and disease and the contribution of medical measures. In H. E. Freeman & S. Levine (Eds.), *The Handbook of Medical Sociology*, (pp. 14–45). Englewood Cliffs, NJ: Prentice Hall.

Minckler, M., & Stone, R. I. (1983). The feminization of poverty. *The Gerontologist, 25*, 351–357.

National Center for Health Statistics (NCHS). (1991). *Health, United States, 1990*. Hyattsville, MD: U.S. Public Health Service.

National Research Council (NRC). (1988). *The aging population in the 21st century*. Washington, DC: National Academy Press.

Older Women's League (OWL). (1989). *Failing America's caregivers: A status report on women who care*. Washington, DC: OWL.

O'Rand, A. (1988). Convergence, institutionalization and bifurcation: Gender and the pension acquisition review. In G. Maddox & P. Lawton (Eds.) *Varieties of aging: Annual review of gerontology and geriatrics*, Vol. 8 (pp. 132–155). New York: Springer Publishing Co.

Ory, M. G., & Duncker, A. P. (1992). Introduction: The home care challenge. In M. G. Ory & A. P. Duncker (Eds.), *In-home care for older people: Health and supportive services*, pp. 1–8. NewburyPark, CA: Sage Publications.

Phillipson, C. (1992). Challenging "the spectre of old age": Community care for older people in the 1990s. In W. Manning and R. Page (Eds.), *Social Policy Yearbook* (pp. 1–22). London: Social Policy Association.

Phillipson, C., & Walker, A. (1986). Conclusion: Alternative forms of policy and practice. In C. Phillipson & A. Walker (Eds.), *Ageing and social policy: A critical assessment*, (pp. 280–281). England: Glower.

Physician Payment Review Commission (PPRC). (1988). *Survey of Medicare beneficiaries*. Washington, DC: Physician Payment Review Commission.

Rice, D. P. (1986). Living longer in the U. S.: Social and economic implications. *Journal of Medical Practice Management, 1*(3), 162–169.

Riley, M. W., & Riley, J. W. (1989). The lives of older people and changing social roles. *Annals of the American Academy of Political and Social Science, 503*, 14–28.

Rodin, J. (1989). Sense of control: Potentials for intervention. *Annals of the American Academy of Political and Social Science, 503*, 29–42.

Rodin, J., & Ickovics, J. R. (1990). Women's health: Review and research agenda as we enter the 21st century. *American Psychologist, 45*(9), 1018–1034.

Rosenthal, C. J., Matthews, S. H., & Marshall, V. W. (1989). Is parent care normal? The experiences of a sample of middle-aged women. *Research on Aging, 11,* 244–260.

Russo, N. F. (1987). Position paper. In A. Eichler and D. L. Parron (Eds.), *Women's mental health: Agenda for research* (pp. 42–56). Rockville, MD: National Institute for Mental Health.

Sofaer, S., & Abel, E. (1990). Older women's health and financial vulnerability: Implications of the Medicare benefit structure. *Women and Health, 16*(3–4), 47–67.

Stone, R., & Kemper, P. (1989). Spouses and children of disabled elders: How large a constituency for long-term care reform? *Milbank Memorial Quarterly, 67,* 485–506.

Taeuber, C. M. (1992). *Sixty-five plus in America.* Washington, DC: U.S. Bureau of the Census.

Tennstedt, S., & McKinlay, J. B. (1989). Informal care for frail older persons. In M. G. Ory & K. Bond (Eds.), *Aging and health care: Social science and policy perspectives* (pp. 145–166). London: Routledge.

Travis, C. B. (1988). *Women and health psychology: Biomedical issues.* Hillsdale, NJ: Erlbaum.

U. S. House of Representatives (Select Committee on Aging). (1990). *Emptying the elderly's pocketbook: Growing impact of rising health care costs.* A Report by the Chairman. Washington, DC: U. S. Government Printing Office.

U. S. Senate (Special Committee on Aging). (1991). *Developments in aging: 1990,* Vol. 1. Washington, DC: U. S. Government Printing Office.

U. S. Senate (Special Committee on Aging), American Association for Retired People, Federal Council on Aging, & U. S. Administration of Aging. (1988). *Aging America: Trends and projections.* Washington, DC: U. S. Department of Health and Human Services.

Verbrugge, L. M. (1989). Recent, present, and future health of American adults. In L. Breslow, J. E. Fielding, and L. B. Lave (Eds.), *Annual review of public health,* Vol. 10 (pp. 333–361). Palo Alto, CA: Annual Reviews, Inc.

Verbrugge, L. M. (1991). Pathways of health and death. In R. D. Apple (Ed.), *Women, health, and medicine: A history handbook* (pp. 41–79). New Brunswick, NJ: Rutgers University Press.

Weissert, W. G. (1991). Home care: Measuring success. In P. R. Katz, R. L. Kane, & M.D. Mezey (Eds.), *Advances in long-term care,* Vol. 1 (pp. 186–199). New York: Springer Publishing Co.

Weissert, W. G., Cready, C. M., & Pawelak, J. E. (1988). The past and future of community-based long-term care. *Milbank Memorial Quarterly, 66,* 309–388.

Chapter 18

Changing the Social Environment to Promote Health

Lennart Levi and Donna M. Cox

Larger cohorts of elderly people, who retire earlier and who are likely to need more health and social care services as they age have focused policy attention on the impending burden of an aging population. Policymakers have become increasingly concerned that modern industrialized nations will have difficulty meeting the needs of older people and, as such will not be able to protect their right to a "life of fulfillment, health, security and contentment" appropriately (United Nations, 1983, p. 9). In 1982 member countries of the United Nations reaffirmed the belief that older people are entitled to the same rights and privileges of other age groups and should be given the opportunity to live full lives as integral members of their families and communities (United Nation, 1983). Ten years later, demographic and social trends prompted the General Assembly to urge the development of practical strategies and programs for maintaining the productivity of the older person, and to provide the elderly with the social and economic resources enabling them to be active members of society (cf. Bulletin on Aging, No. 3/1992).

An emphasis on the social and economic costs associated with aging populations, however, overshadows what could be a potentially positive experience for individuals and the societies in which they live. As recent research suggests, older people do not necessarily grow old and dependent. Many older people live longer and healthier lives following retirement. Therefore, a healthier, more active cohort of older people suggests that the "burden" of aging populations can be turned into "a phenomenon of great social, economic and cultural promise" (cf., Bulletin on Aging No. 3/1992).

Improved Health and Functional Ability of the Elderly: The Swedish Experience

"Last scene of all,
That ends this strange eventful history,
Is second childishness and mere oblivion;
Sans teeth, sans eyes, sans taste, sans everything"
Shakespeare, As You Like It, Act 2, Scene 7

Ultimately, there is no way to escape this "last scene." Yet, it can be postponed considerably, and compressed to a rather brief period of life. In fact, for many people in Western Europe and the United States, the compression of morbidity has already occurred and is likely to continue. For example, in Sweden where the population age 65+ is 71.7% (Official Statistics of Sweden, 1985, 1991, and 1993), the 60-year-old person can expect to do the same things equally well at the age of 80. This was not so in Shakespeare's time, nor as recently as just some five or six decades ago.

Shakespeare lamented about the characteristics of "old age," a time when a person could expect to lose teeth, sight, and other physical and motor functions. Today, due to vast improvements in areas such as nutrition, dental hygiene, and health care in general, these expectations are largely unfounded. Data from Sweden illustrate these changes. In 1971–1972, barely one in two people age 70 had their own teeth. Ten years later, 70% of people in this age group had their own teeth. On average, individuals retained half of their original 32 teeth (William-Olsson & Svanborg, 1984). Moreover, the majority of Swedes over age 65 did not suffer from chewing problems as imagined by Shakespeare. In 1991 of those age 65–74, less than 18% reported impaired chewing ability. Though the percentage who experienced chewing difficulties increased with age, a little over half the population age 85+ reported problems (Official Statistics of Sweden, 1991).

Similarly, the number of elderly in Sweden who reported impaired eyesight has steadily decreased over the years. In 1982 less than 4% of people age 65–74 years reported vision problems. Individuals age 85+ reported more difficulties than younger groups of elderly, but only one quarter to a third of the group reported had problems. Notably, adequate lighting and glasses ameliorate cited difficulties. For example, 95% of citizens in Gothenburg who were age 70 could read the small print in the telephone directory when proper lighting and glasses were available (William-Olsson & Svanborg, 1984).

As for Shakespeare's concern regarding "sans everything," here again Swedish figures are encouraging. Approximately 30% of men and 16% of women aged 65–74 reported hearing impairments. Once again, percentages increased with age, but for males and females age 85+, greater than 40% did not report hearing problems. For those 65–74, less than 10% reported seriously impaired motor function. Even among the oldest segments of the population (age 85+), approximately 40% did not report serious motor function problems (Official Statistics of Sweden, 1991). Furthermore, only 2% of the chronically disabled population 65–84 years are hospitalized in Sweden (Official Statistics of Sweden, 1985). Serious long-term illness was reported by less than 25% of males and females age 65–74, and by less than 40% of those 75–84 years. Among individuals age 85+, serious long-term illness was reported by fewer than 50% of the population. These figures point to the low prevalence of severe disability in the majority of the aged in Sweden, even among the highest age group.

Overall, these figures reflect a rather good state of health and functional ability in the Swedish elderly population. But, the true challenge is to assure that the addition of "years to life" also implies an addition of "life to years." In other words, finding ways to guarantee that the additional years of life in modern times remain productive and satisfying.

Intervention Strategies for Improving Health and Well-Being

The task for the research community is to identify how to promote better health and functioning in older people. More research is needed to identify how to eliminate, buffer or modify influences that counteract healthy aging. Moreover, the objective for maintaining or even improving older people's quality of life should include some consideration of how this improvement will benefit present and future generations worldwide.

Interventions aimed at improving health and functioning in older people are usually focused on the elderly individual, and his or her emotional, cognitive, behavioral, and/or physiological reactions to life conditions. This focus is too limited. A broadened focus is needed to identify pathogenic social conditions that increase older people's risks of illness, disease, and disability. Interventions directed at ameliorating the effects of these conditions are particularly important for older people who may become increasingly vulnerable as they age. Unfortunately, the complementary option for intervening against some of the "slings and arrows of outrageous fortune" is often overlooked.

Social Determinants of Health

Concerns regarding the impact of social determinants of health on the aging process have been noted in recent national and internation policy initiatives. For example, the Swedish Public Health Service Bill (1985, p. 11) declared that, "our health is determined in large measure by our living conditions and lifestyle." The bill enumerates health risks in contemporary society, such as deficient social structures and processes, unemployment and the threat of unemployment, health-related behaviors and life-styles, as well as psychosocial strains, such as the loss or lack of social relationships. These health risks have not been recognized as major determinants of a healthy life and strongly implicated in today's most common disorders and injuries. Thus, policymakers are calling for interventions that represent a holistic approach, that is "people's symptoms and illnesses, their causes and consequences, are appraised in a medical, psychological, and social perspective (Swedish Public Health Service Bill, 1985, p. 18).

The founders of the World Health Organization (WHO) took a visionary view when they unanimously proposed to define health as "not only the absence of disease or infirmity, but also a state of physical, mental, and social well-being" (WHO, 1946; 1981, p. 1). Drawing on this philosophy in their Health for All (HFA) strategy, member states of WHO committed themselves to creating the conditions that will enable all people to enjoy a reasonably healthy life by the year 2000. This strategy changed the predominantly disease-oriented and curative of the health care sector perspective to one that focused on the maintenance and promotion of good health and the prevention of ill health.

Interventions that include related social systems are an essential component of this health-promoting strategy. This broadened perspective requires intersectiorial action among various segments of society. According to the Report of the Technical Discussions of the 39th World Health Assembly (WHO, 1986), health goals can be attained only if service development is based on some collaboration between the health care sector and other development sectors (e.g., food and nutrition, water and sanitation, housing and education, economy and labor).

The formation of services via a socio-medical model is discussed more often than it is applied, however. In both developed and developing countries, governmental action against social, environmental, and health problems in the elderly as well as in other groups, consists of "troubleshooting" and is more reactive than proactive. Action tends to be crisis-oriented, addressing only one or a few immediate, specific problems (e.g., providing meals, housing, or medical care). Not infrequently, governmental responses to the problems of the elderly are acute-care oriented even though many problems are primarily chronic in nature. In such cases, one of many specialized agencies administers the intervention with little or no coordination between other specialized agencies that could assist with the effort. Consequently, social and/or behavioral determinants of health problems are left unattended.

A bird's-eye view of social environment and human health—in the elderly and the general public as well—indicates that the person-environment ecosystem contains many interacting pathogenic, as well as salutogenic factors. Influencing one variable can affect many of the others, with complex interactions and multiple feedback loops. As a result, it is usually impossible to cope successfully with environmental, behavioral, and health problems in any age group by considering—in research, therapy, and/or prevention—just one or two of the components of the total ecosystem. Success at improving health by decreasing risk is more probable if as many of the critical components as possible are examined.

Filling Gaps and Expanding Horizons: Conducting Intervention Studies

Unfortunately, despite many empirical observations, findings have not sufficiently determined which psychosocial environmental factors are trigger symptoms, contribute to disease causation, prevent disease, and/or promote health. Decision makers, often under pressure from the public to act even without evidence that actions will achieve desired goals, initiate interventions without broadly and systematically evaluating how decisions will affect outcomes, or the need for subsequent action. This is why the evaluation of controlled interventions in social systems becomes crucially important. We do not anticipate that all of the policymakers' questions can be answered in this manner. Yet, such studies are an important complement to descriptive and analytic approaches.

Psychosocial medical research is a tool that can provide better answers to questions about the cause, prevention, and treatment of a wide range of ill health and suffering. It should provide important answers to the key questions raised by the President's Commission on Mental Health (1978):

1. Which groups of people are at high (or low) risk of various types of morbidity and mortality?
2. Which individual and social factors contribute to (or counteract) risk, and what is the relative importance of each of those factors?
3. Can the most significant risk factors be effectively reduced or eliminated (and health-promoting factors furthered)?
4. Does eliminating the most significant risk factors (or promoting a salutary factor) effectively lower the rate of various types of morbidity and mortality?
5. If so, are the costs of intervention justified by the benefits obtained?
6. Is the program in accordance with the principles governing the rights of individual and the rights of society?

Answers to these questions may depend on the stage of life under consideration. There may be critical periods of exposure for any risk factor (Ory, 1988). Vulnerability often changes with age, and the most susceptible people may not survive to old age. Furthermore, even when epidemiological links are found between life-style factors and health outcomes, for instance, it does not necessarily follow that eliminating or reducing that factor late in life will improve health and functioning in an elderly person (Kaplan & Haan, 1989). Consequently, age and aging must be considered in these contexts.

In many instances, our current state of knowledge does not provide sufficient information for rational health action, even if combined with evaluation. To provide the necessary data, three complementary forms of research are needed. First, the use of survey techniques and morbidity data can define the problem. These data will describe the magnitude of the problem and identify determinants of health, such as environmental factors, that have important implications for modifying health behaviors. Second, longitudinal, multidisciplinary, intensive studies of the interaction between high-risk situations and high- as compared with low-risk groups, are necessary to identify temporal relationships between and among environmental factors and pathogenic mechanisms as modified by interacting factors. Finally, using data from previously described research, controlled interventions, clinical as well as field experiments, can be developed to reduce risks.

These approaches should include the testing of hypotheses that increase understanding of the psychosocial factors affecting health in populations, young and old. The purpose of the research should be to identify situations that affect health and functioning outcomes, and to conduct projects that utilize some combination of applied and basic research. Strategies for approaching the problems associated with improving care, preventing ill health and increasing well-being are not only desirable but possible. Contrary to popular thought, intervention research that incorporates applied and basic research will not necessarily be more expensive than singular approach strategies, and if long-term costs are considered, may actually produce cost-savings (Kagan & Levi, 1975; Levi, 1987a).

Numerous studies have shown associations between psychosocial and other environmental factors and health, have speculated on ideas for health or social action, or have put forward hypotheses in relation to the spread and control of disease in the community. But, evaluations of community-oriented health action are few. Only on rare occasions have hypotheses been tested and action evaluated to demonstrate that it is possible to carry out controlled, community-oriented social intervention studies (see Kagan, 1981; Levi, Frankenhaeuser & Gardell, 1982; Markides & Cooper, 1989). For the most part, such studies are often considered unethical, technically impossible, too expensive, or too time-consuming. Although there is an element of truth in all four objections, the first three can usually be addressed adequately, and the fourth can be minimized (Kagan, 1981; Levi, 1987b). Of greater importance are the ethical and cost implications of imposing an environmental or health action of unproven value (Kagan, 1981). Illustrating this point, Hazzard (1985) identifies a number of areas for health promotion for the elderly in which the intervention has been hindered by substantial gaps in information. If we are to progress, philosophical and political questions of whether controlled intervention studies should await additional fundamental research, or efforts should be directed at closing these gaps must be addressed.

Integrating Research Approaches

Measures that may prevent disease and promote health can be proposed based on descriptive studies. The characteristics of these measures should be that they are (1) likely to be of causal importance, (2) amenable to change, (3) feasible, (4) acceptable to all concerned, and (5) later evaluated in an interdisciplinary experimental model of study. Then, depending on the outcome in terms of benefits, side effects and costs, a wider application may be implemented, continuously monitored, evaluated, and modified as necessary.

The overall research program should aim at a number of important objectives. First, the research should be systems-oriented. The systems approach can facilitate the analysis of health-related interactions in the human-environment ecosystem (e.g., family, work, hospital, and nursing homes). Second, an interdisciplinary approach should be adopted whereby medical, physiological, emotional, behavioral, social and economic aspects are incorporated. Third, the orientation of the research program should be geared toward problem solving. Epidemiological identification of health problems and their environmental and other correlates should be followed by longitudinal interdisciplinary field studies of exposures, reactions, etc. Fourth, these studies should be followed by experimental evaluations under real-life conditions of presumably health promoting and disease-preventing interventions. The focus of the research program should not be on disease but rather on health. In this way, the aim will be to identify what constitutes and promotes good health, as well as what counteracts ill health.

In addition, the aims of the research should be: (1) intersectorial to promote and evaluate environmental and health actions administered in other sectors (e.g., employment, housing, nutrition, traffic and education); (2) participatory, thereby interacting closely with potential caregivers, receivers, planners, and policymakers; and (3) international to facilitate transcultural, collaborative, and complementary projects with centers in various countries.

Research designed in this way would be of great benefit in distinguishing among stressful social structures and processes, reactions to such stressors, the consequences of such reactions, and the mediators that modify the flow of events. More information is needed on what makes some events and conditions stressful, on the effects of the resulting stress on a potential pathogenic mechanisms, and on the actual health consequences of these processes. Information is similarly needed on the components of health-promoting (salutogenic) processes and their interaction (Antonovsky, 1987; Elliot & Eisdorfer, 1982; Lazarus, 1985; Lazarus & Folkman, 1984).

In the past, most studies have been unifactorial, focusing on a single aspect of the situation (e.g., machine-paced work) or of the individual (e.g., Type A behavior). The single variable is then related to a possibly pathogenic reaction (e.g., catecholamine excretion) and/or morbidity due to a specific disease (e.g., myocardial infarction). Since the mid-1970s, studies have become increasingly multifactorial and even interdisciplinary. The next step is to apply a nonlinear, interactional systems approach (see Miller, 1978) to the entire sequence of events. Research would begin with the life situation and its appraisal, and end with the advantages of having a healthy population that includes intervening and interacting variables and feedback loops. Although this ecosystem approach is admittedly complex, however, attention must also be given to the dynamic influence of changes in social structures that affect the aged and the aging process. Little attention has been paid to stabilities and changes in social structures and processes over an individual's lifetime or to social changes over historical time.

As already indicated, the complementary research projects—epidemiological, intensive longitudinal and intervention studies—should be integrated into long-term research programs based on a continuous exchange of data and interpretations with those concerned (i.e., central and local governments, administrators, caregivers, organizations for retired persons, private enterprise and the general public). Data from other centers, as well as results from ethological and animal studies should be included as well. Therefore, an integrated approach to research becomes more useful and desirable than "one-shot" studies because of the potential for filling existing gaps in knowledge of what influences health and health behavior.

Obstacles Impeding Research Progress

Several methodological issues impede or limit our attempts at social intervention. First, it is often impossible to control all relevant variables in a complex and changing social system. Thus, our assumptions and possibilities for generalization to other institutions and communities become somewhat tenuous (see Thorsland, 1986).

Second, in some cases care-providers and/or policymakers are not inclined to accept an evaluation of a program in which they are involved. A program evaluation may find that changes in behavior are not due to the intervention itself, but rather to the availability of a dedicated and enthusiastic program director, or the extra attention provided to the experimental group. Therefore, a new program may not be necessary and terminated.

Third, additional problems include an identification of what to include in the monitoring process. For example, what aspect of the program should be monitored? How often? Should the focus of the evaluation be on the performance of the care providers, the response of the care receiver, or both? Moreover, age-related factors can affect both the measurement of health indicators and the design and effectiveness of health-promotion interventions (Ory, 1988). This has obvious consequences for the design and interpretation of intervention studies on elderly populations (Backer, 1984; Chiriboga, 1989; Evans, 1983; Hendrikson, 1986; Kivela, 1985; Krause, 1989; Ro, Hendriksen, Kivela, & Thorslund, 1987; Ro & Hjort, 1985; Thorslund, 1986).

Finally, available instruments for measuring interventions and outcomes may lack validity, reliability, and norms with regard to elderly populations. Alternatively, the elderly may find providing information and participating in the intervention to be too difficult (Ory, 1988).

Conclusion

The importance of incorporating social variables in health interventions for workers and pensioners alike is exemplified in studies drawn primarily from the Nordic experience. For example, results from a multidisciplinary longitudinal evaluation of efforts to prevent negative effects of unemployment identified psychosocial and physiological effects of becoming and remaining unemployed. Such results point to the importance of promoting gainful employment for all and rescinding requirements for mandatory retirement of older workers (Arnetz, et al., 1988). Andersson (1984), in his study of lonely female pensioners, demonstrated the physiological benefits to be attained through interventions that seek to increase social contacts and interactions. Similarly, Arnetz (1983) illustrated how health and well-being of institutionalized elderly could be improved with interventions focused on increasing individual autonomy and social interactions. (For reviews of other studies, with particular reference to social interventions to improve health and well-being in older people, see Thorslund [1986], Backer [1984], Rö and Hjort [1985], Hendriksen [1986], and Markides and Cooper [1989].)

In summary, we should strive to identify and modify high-risk reactions, where possible. To achieve this objective, close collaboration is required among and between decision makers who formulate political goals, and researchers who provide the additional knowledge on which to base decisions. If the information provided to decision-makers via basic, applied, and evaluation research assist in the development and refinement of policies and programs, the entire person-environment system becomes cybernetic and self-corrective.

Most importantly, efforts must continue to be directed at expanding our understanding of how interventions early in life (i.e., childhood or adolescence) can help people reach old age with more vigor, as well as how they can postpone disabilities associated with age-related illness or conditions. If we are truly committed to assuring the rights and privileges of all individuals as they age, we must also become committed to research that seeks to understand the dynamic relationships that affect aging, health and behavior.

References

Andersson, L. (1984). Aging and loneliness: An international study of a group of elderly women.

Antonovsky, A. (1987). *Unraveling the mystery of health: How people manage stress and stay well*. San Francisco: Jossey Bass.

Arnetz, B. (1983). Psychophysiological effects of social understimulation in old age. Stockholm: Karolinska Institutet.

Arnetz, B., Brenner, S., Hjelm, H., Levi, L., Petterson, I., Kalner, A., Encroth, P., Kvetnansky, R., & Vigas, M. (1988). Stress reactions in relation to threat of job loss and unemployment. (Stress Research Reports No. 206). Stockholm: Karolinska Institutet.

Backer, P. (1984). Needs of continuous research into care of the elderly. *Scandinavian Journal of Primary Health Care, 2,* 4546.

Bulletin on Aging. (1992). No. 3, pp. 1–2. Vienna, Austria: United Nations Office, Centre for Social Development and Humanitarian Affairs.

Chiriboga, D. A. (1989). The measurement of stress in later life. In: K. S. Markides & C. L. Cooper (Eds.), *Aging, stress and health* (pp. 13–41). Chichester, UK: John Wiley. New York: Van Nostrand Reinhold.

Commission on Mental Health. (1978). *Report to the President* (vol. 1). Washington, DC: U. S. Government Printing Office.

Elliott, G. R., & Eisdorfer, C. (Eds). (1982). *Research on stress and human health* (National Academy of Sciences, Institute of Medicine, report). New York: Springer Publishing Co.

Evans, J. G. (1983). Evaluation of geriatric services. In W. W. Holland (ed.), *Evaluation of health care.* New York: Oxford University Press.

Hazzard, W. R. (1985). A state of the art review of preventive strategies and health promotion for the elderly (Report submitted by Geriatrics and Gerontology Advisory Committee).Washington, DC: Veterans Administration.

Hendriksen, C. (1986). An intervention study among elderly people. *Scandinavian Journal of Primary Health Care, 4,* 39–42.

Kagan, A. R. (1981). A community research strategy applicable to psychosocial factors and health. In L. Levi (Ed.), *Society Stress and Disease*: Vol. 4, Working Life (pp. 339–342). Oxford: Oxford University Press.

Kagan, A. R., & Levi, L. (1975). Health and environment-psychosocial stimuli: A review. In L. Levi (ed.), *Society Stress and Disease*: Vol. 2, Childhood and Adolescence (pp. 241–260). London: Oxford University Press.

Kaplan, G. A. & Haan, M. N. (1989). Is there a role for prevention among the elderly? Epidemiological evidence from the Alameda County Study. In M. Ory & K. Bond (Eds.), *Aging and health care.* (pp. 27–51). New York: Routledge.

Kivela, S. L. (1985). Problems in intervention and evaluation. *Scandinavian Journal of Primary Health Care, 3,* 137–140.

Krause, N. (1989). Issues of measurement and analysis in studies of social support, aging and health. In K. S. Markides & C. L. Cooper (Eds.), *Aging, stress and health* (pp. 43–66). Chichester, UK: John Wiley.

Lazarus, R. S. (1985). Stress: Appraisal and coping capacities. In A. Eichler, M. M. Silverman, & D. M. Pratt (Eds.), *How to define and research stress*

(Administrative document; pp. 59). Rockville, MD: Department of Health and Human Services, National Institute of Mental Health.

Lazarus, R. S. & Folkman, S. (1984). *Stress, appraisal and coping*. New York: Springer Publishing Co.

Levi, L. (Ed.). (1987a). *Society, stress and disease*: Vol. 5, Old Age. Oxford: Oxford University Press.

Levi, L. (Ed.). (1987b). Future research. In R. Kalimo et al. (eds). *Psychosocial factors at work and their relation to health* (pp. 239–45). Geneva: World Health Organization.

Levi, L., Frankenhaeuser, M., & Gardell, B. (1982). Work stress related to social structures and processes. In G. R. Elliott & C. Eisdorfer (Eds.), *Stress and human health: Analysis and implications of research* (pp. 119–146). New York: Springer Publishing Co.

Makides, K. S., & Cooper, C. L. (Eds.) (1989). *Aging, stress and health*. Chichester, UK: John Wiley.

Miller, J. (1978). *Living systems*. New York: McGraw-Hill.

Official Statistics of Sweden (1985). *Living conditions*. Report No. 43. Old People. Stockholm: Statistics Sweden.

Official Statistics of Sweden (1991). Living Conditions. Report No. 68. Ill health and Medical Care 1988–1989. Stockholm Statistics Sweden.

Official Statistics of Sweden (1993). *Statistical yearbook '93*. Stockholm: Statistics Sweden.

Ory, M. (1988). Considerations in the development of age sensitive indicators for assessing health promotion. *Health Promotion, 3*, 2.

Ory, M. G., Abeles, R. P., & Lipman, P. D. (Eds). (1992). *Aging, health and behavior*. Newbury Park: Sage.

Rö, O. C., Hendriksen, C., Kivelä, S., & Thorslund, M. (1987). Intervention studies among elderly people. *Scandinavian Journal of Primary Health Care, 5*, 163–168.

Rö, O. C., & Hjort, P. F. (1985). Interventional research in primary health care for the elderly. *Scandinavian Journal of Primary Health Care, 3*, 133–136.

Swedish Public Health Service Bill No. 1984/85:181. (1985). Stockholm: Ministry of Social Affairs.

Thorslund, M. (1986). Evaluation research in care of the elderly: Some Swedish experiences. *Scandinavian Journal of Primary Health Care, 4*, 33–38.

United Nations (1983). *Vienna international plan of action on aging*. New York: United Nations.

William-Olsson, M., & Svanborg, A. (1984). *Health and vitality*. Malmö: Utbildningsproduktion and the Swedish National Board for Health and Welfare.

World Health Organization. (1946). *Definition of health* (Preparatory Committee of the International Health Conference). Geneva: Author.

World Health Organization. (1986). *Report of the technical discussions of the 39th World Health Assembly* (A39/Technical Discussions/4;15. May 1986). Geneva: Author

World Health Organization (1998). *Basic Documents*, 31st Edition. Geneva.

Chapter 19

Exploring the Future of Health Care for Older People

Robert H. Binstock, Dennis W. Jahnigen, and Stephen G. Post

Predictions regarding the future of health care for older people in the United States are frequently constructed through the practice of "apocalyptic demography" (Robertson, 1991). Typically, demographic projections are plugged into a model constructed from: presently high morbidity rates at older old ages; current modalities of disease prevention, diagnosis, and treatment; spiraling health care costs; and existing structures, policies, and technologies for organizing, financing, and delivering health care. The resulting extrapolations generate foreboding scenarios, such as one that has depicted the elderly population as "a demographic, economic, and medical avalanche...that could ultimately...do great harm" (Callahan, 1987, p. 20).

Such bleak assumptions, however, may be unwarranted. The older population is changing, research advances on processes of aging and age-related health issues are proliferating, and the health care environment is rapidly evolving.

This chapter explores the future of health care for older persons by outlining some of the changes that are emerging now and likely to take place in the decades immediately ahead, and some of the issues that they will generate for older persons, health care providers, researchers, and societal values. These changes will range from those that will be manifested in the "new-old"—the population cohort that will be joining the ranks of older Americans in the next few decades—through shifts in patient–physician relations, alterations in geriatric acute care, challenges in rehabilitation and long-term care, and legal and ethical dilemmas, to issues of political economy.

The New-Old and their Physicians

The population cohort that will reach old age in the early decades of the twenty-first century will be substantially different from those in recent decades. On average, these new-old will have greater life expectancy, be more educated, and have higher incomes (Taeuber, 1992). They will also experience better health at younger old ages and higher levels of function and independence in later life than do present old-age cohorts. Their health status characteristics will be due to numerous factors, including: (1) generally better prenatal care, optimum childhood preventive practices such as immunization for common serious illnesses, better nutrition, and lower childhood accident rates; (2) more healthful work environments with lower work-related injury rates, reduced exposure to known carcinogens, the spread of employer-related wellness and stress-reduction programs, and improved schemes for retirement preparation; and (3) better health practices throughout adult life such as lower rates of smoking, more participation in exercise programs, and greater attention to preventive measures relevant to many chronic diseases (Bortz, 1991).

The new-old will also be likely to have higher expectations regarding health status and their responsibility for it. A 1992 survey revealed, for example, that two-thirds of adults aged 18 and older would like to live to be 100, and expect to undertake personal action for achieving this goal. Over 70% indicated that they have already changed to healthier diets, 50% actively work to reduce stress, 18% have quit smoking, and 35% drink less alcohol than previously (Alliance for Aging Research, 1992).

The new-old will also be likely to have different views regarding the provision of health care, including greater expectations regarding consumer participation in decision making. Due to changing social expectations during the past few decades, they will be more likely than their predecessors to question the decisions of health-care providers, view health care as a basic right of citizenship, and expect expanded government financing of both acute and chronic care services (Surgeon General's Workshop, 1988).

What impact will the sizable cohort of new-old persons have on the practice of medicine, and on the education of health care professionals? Will there be a change in the balance among geriatricians, primary care physicians, and specialists? How will increased patient desires for active participation in health care decisions affect physician–patient relations?

Geriatricians will not be available in large supply for clinical practice with older persons at any time in the foreseeable future. Fellowship-trained specialists in geriatric care only number about 400 at present, with an additional 60 or so produced annually, nationwide (Reuben et al., 1991). The impact of geriatric physicians during the next several decades will be felt primarily through their leadership and education roles in academic medical centers. In the latter half of this decade, for instance, initiatives will be implemented to include formal geriatric education in the training of residents in many medical disciplines, including general surgery, orthopedic surgery, gynecology, and emergency medicine (Friedman, Kazis, Kern, Moskowitz, & Steel, 1991).

Such initiatives in geriatric education will have their largest impact through an increasing number of family doctors and general internists who will provide the bulk of medical care for the new-old. At present such generalists constitute only about 30% of U.S. physicians, as compared with a 50/50 ratio in most western nations (Colwill, 1992). But major efforts are underway in the mid-1990s—through the Physician Payment Review Commission, the Association of American Medical Colleges, the American Council on Graduate Education, and several foundations—to increase the supply of generalists through a series of financial and educational incentives offered to medical students (see, e.g., Council on Graduate Medical Education, 1992).

Interwoven with these changes in medical education is an evolving paradigm of medical practice that is responsive to increasing consumer expectations for more central involvement in medical decision-making processes. This patient-centered or "geriatric-sensitive" paradigm involves extensive data gathering and doctor–patient–family discussions comprised of a five-step process that includes: (1) a search for the patient's objectives (cure, symptom relief, palliation, information, sympathy, or some combination of these); (2) an inventory and ascertainment of the patient's values and perceptions of his or her own quality of life; (3) use of the very best diagnostic techniques and full consideration of therapeutic options; (4) thorough discussions and negotiations with the patient and family members (when indicated) regarding therapeutic options and reasonable objectives; and (5), agreement with the patient and family on the strategy of the medical interventions to be chosen, and their likely outcomes (see Jahnigen & Binstock, 1991).

More widespread use of this geriatric-sensitive model of practice, increasingly taught to medical students, will enhance the probabilities that physicians will make recommendations and decisions that respect the values and preferences of their older patients, while making effective use of health care resources. This undramatic approach contrasts sharply with the more traditional biomedical/disease model of practice, in which the patient's values have customarily remained secondary to biomedical facts, and it has been assumed that the patient's objective is to be cured through any treatment needed for survival. The geriatric-sensitive paradigm will represent an opportunity to minimize unwanted health care without sacrificing the potential benefits of aggressive and sophisticated interventions.

The Evolution of Geriatric Acute Care

The hospital environment for acute care of geriatric patients is already changing in a number of tangible fashions. Some of these developments are due to changes in reimbursement policies for hospital care. Others can be traced to improved understanding of biological and clinical aspects of aging, as well as the familial, social, and economic contexts in which geriatric patients function. Geriatric emergency medicine is developing as a specialty in recognition of the complex challenges frequently involved in treating older patients beset by multiple clinical disorders (Bosker, Schwartz, Jones, & Siqueira, 1990). Multidisciplinary geriatric assessment teams have been established in the belief that they will improve the choice of treatment goals as well as discharge objectives (Gallo, Reichel, & Andersen, 1988).

The adoption of prospective payments for reimbursing hospitals has not only shortened the average length of hospital stays (Russell, 1989), but also has had the salutary effect of heightening the importance of responsible discharge-planning. Nearly one-fifth of elderly patients discharged from hospitals require nursing-home placement for either short-term or long-term care, and in one study over 50% of patients aged 75 and older needed home health care (Rubin, Sizemore, Loftis, Adams-Huet, & Anderson, 1992). The inadequacies of posthospital care plans is one of the more common reasons for unexpected hospital readmissions. Hospitals are becoming increasingly skilled in anticipatory discharge planning, even to the extent of planning prior to a patient's elective admission for such procedures as hip or knee surgery.

More and more diagnostic and therapeutic interventions traditionally undertaken on an inpatient basis—such as cataract surgery, herniorrhaphy, bronchosopy, colonoscopy, and coronary angiography—are now being done as outpatient procedures (Macaluso & Thomas, 1991).

As these trends continue, hospitals will become increasingly populated by patients who are severely ill, requiring intensive and/or high-risk interventions, and more nursing support. In larger hospitals, intensive care unit beds now constitute as much as 20%–25% of the total bed inventory.

At the same time, new "observational" units, attached to hospitals, are likely to be developed for the purpose of providing geriatric patients with brief assessments at relatively low cost. In such units patients who have nonspecific symptoms that may reflect either trivial illness or life-threatening conditions, for example, tiredness, repeated falling, weight loss, or confusion, can receive close observation without the intensity of the inpatient setting. Within one to two days a determination can be made as to whether a patient is well enough to return home, or severely enough ill to require hospitalization.

Special acute care geriatric wards are being established as environments designed to facilitate functional recuperation and independence of older patients. The emphasis is on minimizing the adverse effects of hospitalization, and establishing a milieu that promotes overall physical and mental function. Staffed by nurses who are oriented to the relative frailties of elderly patients, such units undertake such measures as: rehabilitation planning at the time of hospital admission; minimization of a patient's time in bed; provision of congregate meals; and encouragement of active participation of family members in daily care, even allowing families to stay overnight with a patient if they so desire. Preliminary evidence indicates that patients in these acute care geriatric wards have shorter lengths of stay, and experience fewer falls, adverse drug reactions, pressure ulcers, and other iatrogenic events during hospitalization (Rubenstein, Struck, Sui, & Wieland, 1991).

Amid these new developments, however, perhaps the most fundamental element of medical practice in acute-care settings has become increasingly ambiguous. As finances have become a central concern, and more and more physicians function in the context of managed care structures rather than the traditional fee-for-service context: What or who determines the appropriate course of treatment? The third-party payers—Medicare, Medicaid, and insurance companies? Hospital administrators? How authentic is the patient's right to decide in this context? Will the physician's traditional role in determining "good care" become tenuous? What impact will ambiguity in the locus of responsibilities for medical decision-making have on doctor–patient relationships and, most importantly, on the quality of care provided to geriatric patients?

Issues in Rehabilitation and Long-Term Care

For a variety of reasons rehabilitation of older persons has been comparatively neglected in the overall scene of American health care (S.J. Brody & Ruff, 1986). Within recent years this traditional picture has begun to change, in considerable measure due to the initiatives of a handful of professional leaders (e.g., Williams, 1984), who have focused attention on the importance of functional capacities for the quality of life. Increased attention to geriatric rehabilitation is also a side effect of the implementation of Medicare's prospective payment reforms. Now that hospitals have every incentive to discharge patients from acute care beds quickly, rehabilitation operations owned by hospitals are a responsible venue in which to place recuperating patients and receive additional revenue.

In our contemporary political economy, however, newly heightened interest in geriatric rehabilitation may not be accompanied by concomitant increases in financial resources for this purpose. Indeed, rehabilitation is becoming subject to greater analytical scrutiny than ever before, in anticipation of public policy changes that may limit financing for it.

As the sparse data on the efficacy and costs of geriatric rehabilitation are increasingly evaluated, highly sophisticated, complex research efforts will need to be undertaken if adequate resources for geriatric rehabilitation are to be available in the years ahead. Consider just two such challenges. One is the arduous task of subdividing into relatively discrete categories the many diverse types of rehabilitation and patient conditions, so that issues of efficacy and cost can be traced through in a highly differentiated fashion. Another challenge, following from these, will be the need to develop a genuine conceptual merging of rehabilitation and long-term care as parts of the same set of activities, so that they can serve as a unit of analysis for documenting the cost-effectiveness of rehabilitation. For instance, even to the extent that a rehabilitative effort is successful only 10% of the time, it might render unnecessary what would have been required in long-term care costs for these patients. Thus, the amount of unneeded long-term care expenditures on these successfully rehabilitated patients could more than offset the investment in the 90% of similar types of rehabilitative efforts that have failed.

The economic challenges of owning and operating nursing homes that provide a decent standard of quality care are becoming increasingly difficult. Most American nursing homes are becoming heavily dependent on Medicaid financing, which generally provides less revenue than private sources of payment. Medicaid spending on nursing homes increased an estimated 50% between 1989 and 1992, whereas the proportion of nursing home costs paid for out-of-pocket declined, slightly, from 44.4% to 43.7% (Sonnefeld, Waldo, Lemieux, & McKusick, 1991). Moreover, it is becoming harder to recruit and maintain a quality work force of nurses aides and other providers of direct patient care, both in nursing homes and in residential environments (Feldman, 1990). Such pressures are likely to lead to substantial innovations in the nature of care provided in such institutions, and the ways in which it is financed.

Will nursing home patients in the twenty-first century be segregated, physically, and in quality of care and amenities, according to their abilities to pay and the sources of their payments? What ethical issues will be raised by the introduction of architectural and substantial technological innovations (perhaps robotics) in the delivery of care? What will be the implications of reconceptualizations in the roles of nursing home personnel, including physicians?

Health issues for older persons in residential environments are in flux, and will continue to evolve. Although the issues of aging in place have been studied for some years, the stresses and coping mechanisms associated with retirement migration and return migration are just beginning to be investigated systematically.

The types of residential settings in which older persons receive long-term care are rapidly proliferating. In addition to traditional home settings—involving spouses, adult children, siblings, and other family members as caregivers—responsibility for providing care is increasingly undertaken in: assisted living projects; board and care operations; foster care settings; life-care (or continuing-care) communities; and retirement homes. Older persons of the twenty-first century will have fewer adult children, and greater proportions of their potential caregivers (particularly daughters and daughters-in-law) will be in the labor force (E. Brody, 1990).

How will senses of obligation and capacities to provide family care undergo change? What are the origins of elder abuse, and what can be done about it? Will prenegotiated caregiving obligations undertaken by life-care communities and other residential entities be financially viable in the long run, and responsible in terms of the quality of care provided (including respect for the patient's autonomy)? What standards of public policy are appropriate for such long-term care arrangements in private sector and nonprofit settings, as well as in the provision of home care by family members?

Health, Law, and Ethics

The aging of the aged population, high rates of morbidity at advanced ages, the continuous development of technologies for sustaining life, and the high costs of health care have combined to bring a number of legal and ethical issues to the fore.

The Supreme Court's ruling in the case of *Cruzan v. Missouri* (1990) upheld the principle that patients have a "right to die" when such a right has been statutorily expressed by their state governments, and the circumstances of the case meet the criteria set forth by the state. State laws authorizing the use of advance directives—living wills and durable powers of attorney—have been designed in the name of enhanced autonomy for critically-ill patients in controlling their medical care. And they have been buttressed by the implementation of the federal Patient Self-Determination Act (Omnibus Reconciliation Act of 1990, 1990), which requires hospitals, nursing homes, and home health agencies to offer each patient information regarding their particular state's regulations regarding advance directives, and to ask if the patient has executed such a document or now wants to.

These legal instruments, however, are far from self-implementing (Lynn & Teno, 1993; Mezey & Latimer, 1993). A recent study found, for instance, that changes in the care of dying patients have not kept pace with national recommendations regarding the rights of patients to forego life-sustaining medical treatments and receive adequate pain control. Fully 70% of hospital house officers who were surveyed reported that they had acted against their conscience by providing aggressive care to the terminally ill (Solomon et al., 1993).

One effect of the spread of advance directives will be that physicians will be expected to decide, more explicitly and publicly than in the past, what treatments are medically futile. Ethicists, health care providers, and the courts are heavily involved in attempts to define the concept of "futility" in medical care. When is life-saving care futile? How and when should futility be operationalized as a limit on what patients and/or patient surrogates can require of the health care system?

The very definition of when life-saving care is futile is debated actively in the biomedical ethics literature, with definitions ranging from total physiological ineffectiveness of a medical intervention to its improbable success (Youngner, 1988; Schneiderman, Jecker, & Jonsen, 1990). Meantime, hospitals are developing policies regarding futile treatment. And a distinguished panel of professional experts and public figures has proclaimed that "Neither patients nor surrogates have the right to insist on physiologically futile treatment" (New York State Task Force on Life and Law, 1992, p. 204).

Even if ethicists, physicians, and health care organizations reach a consensus on operational definitions of futility, however, withdrawal of life-saving interventions in cases deemed medically-futile may be precluded by courts. In a Minnesota case decided shortly after the Cruzan decision, a hospital wanted to terminate what it regarded as futile care for an 87-year-old woman. But the court denied this request, ruling in favor of the woman's husband who asserted that she had long ago expressed a strong preference, because of her religious convictions, to live in such circumstances (Cranford, 1991).

Also at issue in health care decisions is the "quality of life." In what ways do perceptions of a patient's prospective quality of life affect medical judgments and interpretations of futility? For example, is the use of technology-intensive life-saving measures for severely demented elderly patients to be deemed more futile than comparable efforts for patients who are cognitively intact?

Because quality of life in old age obviously has subjective dimensions, scholarly attempts to define it have been wide-ranging and disparate (S.J. Brody, 1992). Sole reliance on relatively objective measures tends to create an endemic bias against older patients (Avorn, 1984). Nonetheless, for both humane and financial reasons, the effort to use quality of life as a reason for limiting aggressive medical intervention will persist. One of the more readily acceptable applications of such limits, perhaps, might be with respect to patients suffering from severe, terminal dementias (Post & Whitehouse, 1992).

The phenomenon of medical aid in dying (or assisted suicide) has emerged in public view in the past year or two, and is clearly generating major public and professional issues regarding appropriate standards of behavior and public policy. State governments confront issues of how to deal with widely publicized undertakings of assisted suicide. Voters in state referenda are deciding whether to legalize medical assistance in dying. The House of Delegates of the American Bar Association is actively dealing with resolutions on the topic.

The implications for medical practice and social ethics are being hotly debated. One writer has argued that "pre-emptive suicide" is a morally valid response to the reality of growing old (Prado, 1990). Certain physicians have argued that medical assistance in dying should be legalized when requested by competent patients who meet specific clinical criteria (Quill, Cassel, & Meier, 1992). Some ethicists have strongly opposed the practice on moral grounds, and argued that its widespread acceptance might engender a social expectation that patients should undertake suicide (e.g., Jonsen, 1991).

As of now, a social movement favoring medical aid in dying appears to be gathering substantial momentum (Glick, 1992). As it does, will patients be subject to implicit and explicit pressures to seek aid in dying? What will the implications be for health care providers, their professional ethics, and their relationships with patients? What standards of public policy will be appropriate?

A host of ethical and moral issues are implied by biomedical research efforts focused on such matters as: extension of the human species life span (e.g., through nutritional modulation); rejuvenation or reduction of deteriorations associated with normal aging (e.g., through human growth hormone); identification of genetic markers for Alzheimer's and other diseases, and discoveries that the genetic basis of some diseases gets worse with each succeeding familial generation; enhanced procedures (and, possibly, supplies) for undertaking organ transplantation; development of additional artificial organs and anatomical prosthetic devices; and improved methods of preventing, detecting, and treating many diseases and disabilities that are common at older ages.

Should limitations be imposed on these and other scientific frontiers, on moral, financial, or other grounds? What standards of genetic counseling are appropriate for late onset diseases? What principles of allocation should govern the implementation of new technologies? What ethical challenges will be posed for health care providers?

Issues of Political Economy

Since the late 1970s, in the context of growing federal deficits and spiralling health care costs, an artificially homogenized group—"the elderly"—has become a scapegoat for a variety of American problems that have been rhetorically unified as issues of intergenerational conflict and equity. As expenditures on benefits to the aging have climbed to 30% of the annual federal budget, about $450 billion in 1992 (Congressional Budget Office, 1992), older people have become increasingly stereotyped as prosperous, hedonistic, selfish, and politically controlling "greedy geezers." They have been blamed for problems of children, the declining strength of the U.S. economy, and the nation's general inability to free up resources for use in a variety of worthy causes (see Binstock, 1992a).

Especially prominent among the problems for which elderly people have been made scapegoat is spiraling health care costs. A prominent biomedical ethicist, Daniel Callahan, has depicted health care costs for older persons, which constitute about one-third of the nation's annual health care expenditures, or $270 billion out of an estimated $809 billion in 1992 (Sonnefeld et al., 1991), as "a great fiscal black hole" that will absorb an unlimited amount of our national resources (Callahan, 1987, p. 17). He and a number of other academicians and public figures—including politicians—have argued that U.S. society should set limits to health care for older people. Among their proposals, Callahan's is the most drastic in that he has urged that life-saving care be categorically denied to persons who are aged in their late 70s or early 80s.

Putting aside the considerable moral implications and issues of political feasibility involved in Callahan's and other drastic ideas put forth for rationing the health care of older people (see Binstock & Post, 1991), such proposals do not appear to be significant in terms of their potential impact on aggregate health care costs. Analyses of the more extreme scenarios for implementing such proposals suggest that they would save about 5% of annual national health care expenditures (see Jahnigen & Binstock, 1991). It is doubtful that the American public, if reasonably informed about the negligible fiscal impact that could be achieved, will support policy proposals for drastically rationing acute health care for older people.

More plausible, if not desirable, in the years ahead may be limitations on the availability to older persons of selected treatments, because a very specific issue of health care costs—how to pay for Medicare—is relatively urgent. It is estimated that Medicare's Part A Hospital Insurance (HI) costs will exceed tax revenues by 1995, and just after the turn of century the HI trust fund reserves will be exhausted and annual costs will exceed revenues by $66 billion (Ross, 1991). An approach for dealing with this problem might be to limit Medicare (and, by customary practice, private insurance) reimbursement for the application of selected high-cost treatments to older persons—such as newly developed techniques for organ transplantation, or the use of artificial organs, joints, and limbs.

The most likely responses to the challenge of paying for Medicare, however, would involve redistribution of financial burdens among persons eligible for Medicare in accordance with their economic status. Higher rates of out-of-pocket deductibles and co-payments could be established for wealthier Medicare patients on a sliding-scale basis. And Medicare's Part B premiums for Supplementary Medical Insurance, which are now set at a flat rate, could be increased progressively for higher income program participants and partially applied to Part A.

Such measures to redistribute financial burdens among elderly program participants would simply extend a 10-year incremental trend. The Social Security Reform Act of 1983 began this trend by taxing 50% of the Social Security benefits of individuals with incomes exceeding $25,000 and of married couples with over $32,000. The Tax Reform Act of 1986, even as it eliminated an extra personal exemption that had been available to all persons aged 65 and older when filing their federal income tax returns, provided new tax credits to very-low-income older persons on a sliding scale. The Older Americans Act programs of social services, for which all persons aged 60 and older are eligible, have been gradually targeted by Congress to low-income older persons. And the Medicare Catastrophic Coverage Act of 1988 continued this legislative approach in two respects, through its progressive taxation provisions and its requirement that Medicaid must pay Part B premiums and certain out-of-pocket expenses for Medicare enrollees who qualify for Medicaid eligibility. (Although the former provision was repealed in 1989, the latter remains in effect.)

A positive political development regarding health care for older people is that expanded public financing for long-term care has become an issue on the national policy agenda. Adoption of such a policy would not only enhance the array of services available, and perhaps their quality and continuity, but also alleviate the anxiety that many older persons feel when they experience or consider the prospect of spending their lifetime accumulation of assets for nursing home or home care.

A number of major long-term care bills have been introduced in Congress since 1989, with projected expenditures in the first year ranging from $21 to $50 billion depending upon varied details regarding eligible populations and the timing, nature, and extent of coverage (U.S. Senate, 1992). Because of such cost estimates most analysts of Congressional health policies and politics do not expect a major long-term care bill to be enacted within the immediate future. Moreover, the relatively recent political experiences of enacting the Medicare Catastrophic Coverage Act (MCCA) in 1988, and then repealing it in 1989 because of constituent complaints about having to pay new taxes to finance it, have made many members of Congress particularly wary of undertaking a major expansion of health care benefits that centrally involve older persons.

Enactment of an enduring and comprehensive long-term care policy will require the development of widespread popular understanding and political support for the legislation—a lesson that can be learned from the passage and swift repeal of the MCCA (see Binstock, 1992b). Such support will need to be developed through extensive grass-roots consideration of fundamental issues regarding the role of government in financing long-term care. Such issues include: Why should moderately well-off and wealthy persons be protected by government from having to spend their income and assets on long-term health and social care? Which citizens might be taxed to preserve the income and assets—and ultimately the legacies—of others? Do we want to have our government undertake more active steps than at present to preserve economic status inequalities from generation to generation? And, are there any sound reasons for not including chronically-ill and disabled persons of all ages? Without a conscious dialogue on such issues, any new policy on long-term care is likely to suffer the same fate as the short-lived MCCA—a policy developed by public elites in Washington, without any grass-roots understanding, feedback, and popular political support.

Widespread debate on such matters, moreover, may also help most Americans to appreciate better the pivotal role of health status in the quality of life, and to clarify some of the broader issues of distributive justice that are embedded in strategies for reforming the availability and provision of health care in the United States. Is there a morally relevant difference between one group—be it the aged, the demented, the poor, or any other—that justifies unequal treatment in the provision of acute or long-term health care? Should different standards of equity be applied to the health care arena from those applied to other spheres of activity in our society? As political philosopher Michael Walzer (1983) has argued, in a democratic society the answers to such questions are appropriately and most likely to be resolved through a process of widely shared decision making that is attentive to both the particular nature of the goods and services being distributed and the society's most deeply held values.

References

Alliance for Aging Research. (1992). *Americans view aging.* Washington, DC: Alliance for Aging Research.

Avorn, J. (1984). Benefit and cost analysis in geriatric care. *New England Journal of Medicine, 310,* 1294–1301.

Binstock, R.H. (1992a). The oldest old and "intergenerational equity." In R. Suzman, D. Willis, & K. Manton, (Eds.), *The oldest old* (pp. 394–417). New York: Oxford University Press.

Binstock, R.H. (1992b). Aging, disability, and long-term care: The politics of common ground, *Generations, XVI*(1), 83–88.

Binstock, R.H., & Post, S.G., (Eds.) (1991). *Too old for health care: Controversies in medicine, law, economics, and ethics.* Baltimore, MD: Johns Hopkins University Press.

Bortz, W.M. (1991). *We live too short and die too young.* New York: Bantam Books.

Bosker, G., Schwartz, G.R., Jones, J.S., & Sequeira, M. (1990). *Geriatric emergency medicine.* St. Louis, MO: Mosby Year Book Publishers.

Brody, E. (1990). *Women in the middle: Their parent care years.* New York: Springer Publishing Co.

Brody, S.J. (1992). The pursuit of quality. *The Gerontologist, 32,* 867–869.

Brody, S.J. & Ruff, G.E. (1986). *Aging and rehabilitation: Advances in the state of the art.* New York: Springer Publishing Co.

Callahan, D. (1987). *Setting limits: Medical goals in an aging society.* New York: Simon and Schuster.

Colwill, J. (1992). Where have all the primary care applicants gone? *New England Journal of Medicine, 326,* 387-393.

Congressional Budget Office, U.S. Congress. (1992). *The economic and budget outlook: Fiscal years 1993-1997.* Washington, DC: U.S. Government Printing Office.

Council on Graduate Medical Education. (1992). *Improving access to health care through physician workforce reform.* Washington, DC: U.S. Department of Health and Human Services.

Cranford, R.E. (1991). Helga Wanglie's ventilator, *Hastings Center Report, 21*(4), 23-24.

Cruzan v. Director, Missouri Department of Health. (1990). US 110 S Ct (1990) 2841.

Feldman, P.H. (1990). *Who cares for them? Workers in the home care industry.* Westport, CT: Greenwood Press.

Friedman, R.H., Kazis, L., Kern, D., Moskowitz, M., & Steel, K. (1991). *Geriatric graduate medical education.* Washington, DC: Health Services Research Administration, 240-BHPR-5.

Gallo, J.J., Reichel, W., & Andersen, L. (1988). *Handbook of geriatric assessment.* Rockville, MD: Aspen Publishers.

Glick, H.R. (1992). *The right to die: Policy innovation and its consequences.* New York: Columbia University Press.

Jahnigen, D.W., & Binstock, R.H. (1991). Economic and clinical realities: Health care for older people. In R.H. Binstock & S.G. Post, (eds.), *Too old for health care?: Controversies in Medicine, Law, Economics, and Ethics* (pp. 13-43). Baltimore, MD: Johns Hopkins University Press.

Jonsen, A. (1991). Initiative 119: What is at stake? *Commonweal, 118,* 466-472.

Lynn, J., & Teno, J.M. (1993). After the Patient Self-Determination Act: The need for empirical research on advance directives. *Hastings Center Report, 23*(1), 20-24.

Macaluso, J., & Thomas, R. (1991). Extracorporeal shock wave lithotripty: An outpatient procedure. *Journal of Urology, 146,* 714-717.

Mezey, M., & Latimer, B. (1993). The Patient Self-Determination Act: An early look at implementation. *Hastings Center Report, 23,* 16-20.

New York State Task Force on Life and Law (1992). *When others must choose: Deciding for patients without capacity.* New York: New York State Task Force on Life and the Law.

Omnibus Reconciliation Act of 1990 (1990). P.L. 101-508, Secs. 4206 & 4751.

Post, S.G., & Whitehouse, P.J. (1992). Dementia and the life-prolonging technologies used: An ethical question. *Alzheimer Disease and Associated Disorders, 6*(1), 3–6.

Prado, C.G. (1990). *The last choice: Pre-emptive suicide in advanced old age.* New York: Greenwood Press.

Quill, T.E., Cassel, C.K., & Meier, D.E. (1992). Care of the hopelessly ill: Proposed clinical criteria for physician-assisted suicide. *New England Journal of Medicine, 327,* 1380–1383.

Reuben, D.B., Bradley, T.B., Zwanziger, J., Fink, A., Hirsch, S. H., & Beck, J.C. (1991). Geriatrics faculty in the United States: Who are they and what are they doing? *Journal of the American Geriatric Society, 39,* 799–805.

Robertson, A. (1991). The politics of Alzheimer's disease: A case study in apocalyptic demography. In M. Minkler & C.L. Estes, (eds.), *Critical perspectives on aging: The political and moral economy of growing old* (pp. 135–150). Amityville, NY: Baywood Publishing Company.

Ross, S. G. (1991). The financial status of the Social Security and Medicare programs (paper presented at the annual meeting of the Gerontological Society of America, San Francisco, CA, November 23).

Rubenstein, L.Z., Struck, Sui, A.L, & Wieland, (1991). Impacts of geriatric evaluation and management programs on defined outcomes: Overview and evidence. *Journal of the American Geriatrics Society, 39*(Suppl.), 8S–16S.

Rubin, C., Sizemore, M., Loftis, P., Adams-Huet, B., & Anderson, R. (1992). The effect of geriatric evaluation and management on Medicare reimbursement in a large public hospital: A randomized clinical trial. *Journal of the American Geriatrics Society, 40,* 989–995.

Russell, L.B. (1989). *Medicare's new hospital payment system: Is it working?* Washington, DC: The Brookings Institution.

Schneiderman, L.S., Jecker, N.S., and Jonsen, A.R. (1990). Medical futility: Its meaning and ethical implications, *Annals of Internal Medicine. 112,* 951–952.

Solomon, M.Z., O'Donnell, L., Jennings, B., Guilfoy, V., Wolf, S. M., Nolan, K., Jackson, R., Koch-Weser, D., & Donnelley, S. (1993). Decisions near the end of life: Professional views on life-sustaining treatments. *American Journal of Public Health, 83*(1), 14–23.

Sonnefeld, S.T., Waldo, D.R., Lemieux, J.A., & McKusick, D.R. (1991). Projections of national health expenditures through the year 2000. *Health Care Financing Review, 13*(1), 1–27.

Surgeon General's Workshop (1988). *Health promotion and aging.* Washington, DC: U.S. Department of Health and Human Services.

Taeuber, C.M. (1992). *Sixty-five plus in America.* U.S. Bureau of the Census,

Current Population Reports, Special Studies, P23–178. Washington, DC: U.S. Government Printing Office.
U.S. Senate, Special Committee on Aging. (1992). *Developments in aging: 1991, volume I.* Washington, D.C.: U.S. Government Printing Office.
Walzer, M. (1983). *Spheres of justice.* New York: Basic Books.
Williams, T.F., (Ed.). (1984). *Rehabilitation in the aging.* New York: Raven Press.
Youngner, S.J. (1988). Who defines futility? *Journal of the American Medical Association, 260,* 2094–2095.

Index

Acquired immune deficiency syndrome (AIDS), 137
Active life expectancy, 2, 62, 71, 86–87, 107
   sex differences in, 86
Activities of daily living, 11, 28, 102, 110, 290
   Activities of Daily Living Index (ADL), 46, 47, 85, 107, 108, 111
   and definition of quality of life, 29, 32
   in developing countries, 290
   in minorities, 303–304
   Instrumental Activities of Daily Living Index (IADL), 46, 107, 108, 204–205
Acute care, 353–355
Advance directives, 357–360
African Americans. *See* Minorities.
Age and social structure. *See* Social structure and aging.
Age distribution of population
   disability prevalence and incidence, 91, 107
   Indonesia, 287–288
   public policy and, 13
   social change and population aging, 11, 22
   United States, 1
   world elderly population growth, ix–x
Ageism, 239, 263, 269

Aging, 21
   biological changes in, 121, 148
   normal process vs. disease, 22, 57, 106, 121, 148
Alameda County Study, 60, 164
Alzheimer's disease, 9, 22, 24, 79, 123, 133, 137, 359
   caregiver burden, 145–155. *See also* Caregivers.
   Alzheimer's support groups, 154
   prevalence, 145
American Association of Retired People, 24
Arthritis, 9, 79, 108, 123, 125–126, 205, 304
Asian Americans. *See* Minorities.
Assisted suicide, 359
Assistive technology. *See* Self-care and Human factors.
Autonomy. *See* Dependency, Institutionalization, Sense of control.

Bereavement and widowhood, 175, 178, 282–283
Biomedicalization of aging and disability, 13, 88–89, 320, 321
Blacks. *See* Minorities.

Cancer, 9, 133–142, 164, 171, 303, 304
   age and therapies/treatments, 9, 134, 137–138
   age and, 9, 133
   and disabilities, 139

INDEX

breast cancer, 139–140
  coping styles and, 9
  quality of life for cancer patients, 140–142
  subjective meaning of, 136–137
Cardiovascular (CVD) and coronary heart disease (CHD), 9, 22, 108, 133, 164, 220, 303, 305
  age and, 148–149
  prevention of, 153–155
  risk factors for CVD, 151–152, 165
Care-givers
  biobehavioral vulnerabilities and CVD, 152
  physical health of, 150–151
  stress on caregivers, 9, 146
  women as, 324–326
Chronic illness and conditions, 2, 62–64
  and measuring quality of life, 38, 141
  definition, 79
  in minorities, 302–305
  late-life disabilities and, 89, 104
  prevalence and incidence of, x, 107, 123
  self-care for, 102
  sex differences, 2
Cognitive functioning, 4, 28, 32, 205–206, 208, 210, 219, 236
Cohorts, 242–243
Comorbidity. *See* Morbidity.
Comparative international research. *See* Cross-national research.
Conference on Aging: The Quality of Life, 5
Coping, 9, 102
Cross-national research, 12, 287–293

Dependency, 11, 108, 192–193, 217, 321. *See also* Institutionalization.
Depression, 71, 126, 149, 150, 174, 219
Disability, 2, 8, 11
  behavioral competence and quality of life, 4
  definition, 79, 81, 87–88
  disablement process, 81–84
    life-long vs. late-life disability, 89–91

  epidemiology of, 8, 80–81, 91, 108
  impairment, 81, 85
  measurement issues, 85–86, 89
  prevalence and incidence of, 2–3, 106–108, 123–124
  prevention of, 84–85, 91–92, 93
  race and ethnic differences in, 3, 109
  rehabilitation of. *See* Rehabilitation.
  sex differences in, 109
Disease prevention. *See* Prevention of disease or disability.

Economic well-being. *See* Poverty and Socioeconomic status.
Education, 240. *See also* Socioeconomic status.
Established Populations for the Epidemiologic Study of the Elderly (EPESE), 69
Estrogen replacement therapy, 22

Frailty, 8, 23, 236. *See also* Disability.
Framingham Study of Heart Disease, 165

Gerontology and geriatrics, 6, 20
  fields of, 22
  future directions in, 23–24
  number of geriatricians, 352

Health
  and wealth, 264, 281–284, 322
  gender differences in, 290–291. *See also* Women.
  of future cohorts, 351
  perceived, 34
  promotion of, 2, 14. *See also* Interventions.
Health and Retirement Study, 23, 275, 285–286
Health care, 14. *See also* Long-term care.
  acute care, 14
  barriers among minorities to, 304–306, 319
  costs of, 360–363
  doctor–patient interactions, 352–353
  public policy for, 13, 350–363
  socioeconomic status and, 258–260

Health promotion, 112, 225, 267–268.
  See also Prevention of disease
  and disability.
Healthy aging, 7, 100, 338–339. See also
  Successful aging.
  defined, 57–59
  environmental factors in, 66–69, 102,
    129, 204
Healthy life expectancy. See Active life
  expectancy.
Hip fractures, 9, 68, 108, 127–128
Hispanic Americans. See Minorities.
Human factors, 11, 23, 202–211
  and activities of daily living, 11
  and aging, 203
  and Instrumental Activities of Daily
    Living, 204–205
  computers, 209–210
  definition, 11, 203
  driving, 206–208
  medication adherence, 205–206
  work, 209–211

Independence. See Dependency, Institutionalization.
Institutionalization. See also Long-term
  care.
  decision to institutionalize, 150–151
  independence and, 11, 192–193
Internal and external control. See Sense
  of control.
Intervention research, 341–343
  barriers to, 345
  research design issues, 343–345
  socioeconomic status and, 267
Isolation, social. See Social networks
  and support.

Job characteristics and design, 209–211,
  241

Life events. See Stress.
Life expectancy, 1, 2, 8, 19, 23,
    135–136, 283
  and public health, 22
  for Baby Boomers, 25
  of minorities, 304–305
  quality adjusted life years, 45

Life satisfaction, 4, 27, 30–31, 34, 150,
    174, 187
Life style, 2, 7, 102, 105, 122, 123, 133,
    282, 298, 341–342, 351
  socioeconomic status and, 260–262
Long-term care, 11, 13, 14, 107,
    185–198, 319–331, 356–357
  acute care and, 327
  and dependency, 192–193
  costs of, 321, 356, 362–363
  demographic influences on, 320–321
  informal care, 324–326
  projecting need for, 322–323, 326–329
Longevity. See Active life expectancy,
  Life expectancy.
Longitudinal Study of Aging, 65

Marital status. See Social networks and
  support.
Medication adherence, 205–206
Memory, 10, 205–206. See also Cognitive functioning.
  and sense of control, 219, 225,
    226–228
Middle age, 236–237, 241, 244
Minorities, racial and ethnic, 13, 23,
    109, 130, 170, 224, 237, 280,
    285
  definition of minority status, 296
  demographics of, 296–297
  diversity within and among, 298–299
  health and socioeconomic status
    among, 295–311
  poverty and, 299–302
Morbidity, 2, 8, 218–219, 220, 288–289
  and socioeconomic status, 254–255
  comorbidity, 108, 139
  compression of, 2, 62, 66, 93, 107,
    253, 337–338
  disability rates and, 91–92
Mortality, 1, 11, 20, 91, 92–93, 283,
    288–289
  and socioeconomic status, 254–255

National Cancer Institute, 134
National Health Interview Survey, 108,
  204
  Supplement on Aging (SOA), 108

National Institute on Aging, 22, 64, 102
National Institutes of Health, 5, 22
National Long Term Care Survey, 107
Native Americans. *See* Minorities.
Nursing homes. *See* Institutionalization, Long-term care.

Older drivers, 206–208
   accident rates, 207
Oldest-old, 1, 107, 185, 236. *See also* Active life expectancy, Life expectancy.
   Health and Asset Survey of, 275
   projected numbers of, 1
Osteoporosis, 22, 108, 123

Pain, 33, 125
Panel Study of Income Dynamics, 275, 284–285
Personal control. *See* Sense of control.
Poverty, 12, 13, 62, 268–269. *See also* Socioeconomic status.
   and minorities, 13, 300–303
   in old age, 279–281
Prevention of disease or disability, 84–85, 91, 111, 153–155
Productive aging. *See* Successful aging.
Public health
   and "longevity revolution," 22

Quality of life. *See also* Life satisfaction.
   aging and, 4, 140
   behavioral competence, 4
   definitions, 4–7, 27–31, 122
     predictors vs. components, 28
     subjective vs. objective, 27–28
   determinants of, 36, 37
   dimensions or domains of, 4, 7, 28–29
     content areas, 29, 122
     response dimensions, 29–30
   health-related, 4, 122
   interventions to improve, 6, 8
   measurement of, 6–7
     issues in, 36–45
       global vs. specific, 39, 43–44
       proxy respondents, 41
       self-report vs. interviews, 39–41
       sensitivity to change, 43
     scales and instruments for, 44–46
       appropriateness of, 46–48
   psychological well-being, 4, 140

Rehabilitation, geriatric, 9, 14, 68, 124–125, 139–140, 355–357
   arthritis and, 125–126
   deconditioning and muscle strength, 128
   goal of, 124
   hip fracture and, 127–128
   NIH Task Force on Medical Rehabilitation Research, 129–130
   principles of, 128
   stroke and, 126–127
Relocation, residential, 176–177
Retirement, 23, 176, 236, 240, 241, 244
   pensions and retirement trends, 276–278, 293
   work after, 241–242, 243
Risk factors, 7, 8, 59–66, 260–262, 265, 341. *See also* Life styles, Social networks and support.
   among African Americans, 306
   for cardiovascular disease, 9, 149, 151–153
   caregiver burden as risk factor, 146, 149–153
   for disability, 83
   physical activity, 60–61, 64, 71, 122
   quality of life as, 153
   smoking, 7, 59–60, 64, 71, 122
   social, 61–62

Science, development of, 20–21, 94–95
Self-care, 8, 29, 32, 35, 110–111, 194, 322
   aging and, 103, 104, 105
   definition of, 100–101, 103–105
   disabilities and, 8
   domains of, 102
   need for, 105
   relation to professional care, 99–100, 112, 113
Self-efficacy. *See* Sense of control.
Sense of control, 10, 28, 34, 104, 187, 194, 216–229, 260, 321, 329

INDEX

age, disease and, 148, 218–219
aging and, 220–226
and social support, 219–220
correlates of, 218–220
definition of, 217–218
dependency in nursing homes, 192–195, 197
fear of, 217
gender, minority, and SES differences in, 224
intervention to improve, 226–228
measurement of, 218, 219
memory, cognitive functioning and, 10, 219
negative consequences of, 228
quality of life and, 217
social support and, 179–180
Services for health-care, 3
Social change. *See* Social structure and aging.
Social functioning, 32, 35, 109
Social networks and support, 10, 61, 65–66, 68–69, 71, 103, 110–111, 139, 153, 163–180, 260, 293, 346
age and, 169–170
and morbidity, 165–166, 171
and mortality, 164–165
and sense of control, 219–220
buffering hypothesis, 173–174
convoy of social support, 166–169
gender and, 170
interventions to improve, 177–179, 195
marital and familial status and, 170, 283, 293
minorities and, 306–309
types of social support, 171–173
Social Security Insurance, 275, 275–278, 299, 361
Social structure and aging
age structures, 11, 262–265, 266
age-differentiated vs. age-integrated, 11–12, 238–239
age-integrated society
evidence for, 240–242
obstacles to, 244–250
health and, 339–340

social change, 11
structural lag, 237–238
Socioeconomic status, 7, 11, 12, 61, 64–65. *See also* Poverty.
and cardiovascular disease, 153
and life chances, 321
and risk factors, 260–262
and self-care, 111
and sense of control, 219–224
education and health, 288–290
health and wealth, 258–260, 264, 281–284, 291, 302
income in old age, 279–280
mortality and morbidity, 254–255
of minorities, 300–302
of widows, 282–283
social mobility, 255–257, 265
Special populations. *See* Minorities, Oldest old.
Stress, 146, 148, 165–166, 260
life events and, 174–175, 177. *See also* Bereavement, Relocation, Retirement.
social support and, 173–174
Stroke, 9, 126–127
Successful aging, 10, 11, 12, 23, 58, 197, 258. *See also* Healthy aging.
in long-term care facilities, 191–195
model of, 186–191
productive roles, 240, 242

Type A behavior. *See* Risk factors for cardiovascular disease.

Women, 2, 109, 111, 127, 164, 170, 204, 206, 224, 280, 282–283, 290, 296, 300, 303, 322
and active life expectancy, 86
as care-givers, 324–326
breast cancer, 139–140
gender roles, 246–247, 248
labor force participation, 237, 245–246
sex differences in health, 290–291, 323–324
women's movement, 240
World Health Organization (WHO), 101, 102, 124, 339–340

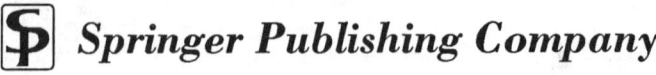 *Springer Publishing Company*

CONTEMPORARY GERONTOLOGY

JOURNAL

A Journal of Reviews and Critical Discourse

Editor: **Robert C. Atchley**, PhD

Associate Editors: **W. Andrew Achenbaum**, PhD, **Elizabeth A. Kutza**, PhD, **M. Powell Lawton**, PhD, **George L. Maddox**, PhD, and **Robert M. Schmidt**, MD, MPH, PhD

This quarterly journal features book reviews to assist gerontologists and other professionals in keeping up with the growing literature on aging. The current provisions for book reviews are limited. Too often, important books go unreviewed, and published reviews are usually two years behind the book publication date, thus hardly relevant for decisions to purchase or adopt new books. In our journal, book reviews are published in less than a year from the date of receiving the book for review, since timeliness is a major value of any scholarly book review.

CONTEMPORARY GERONTOLOGY includes 12-15 reviews per issue, as well as timely essay articles, and letters to the editor. The journal also provides timely essay articles contributing to the critical self-awareness of gerontology in such ways as to clarify concepts and theories, to reflect on the state of the literature in specific areas, and contribute to significant debates and controversies in the field. Editorials, letters to the editor, and a list of books received appears in the journal.

ISSN 1069-0840   (4 annual issues)

536 Broadway, New York, NY 10012-3955 • (212) 431-4370 • Fax (212) 941-7842

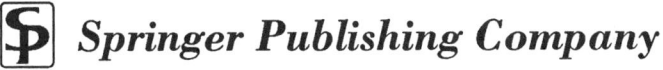 *Springer Publishing Company*

RETIREMENT COUNSELING
A Handbook for Gerontology Practitioners

Virginia E. Richardson, PhD

With the steadily increasing number of individuals approaching retirement age, many more will require counseling to cope with both the social and economic problems that arise, both in pre- and post-retirement. This book is intended to increase the practitioner's awareness of such problems and to recommend intervention strategies for dealing with them.

Richardson addresses social factors that affect the retirement experience such as gender, ethnic background, and poverty, and offers an integration of theory and practice about retirement as well as a unique conceptualization of retirement problems. This book is invaluable to psychologists, social workers, career and retirement counselors, and any clinician working with older adults.

Contents:

I. **Conceptual Issues in Retirement:** The Meaning of Retirement Theories of Retirement Adjustment • The Phases of Retirement
II. **Retirement Intervention:** Retirement Intervention: Generic Model • Preretirement Counseling • Retirement Decision Counseling • Retirement Adjustment Counseling
III. **Gender, Ethnicity, and Retirement:** Intervention • Women and Retirement • Retirement Among African Americans Retirement Among Other Ethnic Minority Groups
IV. **The Future of Retirement:** The Future of Retirement and Retirement Counseling

Springer Series on Life Styles and Issues in Aging
1993   224pp   0-8261-7020-X   hardcover

536 Broadway, New York, NY 10012-3955 • (212) 431-4370 • Fax (212) 941-7842

Springer Publishing Company

HANDBOOK OF THE HUMANITIES AND AGING

Thomas R. Cole, PhD, **David Van Tassel,** PhD, and **Robert Kastenbaum,** PhD, Editors

Serves as a major resource for research into the contributions of the humanities to our understanding of aging and the aged. Offers an authoritative examination of humanistic perspectives on aging spanning history, the arts, religious/spiritual studies, and philosophy. The text is notably free of jargon, and thus equally useful to researchers from the broad range of fields it encompasses.

Contents:

A View from Antiquity: Greece, Rome and Elders, *T.M. Falkner & J. de Luce* • The Older Person in the Western World: From the Middle Ages to the Industrial Revolution, *D.G. Troyansky* • Old Age in the Modern and Postmodern Western World, *C. Conrad* • Aging in Eastern Cultures, *C.W. Keifer* • Aging and Meaning: The Christian Tradition, *S.G. Post* • Aging in Judaism: "Crown of Glory" and "Days of Sorrow," *S. Isenberg* • Islamic, Hindu, and Buddhist Conceptions of Aging, *G.R. Thursby* • Fairy Tales and Spiritual Development in Later Life: The Story of the Shining Fish, *A.B. Chinen* • Images of Aging in American Poetry, 1925–1985, *C.H. Smith* • Old Age in Contemporary Fiction: A New Paradigm of Hope, *C. Rooke* • Walking to the Stars, *M.G. Winkler* • The Creative Process: A Life-Span Approach, *R. Kastenbaum* • Story of the Shoe Box: The Meaning and Practice of Transmitting Stories, *M. Kaminsky* • Literary Gerontology Comes of Age, *A.M. Wyatt-Brown* • Aging in America: The Perspective of History, *C. Haber & B. Gratton* • Elders in World History, *P.N. Stearns* • Bioethics and Aging, *H.T. Moody* • Wisdom and Method: Philosophical Contributions to Gerontology, *R.J. Manheimer* • The Older Student of Humanities: The Seeker and the Source, *D. Shuldiner* • Afterword: Integrating the Humanities into Gerontologic Research, Training, and Practice, *W.A. Achenbaum*

512pp   0-8261-6240-1   hardcover

536 Broadway, New York, NY 10012-3955 • (212) 431-4370 • Fax (212) 941-7842